Lecture Notes in Computer Science 16257

The series Lecture Notes in Computer Science (LNCS), including its subseries Lecture Notes in Artificial Intelligence (LNAI) and Lecture Notes in Bioinformatics (LNBI), has established itself as a medium for the publication of new developments in Computer Science research, teaching, and education.

The series enjoys close cooperation with the international research community, publishing the proceedings of many prestigious conferences and collaborating with important societies.

Proposals

A conference or workshop applying for publication in LNCS should have an international program committee, a coherent subject scope limited to related computer science topics, and an appropriate plan for reviewing the submitted papers. To submit a proposal to LNCS please contact lncs@springer.com.

Publishing Service

LNCS offers a full publishing service, including typesetting of papers, making most content available in PDF, HTML, print, and ePub formats. Authors can embed videos in their content, or add electronic supplementary material to be made available in our digital library (SpringerLink).

Open Access

Conference organisers may opt for gold open access of all content in proceedings volumes. Alternatively individual author teams may select gold open access for their proceedings papers. Please contact lncs@springer.com to enquire about terms.

Societies, Communities

LNCS cooperates with prestigious computer science societies and communities, publishing the proceedings of flagship conferences across all major fields. Among the events and associations are ECCV (European Conference on Computer Vision), IACR (International Association for Cryptologic Research), MICCAI (Medical Image Computing and Computer Assisted Intervention Society), the China Computer Federation (CCF), DASFAA (International Conference on Database Systems for Advanced Applications), PRICAI (Pacific Rim International Conference on Artificial Intelligence), IFIP (International Federation for Information Processing), ETAPS (International Joint Conferences on Theory and Practice of Software), ECML PKDD (European Conf. on Machine Learning and Principles and Practice of Knowledge Discovery in Databases), and IAPR (International Association for Pattern Recognition).

Indexing and Distribution

LNCS submits the content and bibliographic metadata of proceedings volumes to the major abstracting and indexing services, including the Conference Proceedings Citation Index (CPCI, part of Clarivate Analytics' Web of Science), DBLP, Scopus, the EI Engineering (Compendex, Inspec), the ACM Digital Library, and Google Scholar. In addition to the indexing services listed above, Springer Nature content is available worldwide through key university and industry library subscription access, and through major distributors such as Amazon and Google Books.

Sublines

The **Formal Methods** subline (https://link.springer.com/series/15554) was established in cooperation with the Formal Methods Europe association, publishing proceedings and tutorials associated with high-quality events. The Advanced Research in Computing and Software Science (**ARCoSS**) subline was established in cooperation with the European Association for Theoretical Computer Science (EATCS) and the International Joint Conferences on Theory and Practice of Software (ETAPS), and it publishes proceedings of high-quality events in theoretical computer science and foundations of programming.

Special Collections

LNCS includes contributed edited works such as **Festschrifts**, dedicated to individuals who have made excellent contributions to the field of computer science, **State-of-the-Art Surveys**, and **Tutorials**. Please contact lncs@springer.com for further details about any of these volume types.

Transactions

We publish the LNCS Transactions in Large-Scale Data- and Knowledge-Centered Systems and the LNCS Transactions in Petri Nets and Other Models of Concurrency (ToPNoC). Please contact lncs@springer.com for further details.

SharedIt

Springer Nature can make shareable links to online PDFs of published proceedings papers available to authors. This encourages reading by users who otherwise don't have subscription access (for example, via a university library). These shareable links can be communicated via social channels, on institutional repositories, on author websites, or on scholarly collaborative networks.

Overleaf

The LaTeX2e Proceedings Templates are available in the scientific authoring platform Overleaf.

Other Benefits of Publishing

By default, conference **organisers and authors are not charged** for publishing in LNCS. Organisers and participants get **free online access** to the SpringerLink-published papers for 4 weeks during and following the conference. LNCS offers readers transparent reviewing data about all published volumes. Authors retain copyright to their papers and **authors can self-archive** their submitted papers. For more information on publishing service and conditions, please contact lncs@springer.com.

Publishing Policies

We require volume editors (conference organisers), authors of proceedings papers, and reviewers engaged to evaluate papers submitted to conferences to follow our publishing policies and respective codes of conduct (https://www.springernature.com/gp/policies/book-publishing-policies).

LNAI (Lecture Notes in Artificial Intelligence)

This subseries (https://link.springer.com/series/1244) was established in 1988 as a topical subseries of LNCS devoted to artificial intelligence. The editors are Wolfgang Wahlster (DFKI, Berlin), Randy Goebel (University of Alberta, Edmonton), and Zhi-Hua Zhou (Nanjing University).

LNBI (Lecture Notes in Bioinformatics)

This subseries (https://link.springer.com/series/5381) was established in 2003 as a topical subseries of LNCS devoted to bioinformatics and computational systems biology. The editors are Sorin Istrail (Brown University), Pavel Pevzner (University of California, San Diego) and Michael Waterman (University of Southern California).

Xiahai Zhuang · Wangbin Ding · Yuanye Liu ·
Yingliang Ma · Jichao Zhao · Bomin Wang
Editors

Comprehensive Analysis and Computing of Real-World Medical Images

Second MICCAI Challenge, CARE 2025
Held in Conjunction with MICCAI 2025
Daejeon, South Korea, September 23, 2025
Proceedings

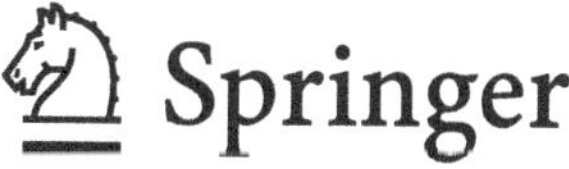

Editors
Xiahai Zhuang
School of Data Science, Fudan University
Shanghai, China

Yuanye Liu
School of Data Science, Fudan University
Shanghai, China

Jichao Zhao
Auckland Bioengineering Institute, University of Auckland
Auckland, New Zealand

Wangbin Ding
School of Imaging, Fujian Medical University
Fuzhou, China

Yingliang Ma
School of Computing Sciences, University of East Anglia
Norwich, UK

Bomin Wang
School of Data Science, Fudan University
Shanghai, China

ISSN 0302-9743 ISSN 1611-3349 (electronic)
Lecture Notes in Computer Science
ISBN 978-3-032-16270-0 ISBN 978-3-032-16271-7 (eBook)
https://doi.org/10.1007/978-3-032-16271-7

This Springer imprint is published by the registered company Springer Nature Switzerland AG
The registered company address is: Gewerbestrasse 11, 6330 Cham, Switzerland

Preface

With the rapid development of artificial intelligence and medical imaging technologies, the field of medical image analysis continues to evolve toward more robust, generalizable, and clinically applicable solutions. Building upon the success of the CARE 2024 Challenge, which emphasized comprehensive analysis and computing of real-world medical images, we were pleased to continue this series with CARE 2025. This year's challenge expanded the scope, diversity, and scale of the tasks, organizing four real-world tracks: CARE-Cardiac, CARE-WHS, CARE-MyoPS, and CARE-Liver. Each track invited solutions for unified cardiac image segmentation, whole-heart segmentation, myocardial pathology segmentation, and liver quantification, respectively. Together, these tracks aimed to advance real-world medical image computing by bridging the gap between AI model development and practical clinical applications.

While popular foundation models such as the Segment Anything Model (SAM) and other vision-language frameworks, have shown remarkable performance on curated datasets, their reliability and generalization in clinical environments remain limited. Real-world medical imaging data are often characterized by motion-induced misalignment, inter-modality variability, and center-dependent distribution shifts. CARE 2025 continued to emphasize robustness, interpretability, and generalizability across diverse modalities and centers, encouraging the development of methods that can adapt to imperfect, heterogeneous data.

Each dataset in CARE 2025 presented its own complexity—ranging from large deformations and small irregular regions of interest, to inconsistencies across modalities and centers. By providing a unified, multi-task platform, the challenge offered an opportunity to benchmark algorithms across diverse clinical settings, fostering progress toward reliable and deployable medical AI solutions.

Following the same rigorous process as in CARE 2024, the peer-review process for this proceedings volume was conducted under a double-blind mechanism to ensure fairness and quality. Each submission was carefully evaluated by at least four reviewers, and only high-quality papers with strong methodological innovation and experimental rigor were accepted for publication. In total, 23 out of 51 submissions were accepted, corresponding to an acceptance rate of approximately 45%.

We hope that the CARE 2025 Challenge will serve as a catalyst for collaboration between academia and clinical research, advancing the mission of comprehensive, interpretable, and trustworthy medical image computing.

For more details about the challenge, datasets, and results, please visit the official website: http://www.zmic.org.cn/care_2025.

October 2025

Xiahai Zhuang
Wangbin Ding
Yuanye Liu
Yingliang Ma
Jichao Zhao
Bomin Wang

Organization

General Chairs

Zhuang, Xiahai	Fudan University, China
Ding, Wangbin	Fujian Medical University, China
Liu, Yuanye	Fudan University, China
Ma, Yingliang	University of East Anglia, UK
Zhao, Jichao	University of Auckland, New Zealand
Wang, Bomin	Fudan University, China

Program Committee

Camara, Oscar	Universitat Pompeu Fabra, Spain
Chen, Bailiang	Université de Lorraine, France
Chen, Zhihao	91360 Med Tech, China
Choi, Hyuntae	Chung-Ang University, South Korea
Dou, Zhi	Fujian Provincial Hospital, China
Frangi, Alejandro F.	University of Manchester, UK
Gao, Shangde	Zhejiang University, China
Gao, Shangqi	University of Cambridge, UK
Gong, Haiyu	Fudan University, China
Gong, Weikang	Fudan University, China
Gu, Yun	University of Auckland, New Zealand
Gunawardhana, Malitha	University of Auckland, New Zealand
Hong, Byung-Woo	Chung-Ang University, South Korea
Huang, Huashan	Fujian Provincial Hospital, China
Huang, Liqin	Fuzhou University, China
Jia, Dengqiang	Macao Polytechnic University, China
Jiang, Suiyang	Fudan University, China
Li, Lei	National University of Singapore, Singapore
Li, Qingya	Northeastern University, China
Li, Yuxin	University of Pennsylvania, USA
Li, Yuzhu	Fudan University, China
Liao, Xuewen	Fujian Provincial Hospital, China
Lin, Xi	University of East Anglia, UK
Lin, Xintao	Fuzhou University, China
Lin, Xingtao	Fuzhou University, China

Sponsors

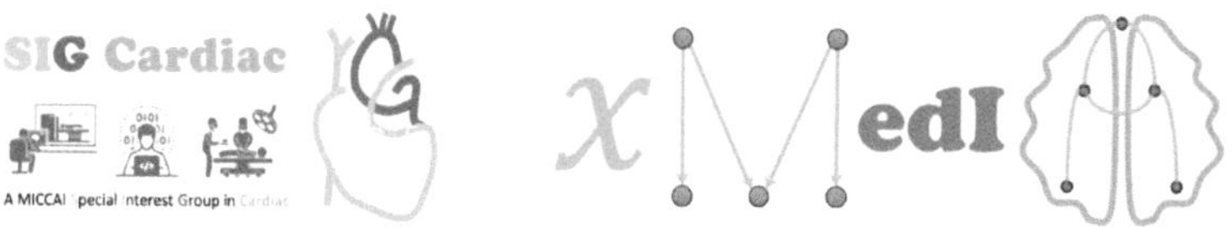

1. MICCAI-SIG Cardiac Imaging, Computational Modelling and Clinical Sciences (SIG-Cardiac)
2. MICCAI-SIG Explainable AI for Medical Image Analysis (SIG-xMedIA)

Keynote

Hippocrates Meets Turing: The Digital Oath—The Imperatives of In Silico Regulatory Science in the Digital Era

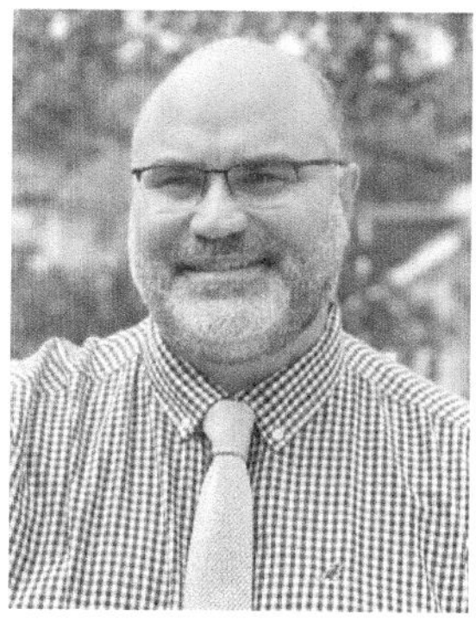

Speaker: Alejandro F. Frangi, FREng, FIEEE
Bicentenary Turing Chair in Computational Medicine, University of Manchester

Abstract The promise of AI-powered medical image analysis has captured the imagination of researchers and clinicians worldwide, yet the journey from laboratory algorithms to real-world clinical deployment remains fraught with challenges that mirror those faced in medical device development. How do we ensure that sophisticated models trained on curated datasets perform reliably across the diverse, unpredictable landscape of clinical practice?

This keynote will explore how the principles of computational regulatory science can address the fundamental challenges facing real-world medical image analysis. We will examine how virtual populations can augment limited clinical datasets, how digital twins can predict algorithmic behavior across diverse scenarios, and how in silico methodologies can establish robust evidence frameworks for safe AI deployment.

Contents

A Unified 3D Cardiac Structure Segmentation Framework for Heterogeneous Medical Data

Zhao Wang, Zheyao Gao, and Qi Dou(✉)

The Chinese University of Hong Kong, Hong Kong, China
qidou@cuhk.edu.hk

Abstract. Segmentation of multiple cardiac structures (e.g., atria, ventricles, myocardium) from multi-center and multi-modality images is crucial for comprehensive cardiovascular disease assessment. However, accurate and unified segmentation remains challenging due to significant data heterogeneity across different imaging modalities (MRI, CT) and anatomical variations among diverse clinical centers. Current methods often rely on separate strategies for specific substructures or modalities, lacking the ability to capture cross-structural correlations and adapt to unseen data distributions, leading to degraded performance in out-of-distribution (OOD) cases. To address these issues, we propose a self-adaptive framework for unified 3D cardiac structure segmentation based self-configuring strategies. It enhances the model's robustness by learning invariant representations across modalities and automatically adjusting segmentation strategies based on data distribution characteristics. In the meanwhile, the structural consistency constraint is introduced to preserve anatomical relationships between cardiac substructures. Experiment results have demonstrated that our method achieved the state-of-the-art performance and alleviated the performance drop on data from unseen centers.

Keywords: Cardiac Structure Segmentation · Unified Framework · Heterogeneous Medical Data

1 Introduction

As a key technical support for the diagnosis, treatment, and assessment of cardiovascular diseases [7,16,22], 3D Cardiac Structure Segmentation [1,2,8] plays an irreplaceable role in clinical practice and medical research. Quantitative analysis of left ventricular and right ventricular volumes, as well as accurate calculation of myocardial thickness and cardiac function indicators, all rely on efficient and precise segmentation of the 3D anatomical structure of the heart. Furthermore, in the early screening, disease staging, and treatment effect monitoring of complex cardiovascular diseases such as coronary heart disease and cardiomyopathy,

X. Zhuang et al. (Eds.): CARE 2025, LNCS 16257, pp. 1–11, 2026.
https://doi.org/10.1007/978-3-032-16271-7_1

this technology provides clinicians with objective quantitative evidence, directly promoting the comprehensiveness and scientificity of disease assessment [6,14].

With the rapid development of medical imaging technology, cardiac data acquired in current clinical practice exhibits prominent "multi-center and multi-modality" characteristics. Multi-center data originates from differences in scanning equipment (e.g., MRI scanners of brands like GE and Siemens), scanning parameters (e.g., sequence selection and slice thickness settings), and patient populations across different medical institutions, leading to inherent heterogeneity in data distribution [25,28]. Multi-modality data, on the other hand, covers various imaging types including MRI (Magnetic Resonance Imaging), CT (Computed Tomography), and ultrasound; differences in grayscale features and tissue contrast among data from different modalities further increase the difficulty of segmentation [29,30,32]. This data characteristic poses severe challenges to accurate cross-center and cross-modal structural segmentation. However, most existing methods adopt the approach of designing independent segmentation strategies for different centers or structures. Although such methods can achieve certain performance on specific data, they struggle to adapt to distribution shift scenarios (e.g., processing data from new centers not involved in training), resulting in a significant decline in segmentation performance on out-of-distribution cases and severely limited generalization ability [15,20,27].

To address these challenges, we propose a self-configuring 3D cardiac segmentation framework that unifies feature extraction and fusion strategies across diverse tasks. By dynamically adapting model architecture, training, and inference strategies to varying data characteristics (e.g., cross-center MRI or mixed-modality CT-MRI data), our approach significantly enhances robustness in out-of-distribution scenarios. Experiments demonstrate that the proposed framework not only mitigates the key limitation of low accuracy on unseen data but also improves segmentation efficiency and precision. It achieves state-of-the-art performance in key metrics (Dice Similarity Coefficient and Hausdorff Distance), offering a novel and effective solution for multi-source cardiac data segmentation.

2 Method

2.1 Unified Segmentation Framework

To enhance the model robustness across multi-center and multi-modality cardiac data, we propose a unified framework tailored for 3D cardiac structure segmentation, by leveraging adaptive design principles consistent with the automated, data-driven configuration paradigm of the nnU-Net [13] framework. As illustrated in Fig. 1, the workflow follows a structured, streamlined pipeline: upon retrieving a 3D cardiac volume from the database, we first determine the target segmentation task (e.g., single cardiac structure segmentation, whole-heart segmentation, or joint structure-pathology segmentation) to align the framework with clinical needs. Next, we construct the segmentation model and configure training/inference strategies in an adaptive manner—drawing on the nnU-Net's

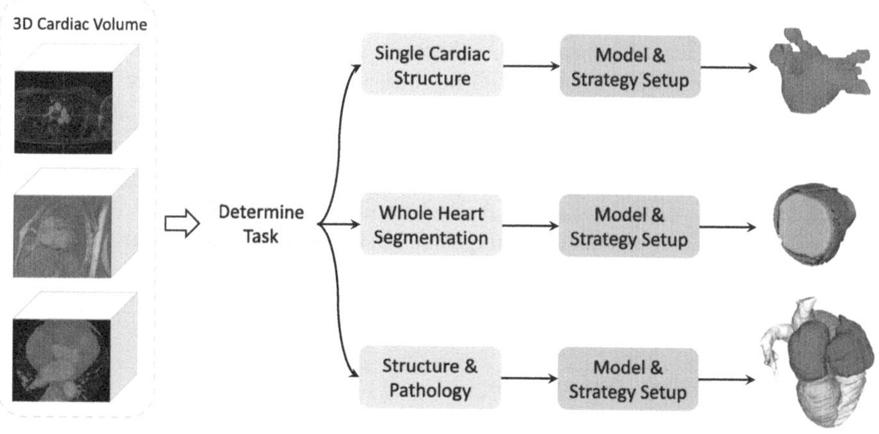

Fig. 1. Our proposed unified framework for 3D cardiac structure segmentation.

core logic of dynamically adjusting parameters (e.g., network topology, patch sampling, and augmentation) to suit data characteristics. Once the model completes training (with validation guided by consistent, reproducible metrics like Dice similarity coefficient, as adopted in the nnU-Net's evaluation pipeline), it enables efficient and accurate generation of 3D cardiac segmentation masks, ensuring reliability across diverse data sources.

2.2 3D U-Net Architecture

The 3D U-Net [4] serves as the foundational model in the nnU-Net framework, designed to handle volumetric medical images. It retains the encoder-decoder structure of the original U-Net [23] but includes minor modifications and dynamic topology adaptation:

Core Structure. The encoder aggregates semantic information via successive pooling operations (at the cost of reduced spatial resolution), while the decoder recovers spatial details by fusing high-resolution feature maps from the encoder (via skip connections) with semantic features from the encoder's bottom layer. This design enables precise segmentation of fine anatomical structures, outperforming networks like FCN [18] or early DeepLab variants [3] for medical tasks, and it incorporates two key modifications distinct from the original U-Net: first, ReLU activation functions are replaced with leaky ReLUs (with a negative slope of 10^{-2}) to mitigate dead neurons; second, instance normalization [26] is employed in place of batch normalization [12], allowing better adaptation to the heterogeneous intensity distributions of medical images.

Dynamic Topology Adaptation. The framework automatically adjusts input patch size, batch size, and number of pooling operations to match dataset-specific image geometries and memory constraints: it starts with a base 3D

U-Net configuration—including an input patch size of $128 \times 128 \times 128$, a batch size of 2, and 30 feature maps at the highest resolution—to establish a consistent baseline. For datasets where the median voxel shape is smaller than 128^3, the framework further refines these parameters by setting the patch size to align with the dataset's median shape and increasing the batch size, ensuring the total number of voxels processed per optimizer step remains stable (with this total capped at $\leq 5\%$ of the dataset). As for pooling operations, they are applied along each axis until the feature map size drops below 8 (with a maximum of 5 pooling steps allowed in total), a design that ensures sufficient aggregation of spatial information to support accurate segmentation.

2.3 Preprocessing Techniques

All preprocessing steps are fully automated (no user intervention) to ensure consistency across datasets, covering three key operations:

Cropping. Data is cropped to the region of non-zero values to reduce computational burden. If cropping reduces the average patient volume by $\geq 25\%$, normalization is restricted to non-zero regions, with out-of-mask values set to 0.

Resampling. CNNs do not natively interpret voxel spacing, so all images are resampled to the dataset's median voxel spacing: third-order spline interpolation is used for image data, while nearest neighbor interpolation is applied to segmentation masks to preserve label integrity.

Normalization. Modality-specific normalization standardizes intensity scales: for CT scans, intensities are first clipped to the [0.5, 99.5] percentiles of values within the segmentation masks of the training set, followed by z-score normalization calculated as

$$I_{\text{norm}} = \frac{I_{\text{clipped}} - \mu}{\sigma},$$

where μ and σ represent the mean and standard deviation of the clipped intensity values, respectively. For MRI and other image modalities, by contrast, per-patient z-score normalization is applied directly without prior intensity clipping.

2.4 Training and Inference Strategy

Loss Function. Models are trained from scratch using a combined loss function to address class imbalance:

$$\mathcal{L}_{\text{total}} = \mathcal{L}_{\text{dice}} + \mathcal{L}_{\text{CE}},$$

where $\mathcal{L}_{\text{CE}}$ is cross-entropy loss, and $\mathcal{L}_{\text{dice}}$ is a multi-class Dice loss:

$$\mathcal{L}_{\text{dice}} = -\frac{2}{|K|} \sum_{k \in K} \frac{\sum_{i \in I} u_i^k v_i^k}{\sum_{i \in I} u_i^k + \sum_{i \in I} v_i^k}.$$

Here, u_i^k is the softmax output of the network for voxel i and class k, v_i^k is the one-hot encoded ground truth, K is the set of classes, and I is the set of voxels in the training patch/batch.

Unbiased Training. As for the difficulty of the structure & pathology task—arising from complex anatomical structures and subtle pathological features that may limit model performance with the current dataset—we aim to enhance training by incorporating additional data from the M&M challenge [19]. However, a notable issue is that the class labels in the M&M challenge do not match those in our used dataset, creating a label mismatch that could introduce noise if not properly addressed. In this scenario, we treat any label from the M&M challenge that does not correspond to our predefined classes as an "unknown" label. For loss computation and model training, we then aggregate the logits of these unknown labels, allowing the model to leverage the meaningful anatomical information from the M&M data without forcing mismatched labels, thus maintaining training stability and improving the model's ability to handle diverse cases.

Optimizer and Learning Rate. The Adam optimizer is used with an initial learning rate of 3×10^{-4}, and an epoch is defined as 250 training batches. Exponential moving averages of training (l_{MA}^t) and validation (l_{MA}^v) losses are tracked: specifically, if l_{MA}^t does not improve by $\geq 5 \times 10^{-3}$ over 30 epochs, the learning rate is reduced by a factor of 5, and training terminates if l_{MA}^v fails to improve by $\geq 5 \times 10^{-3}$ over 60 epochs (or if the learning rate drops below 10^{-6}).

Data Augmentation. On-the-fly data augmentation is used to prevent overfitting in limited medical imaging datasets and enhance training sample diversity, with fixed parameters for the 3D U-Net. The applied techniques include random rotations, scaling, elastic deformations, gamma correction, and mirroring. For 3D U-Nets with a patch aspect ratio > 2, 2D slice-wise augmentation is used instead to avoid distortion issues with 3D augmentation on non-uniform patch shapes.

Patch Sampling. To stabilize training, at least one-third of samples per batch are enforced to contain at least one foreground class. For inference, a patch-based paradigm is adopted to handle large volumes: patches overlap by 50% of their size, with voxels near patch centers weighted more heavily than border voxels to mitigate edge accuracy degradation. Additionally, test-time augmentation is applied, where patches are mirrored along all valid axes—resulting in up to 64 predictions per voxel for the 3D U-Net.

2.5 Postprocessing

Postprocessing is guided by analysis of the training set: first, connected component analysis is performed on all ground-truth segmentation labels, and if a class exhibits a single connected component across all training cases, an observation interpreted as a dataset-specific anatomical property, all but the largest connected component of that class are removed from the final predictions. This step effectively eliminates spurious small regions, ensuring the segmentation results align with anatomical plausibility.

Table 1. Quantitative results of our method compared with previous methods (in-distribution), including CNN and transformer architectures. SCS indicates single structure segmentation. SP indicates structure & pathology. WHS indicates whole heart segmentation. Dice score is reported here.

Method	Architecture	SCS	SP	WHS	Average
3D UNet [4]	CNN	0.9228	0.7289	0.8929	0.8482
STU-Net S [11]	CNN	0.9245	0.7034	0.9109	0.8463
STU-Net B [11]	CNN	0.9278	0.7162	0.9114	0.8518
STU-Net L [11]	CNN	0.9271	0.7120	0.9116	0.8502
STU-Net H [11]	CNN	0.9284	0.7148	0.9103	0.8512
MedNext L k5 [24]	CNN	0.9231	0.6780	0.9108	0.8373
SwinUNETR [9]	Transformer	0.8875	0.6917	0.8542	0.8111
SwinUNETRv2 [10]	Transformer	0.8761	0.6932	0.8659	0.8117
Segformer3D [21]	Transformer	0.8674	0.5972	0.8751	0.7799
nnFormer [31]	Transformer	0.8916	0.6874	0.8845	0.8212
3D UniNet (ours)	CNN	0.9283	0.6925	0.9103	0.8437

Table 2. Quantitative results of our method compared with previous methods (OOD), including CNN and transformer architectures. Dice score and HD are reported here.

Method	SCS		SP		WHS		Average	
	Dice	HD	Dice	HD	Dice	HD	Dice	HD
STU-Net B [11]	0.8881	22.8653	0.7651	9.0646	0.9062	14.5783	0.8531	11.8403
STU-Net H [11]	0.8861	23.5925	0.7627	8.7211	0.9078	11.0341	0.8522	11.0500
3D UniNet (ours)	0.8881	23.9108	0.7754	8.8618	0.9070	12.1432	0.8568	11.4432

3 Experiment

3.1 Experimental Setup

In our experiments, we leverage data from the CARE challenge [5,17,33,34] for both training and evaluation. For the structure-and-pathology task specifically, we incorporate additional training data from the M&Ms challenge [19] to enhance model generalization. Unless otherwise specified, performance is evaluated by splitting the provided training data in a 4:1 ratio (training:validation).

We compare our method against several prior state-of-the-art approaches, including 3D UNet [4], STU-Net [11], MedNext [24], SwinUNETR [9], SwinUNETRv2 [10], Segformer3D [21], and nnFormer [31]. These models are grounded in distinct architectural paradigms—specifically convolutional neural networks (CNNs) and transformers—covering a broad spectrum of state-of-the-art design choices. For quantitative assessment, we adopt the Dice Similarity Coefficient and Hausdorff Distance (HD) as our primary evaluation metrics, which are widely recognized for measuring segmentation accuracy in medical imaging.

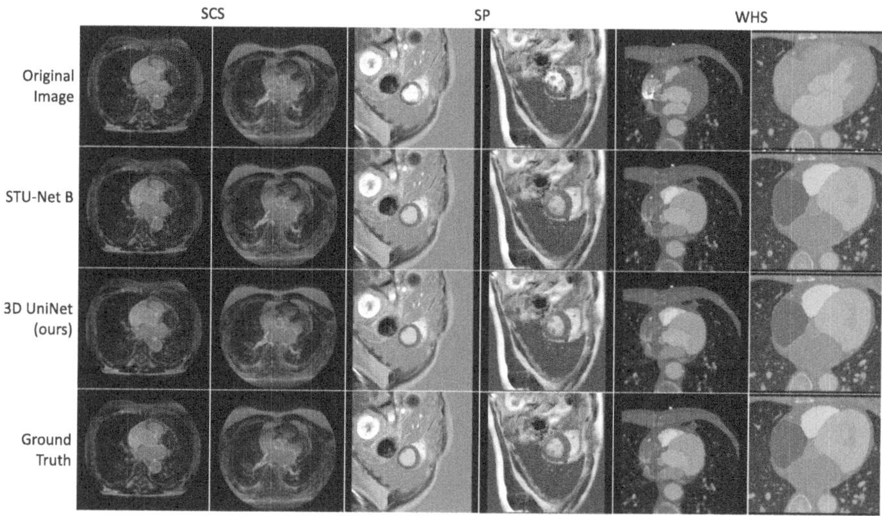

Fig. 2. Qualitative results of cardiac structure segmentation of our 3D UniNet compared with STU-Net B [11].

3.2 Comparison with State-of-the-Art Methods

We compare our method against several prior state-of-the-art approaches, which span diverse model architectural paradigms, encompassing both convolutional and transformer-based designs. We first perform experiments on the training set, using a 4:1 train-validation split to ensure reliable preliminary evaluation, and the corresponding results are presented in Table 1. From these results, it is clear that CNN-based architectures consistently outperform the latest transformer-based alternatives: transformer-based models largely struggle to capture discriminative features from cardiac MRI and CT data, limiting their segmentation accuracy. Specifically, our 3D UniNet outperforms SwinUNETR by 4.60% and

6.57% on the SCS (Single Cardiac Structure) and WHS (Whole-Heart Segmentation) tasks, respectively. The qualitative results are shown in Fig. 2.

Across all evaluated methods, 3D UniNet and STU-Net emerge as the top performers among this diverse set of models. We therefore proceed to further evaluate these two leading models on the official validation set to confirm their generalizability, with results detailed in Table 2. Our findings reveal that 3D UniNet achieves the highest average performance when assessed against the primary evaluation metric: the Dice Similarity Coefficient.

3.3 Ablation Studies

To further validate the role of key components in our framework, we conduct a series of ablation studies and evaluate on the official validation set.

Table 3. Ablation study on utilizing postprocessing techniques.

Method	SCS		SP		WHS		Average	
	Dice	HD	Dice	HD	Dice	HD	Dice	HD
3D UniNet	0.8881	23.9108	0.7754	8.8618	0.9070	12.1432	0.8568	11.4432
3D UniNet post.	0.8881	23.9108	0.7754	8.8618	0.9067	11.8761	0.8567	11.3764

First, we assess the impact of our postprocessing technique by applying it to model predictions, with corresponding results presented in Table 3. These findings clearly indicate that the postprocessing technique fails to yield any positive improvement in model performance—suggesting it does not address the core challenges of the segmentation task in this context.

Table 4. Ablation on utilizing additional data from M&M challenge [19] for structure & pathology task. 3D UniNet naive indicates directly adopt the data for training. 3D UniNet unbiased indicates the extra label is set an unknown class. 3D UniNet reweight indicates the class weight for extra label is set as 0

Method	Dice	HD
3D UniNet	0.7754	8.8618
3D UniNet naive	0.7782	8.3091
3D UniNet unbiased	0.7723	8.7711
3D UniNet reweight	0.7734	9.2524

Next, we investigate the effect of incorporating additional training data (sourced from the M&Ms challenge [19]) specifically for the structure-and-pathology task, with detailed results shown in Table 4. Our analysis reveals that even naive integration of this extra training data—without additional parameter tuning or data alignment—leads to a measurable improvement in the model's performance on the validation set, highlighting the value of expanded data diversity for complex segmentation tasks.

4 Conclusion

In this work, we propose a unified framework to address the multi-structure segmentation challenge in cardiac imaging segmentation tasks. For each individual segmentation task, our framework is capable of determining an appropriate model architecture and tailored training strategy—ensuring it achieves optimal performance aligned with the task's specific demands. Our method outperforms previous state-of-the-art approaches by a significant margin, with a particularly notable advantage over transformer-based models, which often struggle to capture discriminative features in cardiac imaging data. Furthermore, we find that incorporating additional training data for complex, high-difficulty tasks (e.g., the structure & pathology segmentation task) yields a positive effect on enhancing model performance, underscoring the value of data diversity for challenging medical segmentation scenarios. We anticipate our work will serve as a robust baseline and practical solution for advancing 3D cardiac structure segmentation research and clinical applications.

References

1. Baumgartner, C.F., Koch, L.M., Pollefeys, M., Konukoglu, E.: An exploration of 2d and 3d deep learning techniques for cardiac mr image segmentation. In: International Workshop on Statistical Atlases and Computational Models of the Heart, pp. 111–119. Springer (2017)
2. Chang, Q., Yan, Z., Zhou, M., Liu, D., Sawalha, K., Ye, M., Zhangli, Q., Kanski, M., Al'Aref, S., Axel, L., et al.: Deeprecon: joint 2d cardiac segmentation and 3d volume reconstruction via a structure-specific generative method. In: MICCAI, pp. 567–577. Springer (2022)
3. Chen, L.C., Papandreou, G., Kokkinos, I., Murphy, K., Yuille, A.L.: Deeplab: semantic image segmentation with deep convolutional nets, atrous convolution, and fully connected crfs. TPAMI **40**(4), 834–848 (2017)
4. Çiçek, Ö., Abdulkadir, A., Lienkamp, S.S., Brox, T., Ronneberger, O.: 3d u-net: learning dense volumetric segmentation from sparse annotation. In: MICCAI, pp. 424–432. Springer (2016)
5. Gao, S., Zhou, H., Gao, Y., Zhuang, X.: Bayeseg: Bayesian modeling for medical image segmentation with interpretable generalizability. Med. Image Anal. **89**, 102889 (2023)
6. Genereux, P.: Staging of valve disease based on the extent of cardiac damage: ready for the guidelines? (2022)
7. Goldsborough, E., Osuji, N., Blaha, M.J.: Assessment of cardiovascular disease risk: a 2022 update. Endocrinol. Metab. Clin. **51**(3), 483–509 (2022)

8. Habijan, M., Galić, I., Romić, K., Leventić, H.: Ab-resunet+: improving multiple cardiovascular structure segmentation from computed tomography angiography images. Appl. Sci. **12**(6), 3024 (2022)
9. Hatamizadeh, A., Nath, V., Tang, Y., Yang, D., Roth, H.R., Xu, D.: Swin unetr: Swin transformers for semantic segmentation of brain tumors in mri images. In: International MICCAI Brainlesion Workshop, pp. 272–284. Springer (2021)
10. He, Y., Nath, V., Yang, D., Tang, Y., Myronenko, A., Xu, D.: Swinunetr-v2: stronger swin transformers with stagewise convolutions for 3d medical image segmentation. In: MICCAI, pp. 416–426. Springer (2023)
11. Huang, Z., Wang, H., Deng, Z., Ye, J., Su, Y., Sun, H., He, J., Gu, Y., Gu, L., Zhang, S., Qiao, Y.: Stu-net: scalable and transferable medical image segmentation models empowered by large-scale supervised pre-training. arXiv preprint arXiv:2304.06716 (2023)
12. Ioffe, S., Szegedy, C.: Batch normalization: accelerating deep network training by reducing internal covariate shift. In: ICML, pp. 448–456. pmlr (2015)
13. Isensee, F., Jaeger, P.F., Kohl, S.A., Petersen, J., Maier-Hein, K.H.: nnu-net: a self-configuring method for deep learning-based biomedical image segmentation. Nat. Methods **18**(2), 203–211 (2021)
14. Jankowski, J., Floege, J., Fliser, D., Böhm, M., Marx, N.: Cardiovascular disease in chronic kidney disease: pathophysiological insights and therapeutic options. Circulation **143**(11), 1157–1172 (2021)
15. Karimi, D., Gholipour, A.: Improving calibration and out-of-distribution detection in deep models for medical image segmentation. IEEE Trans. Artif. Intell. **4**(2), 383–397 (2022)
16. Khan, S.S., Coresh, J., Pencina, M.J., Ndumele, C.E., Rangaswami, J., Chow, S.L., Palaniappan, L.P., Sperling, L.S., Virani, S.S., Ho, J.E., et al.: Novel prediction equations for absolute risk assessment of total cardiovascular disease incorporating cardiovascular-kidney-metabolic health: a scientific statement from the American heart association. Circulation **148**(24), 1982–2004 (2023)
17. Li, L., Zimmer, V.A., Schnabel, J.A., Zhuang, X.: Atrialjsqnet: a new framework for joint segmentation and quantification of left atrium and scars incorporating spatial and shape information. Med. Image Anal. **76**, 102303 (2022)
18. Long, J., Shelhamer, E., Darrell, T.: Fully convolutional networks for semantic segmentation. In: CVPR, pp. 3431–3440 (2015)
19. Martín-Isla, C., Campello, V.M., Izquierdo, C., Kushibar, K., Sendra-Balcells, C., Gkontra, P., Sojoudi, A., Fulton, M.J., Arega, T.W., Punithakumar, K., et al.: Deep learning segmentation of the right ventricle in cardiac mri: the m&ms challenge. JBHI **27**(7), 3302–3313 (2023)
20. Nguyen, D.M.H., Pham, T.N., Diep, N.T., Phan, N.Q., Pham, Q., Tong, V., Nguyen, B.T., Le, N.H., Ho, N., Xie, P., et al.: On the out of distribution robustness of foundation models in medical image segmentation. arXiv preprint arXiv:2311.11096 (2023)
21. Perera, S., Navard, P., Yilmaz, A.: Segformer3d: an efficient transformer for 3d medical image segmentation. In: CVPR, pp. 4981–4988 (2024)
22. Petersen, K.S., Kris-Etherton, P.M.: Diet quality assessment and the relationship between diet quality and cardiovascular disease risk. Nutrients **13**(12), 4305 (2021)
23. Ronneberger, O., Fischer, P., Brox, T.: U-net: convolutional networks for biomedical image segmentation. In: MICCAI, pp. 234–241. Springer (2015)
24. Roy, S., Koehler, G., Ulrich, C., Baumgartner, M., Petersen, J., Isensee, F., Jaeger, P.F., Maier-Hein, K.H.: Mednext: transformer-driven scaling of convnets for medical image segmentation. In: MICCAI, pp. 405–415. Springer (2023)

25. Song, X., Zhou, F., Frangi, A.F., Cao, J., Xiao, X., Lei, Y., Wang, T., Lei, B.: Multicenter and multichannel pooling gcn for early ad diagnosis based on dual-modality fused brain network. TMI **42**(2), 354–367 (2022)
26. Ulyanov, D., Vedaldi, A., Lempitsky, V.: Instance normalization: the missing ingredient for fast stylization. arXiv preprint arXiv:1607.08022 (2016)
27. Yuan, M., Xia, Y., Dong, H., Chen, Z., Yao, J., Qiu, M., Yan, K., Yin, X., Shi, Y., Chen, X., et al.: Devil is in the queries: advancing mask transformers for real-world medical image segmentation and out-of-distribution localization. In: CCPR, pp. 23879–23889 (2023)
28. Yue, G., Wei, P., Zhou, T., Jiang, Q., Yan, W., Wang, T.: Toward multicenter skin lesion classification using deep neural network with adaptively weighted balance loss. TMI **42**(1), 119–131 (2022)
29. Zhang, S., Zhang, J., Tian, B., Lukasiewicz, T., Xu, Z.: Multi-modal contrastive mutual learning and pseudo-label re-learning for semi-supervised medical image segmentation. Med. Image Anal. **83**, 102656 (2023)
30. Zhang, Y., Yang, J., Tian, J., Shi, Z., Zhong, C., Zhang, Y., He, Z.: Modality-aware mutual learning for multi-modal medical image segmentation. In: MICCAI, pp. 589–599. Springer (2021)
31. Zhou, H.Y., Guo, J., Zhang, Y., Yu, L., Wang, L., Yu, Y.: nnformer: interleaved transformer for volumetric segmentation (2022)
32. Zhu, Z., Wang, Z., Qi, G., Mazur, N., Yang, P., Liu, Y.: Brain tumor segmentation in mri with multi-modality spatial information enhancement and boundary shape correction. Pattern Recogn. **153**, 110553 (2024)
33. Zhuang, X.: Multivariate mixture model for myocardial segmentation combining multi-source images. TPAMI **41**(12), 2933–2946 (2019)
34. Zhuang, X., Shen, J.: Multi-scale patch and multi-modality atlases for whole heart segmentation of mri. Med. Image Anal. **31**, 77–87 (2016)

Uncertainty-Guided Curriculum Learning for Automated Liver Fibrosis Staging on Heterogeneous MRI

Yuxin Jin[1], Fengjun Zhao[1], Yanrong Chen[2], and Xuelei He[1(✉)]

[1] Northwest University, Xi'an, China
{fjzhao,xueleihe}@nwu.edu.cn
[2] The First Affiliated Hospital of Xi'an Jiaotong University, Xi'an, China
yanrong_chen415@163.com

Abstract. Liver fibrosis, a major global health issue induced by chronic liver diseases, requires accurate staging for prognosis, treatment planning, and prevention of cirrhosis progression. Automated staging using MRI has emerged as a promising solution, but heterogeneity across multi-center and multi-phase MRI data—caused by variations in imaging protocols, device types, and image quality—significantly limits the generalizability and clinical transferability of deep learning models. Given such distributional discrepancies, a single model struggles to adequately capture all key features. To address this challenge, we propose an uncertainty-guided curriculum learning framework that progressively incorporates samples with higher uncertainty, thereby improving robustness in fibrosis staging. Experimental results demonstrate superior modeling of hard cases and enhanced cross-modal generalization in both cirrhosis and substantial fibrosis detection tasks. Our framework offers a clinically viable pathway to improving automated fibrosis staging on heterogeneous MRI data. The code is available at https://github.com/pazjin/FibUCL.

Keywords: Liver fibrosis staging · MRI heterogeneity · Uncertainty estimation · Domain generalization · Deep learning · Medical image analysis · Cross-modal robustness

1 Introduction

Liver fibrosis, a common outcome of chronic liver disease, can progress to cirrhosis or hepatocellular carcinoma (HCC), making accurate staging essential. Histopathology, the clinical gold standard, is invasive and limited for early screening. MRI provides non-invasive, multi-modal assessment with strong staging potential [18].

Traditional interpretation relies on radiologists' judgment, while deep learning, despite recent advances [3,16], faces challenges with multi-modal MRI due to inter-center heterogeneity and modality redundancy or conflict.

X. Zhuang et al. (Eds.): CARE 2025, LNCS 16257, pp. 12–22, 2026.
https://doi.org/10.1007/978-3-032-16271-7_2

We propose an **uncertainty-guided progressive learning framework**. Slice-level prediction entropy identifies challenging samples for progressive training, improving robustness and generalization. Domain shifts are mitigated via Maximum Mean Discrepancy (MMD), and an attention-gated Mixture-of-Experts (MOE) enables adaptive modality fusion.

Contributions:

- Entropy-based curriculum for progressive incorporation of high-uncertainty samples.
- Attention-gated MOE with MMD for robust cross-modal and cross-center learning.
- Extensive multi-center, multi-modal validation achieving state-of-the-art fibrosis staging.

2 Related Work

Uncertainty modeling (MC Dropout, ensembles, entropy-based sampling [6, 14, 15, 19, 25]) improves robustness and hard-sample handling, yet cross-center overconfidence remains a challenge [10]. Curriculum learning and hard-sample mining [2, 7, 8, 11, 17, 23] enhance convergence, but fixed-threshold approaches lack flexibility. Domain shifts are typically addressed via MMD, CORAL, or adversarial alignment [4, 12, 20], and multi-modal fusion (attention, gated fusion, MOE [1, 9, 21]) exploits complementary information. Our method unifies entropy-guided curriculum, MMD alignment, and MOE-based fusion to robustly handle cross-modal heterogeneity and challenging samples.

3 Methodology

3.1 Problem Formulation

Let the multi-modal MRI slice set be denoted as $\mathcal{X} = \{x_i^m\}_{i=1,m\in\mathcal{M}}^N$, where N represents the total number of slices and $\mathcal{M}$ denotes the set of modalities. We define a discriminative mapping function $f_\theta : \mathcal{X} \rightarrow \{0, 1\}$, aiming to solve the following two binary sub-tasks simultaneously:

$$y_i^{(1)} = \begin{cases} 1, & \text{if stage is S4} \\ 0, & \text{if stage is S1–S3} \end{cases} \qquad y_i^{(2)} = \begin{cases} 1, & \text{if stage is S2–S4} \\ 0, & \text{if stage is S1} \end{cases} \tag{1}$$

Under the generalization constraints of cross-modality $\mathcal{M}$ and cross-domain $\mathcal{D}$, the overall optimization objective is formulated as:

$$\min_\theta \; \mathbb{E}_{x\sim\mathcal{D}_{\text{train}}} \, \ell\big(f_\theta(x), y\big) \; + \; \lambda \cdot \text{Dist}\big(\mathcal{D}_{\text{train}}, \mathcal{D}_{\text{test}}\big), \tag{2}$$

where $\ell(\cdot)$ denotes the classification loss, $\text{Dist}(\cdot, \cdot)$ measures the cross-domain feature distribution discrepancy, and λ is a balancing coefficient.

3.2 Entropy-Guided Progressive Curriculum

We quantify sample-level uncertainty using predictive entropy:

$$u_i = - \sum_{c \in \{0,1\}} \hat{p}_i^{(c)} \log \hat{p}_i^{(c)}, \tag{3}$$

where higher u_i indicates greater uncertainty.

Sample Stratification. Entropy values $\{u_i\}$ are clustered (K=3) in a one-dimensional space to adaptively partition samples without manual thresholds. The clusters are ranked by average entropy, yielding three cohorts:

- **Reliably-Predicted Cohort (RPC)**: low-entropy cluster, stable predictions with high confidence;
- **Ambiguously-Predicted Cohort (APC)**: medium-entropy cluster, mostly correct but with noticeable uncertainty;
- **Challenging-Predicted Cohort (CPC)**: high entropy cluster, misclassified or highly uncertain samples representing the most challenging cases.

Progressive Training. The ordering of cohorts follows principles of curriculum learning, where tasks of intermediate difficulty are introduced prior to the easiest or hardest cases to stabilize optimization. Specifically, beginning with the **APC** cohort provides sufficiently informative yet tractable samples, enabling the model to establish discriminative decision boundaries without being overwhelmed by noise or trivial patterns. Once a reliable representation is formed, exposure to the **CPC** cohort introduces the most challenging samples, encouraging adaptation to rare but critical failure modes. Finally, training on the **RPC** cohort consolidates confident predictions, serving as a regularization stage that prevents overfitting to high-entropy cases and reinforces overall robustness. This APC $\rightarrow$ CPC $\rightarrow$ RPC progression balances stability, adaptability, and generalization, and was further corroborated by empirical observations that alternative orders led to unstable convergence or degraded accuracy.

3.3 Multi-modal Fusion & Domain Alignment

To address modality heterogeneity and multi-center domain shifts, we employ a Mixture-of-Experts (MOE) based dynamic fusion strategy. A gating network $G(\cdot)$ generates modality weights $\alpha_m(x)$ as:

$$\hat{y} = \sum_{m \in \mathcal{M}} \alpha_m(x) \cdot E_m(x^m), \quad \alpha_m(x) = \frac{\exp(G_m(x))}{\sum_{m'} \exp(G_{m'}(x))}. \tag{4}$$

Meanwhile, cross-domain feature alignment is achieved via Maximum Mean Discrepancy (MMD):

$$\text{MMD}^2(Z_s, Z_t) = \left\| \frac{1}{N_s} \sum_{i=1}^{N_s} \phi(z_s^i) - \frac{1}{N_t} \sum_{j=1}^{N_t} \phi(z_t^j) \right\|_{\mathcal{H}}^2. \tag{5}$$

As shown in Fig. 1, MOE enables dynamic cross-modality fusion, while MMD facilitates feature consistency across centers.

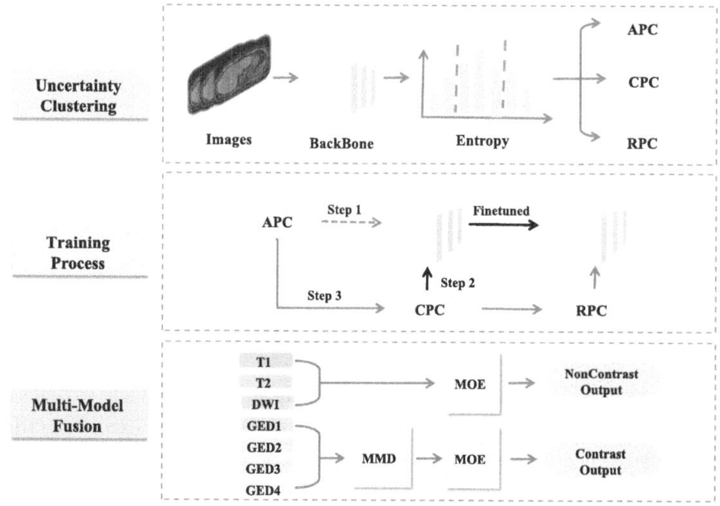

Fig. 1. Entropy-guided curriculum partitioning and multi-modal fusion architecture. **Uncertainty Clustering and Training Process:** Samples are partitioned into RPC, APC, and CPC subsets via predictive entropy, forming a progressive training pathway. **Multi-Modal Fusion:** A mixture-of-experts (MOE) framework adaptively weights modalities, while MMD loss enforces cross-domain feature alignment.

3.4 UPMA Loss: Uncertainty-Guided Progressive Multi-domain Alignment

By integrating classification objectives with cross-domain alignment, we propose an uncertainty-guided composite loss:

$$\mathcal{L}_{\text{UPMA}} = \frac{1}{|\mathcal{S}|} \sum_{i \in \mathcal{S}} \ell_{\text{CE}}(\hat{y}_i, y_i) + \lambda_{\text{MMD}} \cdot \text{MMD}^2(Z_s, Z_t), \tag{6}$$

where $\mathcal{S}$ denotes the current training subset, ℓ_{CE} is the cross-entropy loss, and λ_{MMD} controls the strength of domain alignment. The training proceeds in two stages: (1) $\mathcal{S} = \text{APC}$, focusing on moderately difficult cases; (2) $\mathcal{S} = \text{APC} \cup \text{CPC}$, enhancing robustness and generalization.

4 Experiments

4.1 Dataset

We constructed a multi-center liver MRI cohort of **360 patients** spanning fibrosis stages S1–S4, selected from a larger pool of 610 cases acquired on scanners from Philips and Siemens. The dataset covers **non-contrast** (T1, T2, DWI_800) and **contrast-enhanced dynamic** phases (arterial, portal, delayed, hepatobiliary) from Gd-EOB-DTPA MRI. Each case is stored in Nifty format, with occasional missing phases and without prior spatial registration [5,13,24]. Preprocessing employed `TotalSegmentator` for liver ROI extraction and slice generation.

Slice-level features were extracted by modality-specific ResNet18s and fused via an attention-gated Mixture-of-Experts (MOE) with TENT-based domain adaptation.

4.2 Training Setup

In this study, ResNet18 was employed as the backbone feature extractor to perform slice-wise classification across different modalities (T1WI, T2WI, DWI_800, GED1–GED4). For non-contrast learning tasks (NonContrast), Subtask1_prob_S4 and Subtask2_prob_S1 utilized T1WI, T2WI, and DWI_800 modalities, whereas contrast learning tasks (Contrast) utilized GED1–GED4 modalities.

Training hyperparameters for samples of different entropy categories are summarized in Table 1. All experiments used a batch size of 128. Specifically, all cohort (ALL) were trained with a learning rate of 1×10^{-6} for 100 epochs; APC were trained with a learning rate ranging from 1×10^{-6} to 1×10^{-5} for 100 epochs; APC+CPC were trained with a learning rate of 1×10^{-5} for 50 epochs.

For contrast-enhanced tasks, multi-modal domain generalization using MMD was applied to mitigate distributional differences across scanning sequences: the total loss for liver cirrhosis detection was defined as $\mathcal{L}_{total} = \mathcal{L}_{cls} + 0.1 \times \mathcal{L}_{MMD}$, and for substantial fibrosis detection as $\mathcal{L}_{total} = \mathcal{L}_{cls} + 0.05 \times \mathcal{L}_{MMD}$.

Finally, multi-modal predictions were aggregated using a mixture-of-experts (MOE) framework based on an attention gating network (AttentionGatingNet). MOE was trained using the Adam optimizer with a learning rate of $1e-3$ and binary cross-entropy loss (BCELoss) for 100 epochs, with validation performed every 20 epochs. The dataset was stratified by labels with an 80%/20% train/validation split. The gating network outputs were used to dynamically weight the contributions of each modality expert, enabling adaptive modeling according to sample difficulty.

Table 1. Training hyperparameters for different entropy categories.

Entropy Category	Learning Rate	Batch Size	Epochs
ALL	1×10^{-6}	128	100
APC	$1 \times 10^{-6} \sim 1 \times 10^{-5}$	128	100
APC + CPC	1×10^{-5}	128	50

4.3 Quantitative Results and Analysis

Contrast tasks (Tables 2, 3) showed Std outperforming early, while entropy-guided learning dominated after CPC integration, reaching near-saturation (AUC 0.980–0.998, ACC >0.955). Non-contrast tasks (Tables 4, 5) achieved similar trends: Std nearly perfected T1/T2, while entropy substantially boosted DWI_800 (0.906→0.995).

Table 2. Subtask1_prob_S4 across Contrast sequences

Contrast	**GED1**		**GED2**		**GED3**		**GED4**	
	AUC	ACC	AUC	ACC	AUC	ACC	AUC	ACC
base	0.954	0.899	0.968	0.913	0.915	0.856	0.954	0.892
APC_entropy	0.952	0.940	0.929	0.938	0.902	0.908	0.952	0.961
APC_std	0.992	**0.983**	**0.995**	**0.968**	**0.999**	**0.989**	**0.999**	0.983
APC+CPC_entropy	**0.996**	0.975	**0.995**	0.961	0.996	0.969	0.998	**0.986**
APC+CPC_std	0.995	0.966	0.994	0.961	0.994	0.960	0.998	0.980
all_entropy	0.994	0.964	0.993	0.964	0.996	0.966	0.998	0.983
all_std	0.995	0.969	0.993	0.961	0.980	0.955	0.990	0.972

Table 3. Subtask2_prob_S1 across Contrast sequences

Contrast	**GED1**		**GED2**		**GED3**		**GED4**	
	AUC	ACC	AUC	ACC	AUC	ACC	AUC	ACC
base	0.841	0.835	0.872	0.821	0.874	0.808	0.906	0.833
APC_entropy	0.974	0.946	0.959	0.956	0.962	0.911	0.977	0.936
APC_std	0.985	0.954	**0.992**	**0.975**	**0.996**	**0.976**	0.994	**0.982**
APC+CPC_entropy	**0.998**	0.972	**0.992**	0.933	**0.996**	0.960	**0.998**	0.967
APC+CPC_std	0.993	0.974	0.990	0.950	0.993	0.953	0.994	0.971
all_entropy	**0.998**	**0.980**	**0.992**	0.933	**0.996**	0.966	**0.998**	0.969
all_std	0.963	0.958	0.966	0.952	0.982	0.972	0.980	0.967

4.4 External Validation and Ablation Study

We evaluated generalization on the competition validation set, comparing Adabn_Tent and MOE variants with different MMD weights (Fig. 2). Figure 3 further compares MOE with mean-voting (MIN) across subtasks and modalities.

For *Contrast* sequences, MMD-0.1+MOE achieved the highest Subtask1 AUC (0.8050), while Subtask2 peaked with MMD-0.05+MOE (0.7822), highlighting task-dependent complementarity of domain alignment. In *NonContrast* sequences, standalone MOE reached the highest Subtask2 AUC (0.7541), suggesting limited benefit of MMD regularization under low domain shift. Across all settings, MOE consistently outperformed MIN and Adabn_Tent [22], demonstrating that uncertainty-driven progressive fusion combined with task- and modality-aware domain alignment yields robust and generalizable performance in multi-modal, multi-task fibrosis staging.

Table 4. Subtask1_prob_S4 across Non-Contrast Sequences

NonContrast	T1		T2		DWI_800	
	AUC	ACC	AUC	ACC	AUC	ACC
base	0.966	0.922	0.955	0.888	0.906	0.845
APC_entropy	0.937	0.936	0.961	0.949	0.970	0.903
APC_std	**0.997**	**0.977**	**1.000**	**0.992**	0.963	0.921
APC+CPC_entropy	0.994	0.961	0.998	0.978	0.995	**0.979**
APC+CPC_std	0.995	0.966	0.998	0.975	**0.997**	0.973
all_entropy	0.995	0.964	0.998	0.980	0.995	0.976
all_std	0.992	0.964	0.998	0.980	**0.996**	0.970

Table 5. Subtask2_prob_S1 across Non-Contrast Sequences

NonContrast	T1		T2		DWI_800	
	AUC	ACC	AUC	ACC	AUC	ACC
base	0.823	0.816	0.921	0.905	0.890	0.818
APC_entropy	0.979	0.968	0.962	0.964	0.957	0.796
APC_std	0.993	0.976	**1.000**	**0.997**	0.985	0.980
APC+CPC_entropy	**0.997**	**0.978**	0.997	0.983	**0.998**	**0.985**
APC+CPC_std	0.990	0.962	0.992	0.941	0.974	0.949
all_entropy	**0.997**	0.972	0.997	0.986	**0.998**	0.979
all_std	0.963	0.927	0.979	0.955	0.957	0.948

4.5 Performance on In-Distribution and Out-of-Distribution Test Sets

On the test set (see Table 6 for Subtask1 and Table 7 for Subtask2), *in-distribution (ID)* performance was moderate for both **Subtask1** and **Subtask2** across modalities (ACC 47.5–65.8%, AUC 67–79%). *Out-of-distribution (OOD)* results showed marked drops in AUC, especially for contrast sequences (**Subtask1** AUC 64.1%), while ACC could be misleadingly high (**Subtask2** ACC 92.9%). These results highlight the impact of domain shift and the need for robust generalization across unseen vendors.

Table 6. Test set performance (ACC and AUC) on **Subtask1** (S1–3 vs S4) across Contrast and Non-Contrast modalities. Results are reported on *In-Distribution* (Vendors A, B1, B2) and *Out-of-Distribution* (Vendor C) sets.

Modality	Setting	ACC (%)	AUC (%)
Contrast	ID (Vendors A, B1, B2)	47.50	78.03
	OOD (Vendor C)	32.86	64.11
Non-Contrast	ID (Vendors A, B1, B2)	47.50	79.78
	OOD (Vendor C)	32.86	46.25

Table 7. Test set performance (ACC and AUC) on **Subtask2** (S1 vs S2–4) across Contrast and Non-Contrast modalities. Results are reported on *In-Distribution* (Vendors A, B1, B2) and *Out-of-Distribution* (Vendor C) sets.

Modality	Setting	ACC (%)	AUC (%)
Contrast	ID (Vendors A, B1, B2)	65.83	78.20
	OOD (Vendor C)	92.86	52.62
Non-Contrast	ID (Vendors A, B1, B2)	65.83	67.27
	OOD (Vendor C)	92.86	40.31

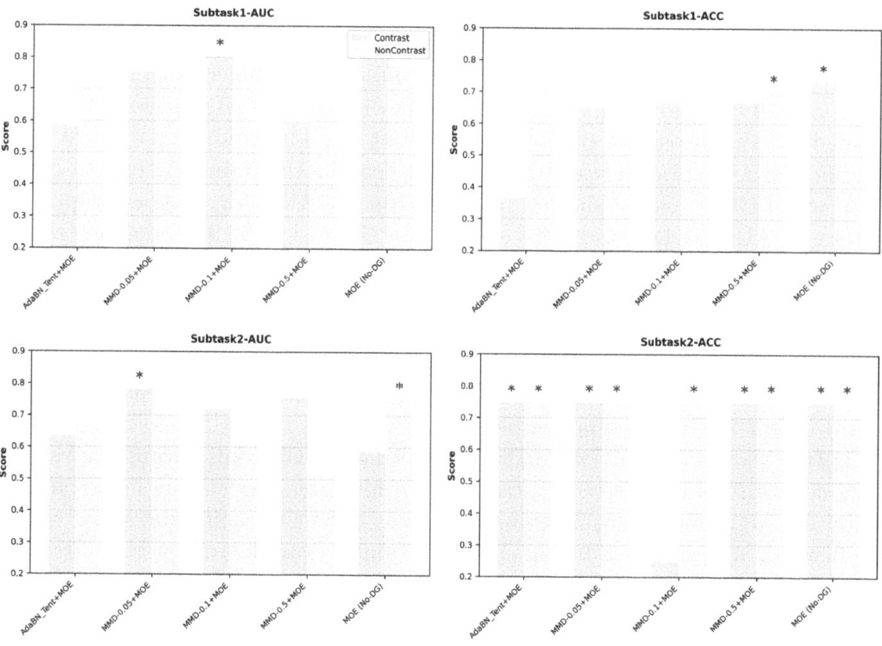

Fig. 2. Validation set performance on the competition platform across two subtasks (Contrast vs NonContrast). Best values are highlighted in *.

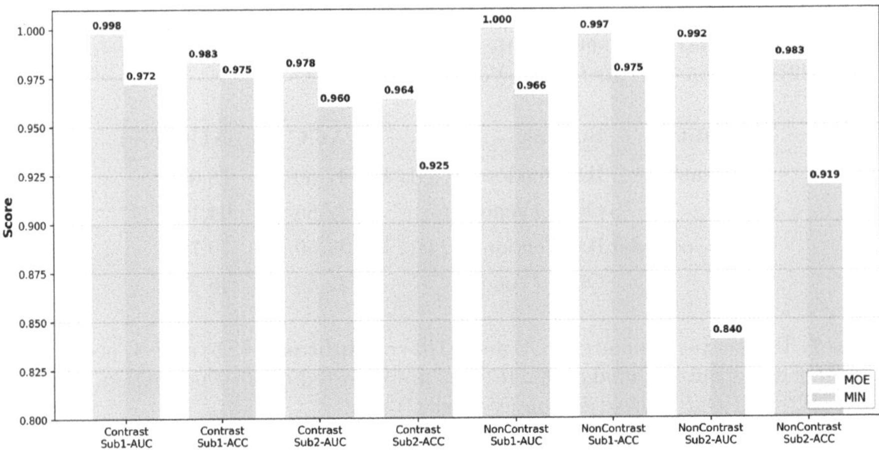

Fig. 3. Comparison of MOE and mean-voting (MIN) ensemble on different subtasks.

5 Conclusion and Future Work

We introduced an entropy-driven curriculum for MRI-based liver fibrosis staging. Progressive integration of high-uncertainty samples, combined with MMD alignment and MOE fusion, achieved moderate in-distribution (ID) performance and highlighted the impact of domain shift on out-of-distribution (OOD) test sets. Specifically, ACC ranged from 47.5% to 65.8% and AUC from 67% to 79% on ID data, while OOD results showed marked drops in AUC for contrast sequences (Subtask1 AUC 64.1%) and inflated ACC for Subtask2 (92.9%), demonstrating both the promise and limitations of our approach across unseen vendors.

These observations underscore the need for robust domain generalization, as well as careful interpretation of ACC and AUC metrics in multi-vendor settings. While the progressive curriculum stabilizes training and enables fusion across contrast and non-contrast modalities, OOD sensitivity indicates room for improvement in vendor-agnostic performance.

Future work will focus on further mitigating domain shift through advanced alignment and self-supervised strategies, evaluating models on larger multi-center datasets, and exploring computationally efficient architectures that retain the benefits of progressive fusion and uncertainty-aware learning. This direction aims to enhance robustness, interpretability, and generalization of automated multi-modal liver fibrosis staging.

Acknowledgments. This study was supported by the National Natural Science Foundation of China (Grants No. 62201459 and 62476218), the General Project of the Key Research and Development Plan of Shaanxi Province (Grants No. 2024SF-YBXM-321 and 2025SF-YBXM-380), the Xi'an Association for Science and Technology (XAST) Youth Talent Support Project (Grant No. 0959202513085), and the Scientific and Technological Projects of Xi'an (Grant No. 201805060ZD11CG44).

Disclosure of Interests The authors have no competing interests to declare that are relevant to the content of this article.

References

1. Arevalo, J., et al.: Gated multimodal units for information fusion. arXiv preprint arXiv:1702.01992 (2017), https://arxiv.org/abs/1702.01992
2. Bengio, Y., Louradour, J., Collobert, R., Weston, J.: Curriculum learning. In: ICML, pp. 41–48 (2009). https://doi.org/10.1145/1553374.1553380
3. Choi, K.J., et al.: Development and validation of a deep learning system for staging liver fibrosis by using contrast agent-enhanced ct images in the liver. Radiology **289**(3), 688–697 (2018). https://doi.org/10.1148/radiol.2018180873
4. Ganin, Y., Lempitsky, V.: Unsupervised domain adaptation by backpropagation. In: ICML (2016). https://doi.org/10.48550/arXiv.1409.7495
5. Gao, Z., Liu, Y., Wu, F., Shi, N., Shi, Y., Zhuang, X.: A reliable and interpretable framework of multi-view learning for liver fibrosis staging. In: International Conference on Medical Image Computing and Computer-Assisted Intervention, pp. 178–188 (2023). https://doi.org/10.1007/978-3-031-43904-9_18
6. Han, Z., et al.: Trusted multi-view classification with dynamic evidential fusion. IEEE Trans. Pattern Anal. Mach. Intell. **45**(2), 2551–2566 (2022). https://doi.org/10.1109/TPAMI.2022.3171983
7. Islam, M., et al.: Paced-curriculum distillation with prediction and label uncertainty for image segmentation. Int. J. Comput. Assist. Radiol. Surg. **18**(10), 1875–1883 (2023). https://doi.org/10.1007/s11548-023-02847-9
8. Iwamoto, S., et al.: Improving reliability of semantic segmentation by uncertainty modeling with Bayesian deep networks and curriculum learning. In: MICCAI Workshop (2021). https://doi.org/10.1007/978-3-030-87735-4_4
9. Jacobs, R.A., et al.: Adaptive mixtures of local experts. Neural Comput. **3**(1), 79–87 (1991). https://doi.org/10.1162/neco.1991.3.1.79
10. Jungo, A., Reyes, M.: Assessing reliability and challenges of uncertainty estimations for medical image segmentation. In: MICCAI (2019). https://doi.org/10.1007/978-3-030-32245-8_6
11. Li, C., et al.: Dynamic curriculum learning via in-domain uncertainty for medical image classification. In: MICCAI (2023). https://doi.org/10.1007/978-3-031-43904-9_72
12. Li, Y., et al.: Domain generalization via conditional invariant representations. In: ICML (2018). https://doi.org/10.48550/arXiv.1807.08479
13. Liu, Y., Gao, Z., Shi, N., Wu, F., Shi, Y., Chen, Q., Zhuang, X.: Merit: multi-view evidential learning for reliable and interpretable liver fibrosis staging. Med. Image Anal. **102**, 103507 (2025). https://doi.org/10.1016/j.media.2025.103507
14. Loftus, T.J., et al.: Uncertainty-aware deep learning in healthcare: a scoping review. PLOS Digital Health **1**(8), e0000085 (2022). https://doi.org/10.1371/journal.pdig.0000085

15. Ma, H., et al.: Trustworthy multimodal regression with mixture of normal-inverse gamma distributions. In: NeurIPS, vol. 34 (2021). https://doi.org/10.48550/arXiv.2111.08456
16. Masugi, Y., et al.: Quantitative assessment of liver fibrosis reveals a nonlinear association with fibrosis stage in nonalcoholic fatty liver disease. Hepatol. Commun. **2**(1), 58–68 (2018). https://doi.org/10.1002/hep4.1121
17. Peng, J., et al.: Self-paced contrastive learning for semi-supervised medical image segmentation with meta-labels. In: NeurIPS, vol. 34 (2021). https://doi.org/10.48550/arXiv.2107.13741
18. Petitclerc, L., et al.: Liver fibrosis: review of current imaging and mri quantification techniques. J. Magn. Reson. Imaging **45**(5), 1276–1295 (2017). https://doi.org/10.1002/jmri.25550
19. Sensoy, M., Kaplan, L., Kandemir, M.: Evidential deep learning to quantify classification uncertainty. In: NeurIPS, vol. 31 (2018). https://doi.org/10.48550/arXiv.1806.01768
20. Sun, B., Saenko, K.: Deep coral: correlation alignment for deep domain adaptation. In: ECCV (2016). https://doi.org/10.1007/978-3-319-49409-8_35
21. Vaswani, A., et al.: Attention is all you need. In: NeurIPS (2017). https://doi.org/10.48550/arXiv.1706.03762
22. Wang, D., Shelhamer, E., Liu, S., Olshausen, B., Darrell, T.: Tent: fully test-time adaptation by entropy minimization. In: International Conference on Learning Representations (ICLR) (2021), https://openreview.net/forum?id=uXl3bZLkr3c
23. Wang, X., Chen, Y., Zhu, W.: A survey on curriculum learning. IEEE Trans. Pattern Anal. Mach. Intell. **44**(9), 4555–4576 (2021). https://doi.org/10.48550/arXiv.2010.13166
24. Wu, F., Zhuang, X.: Minimizing estimated risks on unlabeled data: a new formulation for semi-supervised medical image segmentation. IEEE Trans. Pattern Anal. Mach. Intell. **45**(5), 6021–6036 (2023). https://doi.org/10.1109/TPAMI.2022.3215186
25. Zou, K., et al.: Evidencecap: towards trustworthy medical image segmentation via evidential identity cap. arXiv preprint arXiv:2301.00349 (2023), https://arxiv.org/abs/2301.00349

Uncertainty-Guided Hard–Soft Priors for Myocardial Scar and Edema Segmentation on Multi-sequence CMR Images

Haohao Luan[1], Yilin Lyu[2], Jinwei Dong[1], and Lin Pan[1](✉)

[1] College of Physics and Information Engineering, Fuzhou University, Fuzhou, China
panlin@fzu.edu.cn

[2] Department of Biomedical Engineering, National University of Singapore, University Hall, Singapore

Abstract. Accurate delineation of myocardial scar and edema in multi-sequence cardiac MR (CMR) remains challenging in real-world, multi-centre cohorts owing to boundary ambiguity, artefacts, inter-sequence misalignment or absence, and distribution shift. We present an uncertainty-guided coarse-to-fine framework that couples a hard anatomical prior with a soft uncertainty prior. In Stage-1, a 3D nnU-Net produces a structure-centred coarse mask and per-voxel probability volumes. From these probabilities we compute a Calibrated Ensemble Entropy (CEE) map via temperature-calibrated ensembling with transformation marginalisation, followed by normalised entropy. In Stage-2, a 2D nnU-Net operating within a static, mask-defined ROI receives five channels (C0, LGE, T2, the coarse mask, and the CEE map), and predictions are subsequently restored to the native image space. The ROI suppresses remote false positives, whereas the CEE map highlights uncertain boundaries and artefact-susceptible regions. Experiments on the CARE 2025 MyoPS validation cohort show consistent accuracy gains (higher mean Dice and Precision and lower 95% Hausdorff distance) without modifying the base nnU-Net design or introducing auxiliary augmentation/adaptation networks, with the largest improvements observed for edema.

Keywords: Myocardial pathology segmentation · Uncertainty calibration · Temperature scaling · Hard–soft priors · Coarse-to-fine

1 Introduction

Cardiac magnetic resonance (CMR) provides complementary tissue contrasts: late-gadolinium enhancement (LGE) delineates infarcted scar, T2-weighted imaging depicts edema, and cine bSSFP supplies sharp anatomy. Yet fully automatic delineation across real-world, multi-center acquisitions remains challenging because of ambiguous boundaries, imaging artifacts, sequence misalignment or absence, and distribution shift. The CARE2025 MyoPS track targets this gap by encouraging robust, clinically reliable segmentation of scar and edema under heterogeneous conditions [3, 21].

X. Zhuang et al. (Eds.): CARE 2025, LNCS 16257, pp. 23–32, 2026.
https://doi.org/10.1007/978-3-032-16271-7_3

Coarse-to-fine pipelines are a pragmatic solution: Stage-1 localizes the heart and reduces the search space, and Stage-2 performs ROI-constrained fine segmentation within a mask-defined region (a pattern widely adopted in biomedical and cardiac segmentation, e.g. nnU-Net's 3D cascade, cascaded FCNs for organ/lesion segmentation, and multi-stage cardiac MRI pipelines [15, 25, 26]). However, forwarding only a coarse mask as a hard prior leaves the refinement model unaware of where Stage-1 is uncertain, often producing blurred myocardium–cavity boundaries and remote false positives [16]. We therefore propose an uncertainty-guided coarse-to-fine framework that couples a hard anatomical prior with a soft uncertainty prior [12].

Concretely, Stage-1 (3D nnU-Net) predicts a structure-centered coarse mask and softmax probability volumes [1]. From these probabilities we derive a Calibrated Ensemble Entropy (CEE) map via transformation-marginalised, temperature-calibrated ensembling, and then computing voxel-wise normalized entropy [7, 8]. Stage-2 receives five channels—C0, LGE, T2, the coarse mask, and the CEE map—inside a mask-guided static ROI crop [17, 27]. The mask suppresses background and ventricular false positives, while the entropy highlights ambiguous edges and artifact-prone zones [13, 20]. Predictions are mapped back to the original image space via a two-step restoration [19]. The entire pipeline is plug-and-play with standard nnU-Net training and adds negligible inference cost because uncertainty is computed once from Stage-1 outputs.

The main contributions of this work are as follows:

- We unify hard and soft priors, improving boundary fidelity and reducing spurious predictions under multi-center variability.
- We provide a practical CEE formulation that yields reliable voxel-wise uncertainty via transformation-marginalised, temperature-calibrated ensembling.
- We deliver a simple, reproducible ROI-and-restoration pipeline tailored to CARE2025 that yields consistent gains, particularly for edema where ambiguity is greatest.

2 Method

Figure 1 outlines the proposed uncertainty-guided hard–soft prior framework. Stage-1 uses a 3D nnU-Net to process multi-sequence CMR (C0/LGE/T2) and predicts a structure-centered coarse mask M together with per-voxel class probabilities P [23]. The mask induces a static ROI, and the forward spatial transforms are retained to permit exact inverse mapping to native image coordinates during two-step restoration. From P we derive a calibrated ensemble entropy (CEE) map via temperature-calibrated ensembling with transformation marginalisation, followed by voxel-wise normalised Shannon entropy (Fig. 2) [7]. Stage-2 uses a 2D nnU-Net operating within the mask-defined ROI and receives five channels (C0, LGE, T2, the coarse mask M, and the CEE map) to refine the segmentation. The CEE map highlights ambiguous boundaries, whereas the mask suppresses background and ventricular false positives. The refined prediction is finally restored to the native image space using the recorded transforms.

2.1 Uncertainty-Guided Hard-Soft Prior Framework

Stage-1: Coarse Anatomical Priors.

Given a trimodal CMR volume $X = \{X^{(0)}, X^{(1)}, X^{(2)}\} \in \mathbb{R}^{H\times W\times Z\times 3}$, the Stage-1 3D nnU-Net f_θ produces voxel-wise class probabilities defined as

$$\mathbf{P} = \mathrm{softmax}(f_\theta(X)) \in [0,1]^{H\times W\times Z\times K}, \sum_{k=1}^{K} \mathbf{P}_k = 1 \tag{1}$$

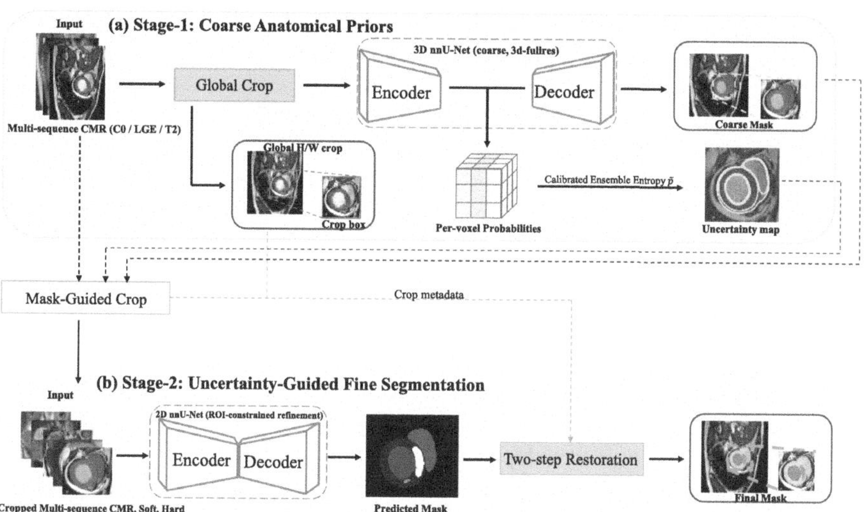

Fig. 1. Overview of our uncertainty-guided hard–soft prior framework. Stage-1 (3D nnU-Net) ingests multi-sequence CMR (C0/LGE/T2) and outputs a structure-centered coarse mask (hard prior) and a CEE entropy map (soft prior). The mask defines a static ROI, and crop metadata are recorded. Stage-2 (2D nnU-Net) takes five channels [C0, LGE, T2, mask, CEE] within the mask-guided crop to refine pathology. Predictions are mapped back by two-step restoration. Black dashed lines denote prior propagation and mask-guided cropping; orange dashed lines carry crop metadata for restoration.

The coarse, structure-centred mask is then given by the voxel-wise maximum a posteriori label,

$$M = \arg \underset{k}{max} \mathbf{P}_k, \tag{2}$$

From M we derive a static region of interest by computing a tight bounding box B (optionally dilated by a margin r) and define a crop operator $\mathcal{C}_B(\cdot)$ that can be applied to any volume or channel; we also record the geometric metadata for two-step restoration, defined as

$$\Gamma = \{\text{origin } o, \text{spacing } s, \text{direction } R, \text{bbox } B\}, \tag{3}$$

These operators ensure consistent ROI extraction across sequences and permit exact inverse mapping to native image coordinates during restoration. The probability tensor $\mathbf{P}$ is forwarded to Sect. 2.2 to construct the calibrated ensemble entropy (CEE) map $U \in [0,1]^{H \times W \times Z}$, which serves as a soft prior complementary to the hard prior M.

Stage-2: Five-channel refinement with ROI constraint and two-step restoration.

Inside the static ROI, the five-channel input is defined as

$$\tilde{X} = \mathcal{C}_B\Big(X^{(0)} \| X^{(1)} \| X^{(2)} \| M \| U\Big) \in \mathbb{R}^{h \times w \times z \times 5}, \tag{4}$$

where "$\|$" denotes channel-wise concatenation and $\mathcal{C}_B$ crops to the mask-defined ROI. The refinement network is a 2D nnU-Net operating within the static, mask-defined ROI; its probabilistic output and hard prediction are given by

$$\mathbf{Q} = \mathrm{softmax}\big(g_\phi(\tilde{X})\big), \hat{Y} = \arg \underset{k}{max} \mathbf{Q}_k, \tag{5}$$

Mapping back to the native image space is performed as a two-step restoration. First, inverse cropping places $\hat{Y}$ on the full canvas via $C_B^{-1}(cdot)$; second, resampling restores physical coordinates as follows

$$\mathbf{x}_{\mathrm{phys}} = R(\mathbf{i} \odot s) + o, \tag{6}$$

where $\mathbf{i}$ is the voxel index, R is the direction matrix, s the spacing vector, o the origin, and "$\odot$" denotes element-wise multiplication (nearest-neighbour for masks; trilinear for probabilities).

The two stages are trained independently without gradient coupling. Stage-1 (3D nnU-Net) outputs a coarse mask and voxel-wise probabilities. Stage-2 (ROI-constrained refinement 2D nnU-Net) operates within the static ROI defined by the coarse mask and refines the segmentation using five input channels [18, 20]. Both stages use the standard compound loss—soft Dice plus cross-entropy—defined as

$$\mathcal{L} = \mathcal{L}_{\mathrm{CE}}(\mathbf{Q}, \mathbf{Y}) + \mathcal{L}_{\mathrm{Dice}}(\mathbf{Q}, \mathbf{Y}), \tag{7}$$

The cross-entropy term is given by

$$\mathcal{L}_{\mathrm{CE}}(\mathbf{Q}, \mathbf{Y}) = -\frac{1}{|\Omega|} \sum_{\mathbf{x} \in \Omega} \sum_{k=1}^{K} Y_k(\mathbf{x}) \log(Q_k(\mathbf{x}) + \epsilon), \tag{8}$$

jlksdjfklis the one-hot ground truth, and $\epsilon > 0$ ensures numerical stability. The soft Dice term is defined as

$$\mathcal{L}_{\mathrm{Dice}} = 1 - \frac{2 \sum_{k=1}^{K} \langle Q_k, Y_k \rangle + \epsilon}{\sum_{k=1}^{K} \|Q_k\|_1 + \sum_{k=1}^{K} \|Y_k\|_1 + \epsilon}. \tag{9}$$

We set $K = 6$ classes (background, LV, RV, myocardium, edema, scar). Final predictions are mapped back to the native image space via two-step restoration using the recorded crop metadata.

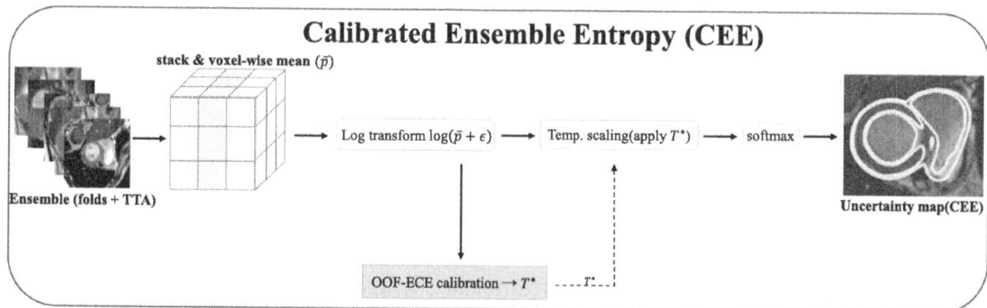

Fig. 2. Calibrated Ensemble Entropy (CEE) pipeline. Predictions produced across cross-validation folds and stochastic test-time augmentations are aggregated to obtain the voxel-wise mean $\overline{p}$. A log transform $z = \log(\overline{p} + \varepsilon)$ is applied, and the temperature T^* is selected by minimising the out-of-fold expected calibration error (OOF–ECE). At inference, temperature scaling z/T^* followed by softmax yields calibrated probabilities $\overline{p}$; their normalised Shannon entropy produces the CEE uncertainty map U. Solid arrows denote data flow; the dashed arrow indicates re-use of T^* estimated once offline.

2.2 Calibrated Ensemble Entropy

To expose prediction ambiguity to the refinement stage, we convert multi-fold, multi-augmentation outputs into a calibrated voxel-wise uncertainty [10]. Given softmax probabilities $p^{(f,a)}(\mathbf{x}) \in [0,1]^K$ from fold $f \in \{1, \ldots, F\}$ and test-time augmentation $a \in \{1, \ldots, A\}$, the transformation-marginalised predictive mean is defined as

$$\overline{\mathbf{p}}(\mathbf{x}) = \frac{1}{FA} \sum_{f=1}^{F} \sum_{a=1}^{A} p^{(f,a)}(\mathbf{x}) \in [0,1]^K. \tag{10}$$

This aggregates variability across folds (epistemic) and augmentations (aleatoric), yielding a single distribution per voxel for calibration. Because probabilities can be miscalibrated, we apply temperature scaling to the log-probabilities as

$$z(\mathbf{x}) = \log(\overline{\mathbf{p}}(\mathbf{x}) + \varepsilon), \tag{11}$$

and select the optimal temperature by minimising the out-of-fold expected calibration error (ECE), given by

$$T^* = \arg \underset{T>0}{min} \mathrm{ECE}\left(\mathrm{softmax}\left(\frac{z}{T}\right), Y_{\mathrm{oof}}\right), \tag{12}$$

Here Y_{oof} denote out-of-fold labels. The ECE over confidence bins $\{S_b\}_{b=1}^{B}$ is defined as

$$\mathrm{ECE} = \sum_{b=1}^{B} \frac{|S_b|}{\sum_j |S_j|} |\mathrm{acc}(S_b) - \mathrm{conf}(S_b)|, \tag{13}$$

where $\mathrm{acc}(S_b) = \frac{1}{|S_b|} \sum_{i \in S_b} 1[\hat{y}_i = y_i]$ and $\mathrm{conf}(S_b) = \frac{1}{|S_b|} \sum_{i \in S_b} \underset{k}{max} \hat{p}_{i,k}$. Using T^*, the calibrated probabilities are given by

$$\tilde{\mathbf{p}}(\mathbf{x}) = \mathrm{softmax}\left(\frac{z(\mathbf{x})}{T^*}\right). \tag{14}$$

When only probabilities (not logits) are stored, the same operation can be written as the power transform

$$\tilde{\mathbf{p}}(x) = \frac{(\overline{\mathbf{p}}(x) + \varepsilon)^{\frac{1}{T^*}}}{\sum_k (\overline{p}_k(x) + \varepsilon)^{\frac{1}{T^*}}}. \tag{15}$$

This softens ($T^* > 1$) or sharpens ($T^* < 1$) the distribution while preserving the arg-max class. Finally, voxel-wise uncertainty is computed as the normalised Shannon entropy of the calibrated distribution:

$$U(\mathbf{x}) = -\frac{1}{\log K} \sum_{k=1}^{K} \tilde{p}_k(\mathbf{x}) \log(\tilde{p}_k(\mathbf{x}) + \varepsilon) \in [0,1], \tag{16}$$

Values near 1 indicate ambiguous voxels (e.g., weak boundaries or artifacts), whereas values near 0 indicate confident predictions [14]. In practice, T^* is estimated once on out-of-fold predictions and fixed at inference, yielding a simple, reproducible soft prior that complements the mask-defined hard prior used by Stage-2 [7].

3 Experiments and Results

3.1 Dataset and Experiment Settings

The data are from the CARE2025 MyoPS Challenge, which provides multi-sequence CMR from 300 patients collected across eight centres in China, France, and the United Kingdom [2]. Each case may contain up to three sequences (LGE, T2, bSSFP) and five target labels (scar, edema, LV cavity, myocardium, RV cavity), with sequence availability and annotation completeness varying by centre. We follow the official split: 235 cases from centres A–H for training, 25 cases from centre D for validation, and 40 test cases (25 out-of-distribution from centre D and 15 in-distribution from centre B) [2, 3]. For preprocessing, volumes are converted to a common orientation, cropped to a uniform in-plane size centred on the heart, and z-score normalised per sequence. All subsequent experiments use these releases without additional manual curation.

Our framework is implemented in PyTorch and trained on a single NVIDIA RTX 3080 GPU. Stage-1 adopts the 3D full-resolution configuration and Stage-2 the 2D high-resolution configuration [1]. We optimize with SGD (Nesterov momentum 0.99) using an initial learning rate 0.01 with polynomial decay and weight decay 3×10^{-5}. Batch sizes are 2 (3D) and 12 (2D). The loss is $\mathcal{L} = \mathcal{L}_{\mathrm{CE}} + \mathcal{L}_{\mathrm{Dice}}$ with equal weights, and data augmentation follows nnU-Net defaults (axis mirroring, rotations/scales, gamma, Gaussian noise/blur). Unless otherwise stated, training follows nnU-Net's default schedule, and the checkpoint with the best mean Dice on the validation center is used for inference.

3.2 Comparison Study

Table 1 compares baselines on the CARE 2025 MyoPS validation set. The proposed hard–soft prior framework (Ours) achieves the best overall performance—mean

Table 1. Baseline comparison on the CARE 2025 MyoPS validation set. Columns report Dice (↑), Sensitivity (↑), Precision (↑), and Hausdorff distance (HD ↓; 95th-percentile, mm) for scar, edema, and their unweighted mean (Mean (S&E)). "nnU-Net" is the canonical 3D nnU-Net baseline; "Ours" is the proposed hard–soft prior framework (Stage-1 hard prior and Stage-2 ROI-constrained 2D refinement with CEE). Bold numbers mark the best performance.

Model	Scar				Edema				Mean(S&E)			
	Dice ↑	Sen ↑	Pre ↑	HD ↓	Dice ↑	Sen ↑	Pre ↑	HD ↓	Dice ↑	Sen ↑	Pre ↑	HD ↓
ResNet	0.555	0.545	0.670	18.906	0.585	0.571	0.740	24.601	0.570	0.558	0.705	21.754
nnU-Net	0.604	0.568	0.697	17.524	0.665	0.611	0.758	22.715	0.634	0.590	0.728	20.120
Ours	**0.634**	**0.574**	**0.752**	**16.287**	**0.687**	**0.631**	**0.788**	**22.065**	**0.661**	**0.603**	**0.770**	**19.176**

Dice 0.661, Sensitivity 0.603, Precision 0.770, and 95HD 19.176 mm—exceeding the canonical nnU-Net (mean Dice 0.634, Sensitivity 0.590, Precision 0.728, 95HD 20.120 mm). Class-wise, scar Dice increases from 0.604 to 0.634 and 95HD decreases from 17.524 mm to 16.287 mm; edema Dice increases from 0.665 to 0.687 and 95HD decreases from 22.715 mm to 22.065 mm. These results indicate that the mask-defined ROI suppresses remote false positives, while the calibrated ensemble entropy sharpens ambiguous boundarie.

3.3 Ablation Study

Table 2 summarises the ablation of the proposed hard–soft prior framework. Starting from the backbone without priors (a), adding the hard prior via a coarse mask and ROI (b) reduces remote false positives and improves mean precision and boundary quality—Precision increases from 0.728 to 0.768 and 95HD decreases from 20.12 mm to 19.55 mm—with only a small drop in Sensitivity (from 0.590 to 0.584). Using the soft prior alone (c)—the CEE entropy map—enhances boundary awareness and slightly increases mean Dice from 0.645 to 0.651 and Sensitivity from 0.584 to 0.591, while keeping 95HD low (19.28 mm). Combining both cues (d) yields the strongest overall performance across scar and edema, with the highest mean Dice (0.661), Sensitivity (0.603) and Precision (0.770), and the lowest 95HD (19.18 mm). Class-wise improvements are consistent: scar Dice increases from 0.604 to 0.634 (95HD from 17.52 mm to 16.29 mm), and edema Dice from 0.665 to 0.687 (95HD from 22.72 mm to 22.07 mm). These trends indicate that calibrated uncertainty sharpens ambiguous edema boundaries, whereas the ROI suppresses ventricular/background false positives [24].

Table 3 compares alternative soft priors under the same backbone and hard prior. Entropy from a single softmax probability volume serves as the baseline (mean Dice = 0.658; 95HD = 19.29 mm). MC-Dropout ($S = 20$) and TTA ($S = 8$) achieve similar mean Dice (0.659) and slightly lower 95HD ($\approx$ 19.00–19.03 mm) but require multiple forward passes. In contrast, the proposed CEE prior aggregates predictions across cross-validation folds and stochastic test-time transformations at Stage-1, applies out-of-fold temperature calibration, and computes voxel-wise entropy of the calibrated distribution; at inference it requires no additional forward passes. This procedure attains the highest mean Dice (0.661) and Precision (0.770), comparable Sensitivity (0.603), and a lower 95HD than the softmax baseline (19.18 mm vs 19.29 mm).

Table 2. Ablation of the proposed uncertainty-guided hard–soft prior framework on the CARE 2025 MyoPS validation set. Columns report Dice (↑), Sensitivity (↑), Precision (↑), and Hausdorff Distance (HD ↓) for scar, edema, and their mean. "Input" indicates five-channel input (C0/LGE/T2 + coarse mask + CEE). $_\mathbf{H}$ denotes the hard prior (coarse mask/ROI), and $_\mathbf{S}$ denotes the soft prior (CEE entropy). Models (a)–(d) progressively add priors: (a) no prior, (b) hard only, (c) soft only, (d) hard-soft (ours). Bold numbers mark the best performance.

Model	Input	H	S	Scar				Edema				Mean(S&E)			
				Dice ↑	Sen ↑	Pre ↑	HD ↓	Dice ↑	Sen ↑	Pre ↑	HD ↓	Dice ↑	Sen ↑	Pre ↑	HD ↓
(a)	√	×	×	0.604	0.568	0.697	17.524	0.665	0.611	0.758	22.715	0.634	0.590	0.728	20.120
(b)	√	√	×	0.615	0.560	0.740	16.800	0.675	0.607	**0.795**	22.300	0.645	0.584	0.768	19.550
(c)	√	×	√	0.620	0.562	0.733	**15.594**	0.682	0.619	0.789	22.962	0.651	0.591	0.761	19.278
(d)	√	√	√	**0.634**	**0.574**	**0.752**	16.287	**0.687**	**0.631**	0.788	**22.065**	**0.661**	**0.603**	**0.770**	**19.176**

Table 3. Study of soft priors $_\mathbf{S}$ for Stage-2. All methods use the same backbone and hard prior; only the uncertainty map differs. Softmax computes voxel-wise entropy from a single probability volume without calibration; *MC-Dropout* and *TTA* average SSS stochastic passes; *CEE (ours)* applies out-of-fold temperature scaling to the aggregated probabilities and computes normalized entropy with no extra test-time sampling. Averaged over scar & edema, CEE yields higher Dice and Precision with comparable Sensitivity and lower HD: + 0.002 Dice, + 0.006 Precision, and – 0.11 HD relative to the Softmax baseline (0.658/0.764/19.29). Per-class gains vs. Softmax are + 0.003 Dice / + 0.007 Precision (scar) and + 0.002 Dice / + 0.004 Precision (edema). MC-Dropout (S = 20) and TTA (S = 8) require multiple passes, whereas CEE is one-shot at inference.

Soft prior $_\mathbf{S}$	Scar				Edema				Mean(S&E)			
	Dice ↑	Sen ↑	Pre ↑	HD ↓	Dice ↑	Sen ↑	Pre ↑	HD ↓	Dice ↑	Sen ↑	Pre ↑	HD ↓
Softmax	0.631	0.573	0.745	16.400	0.684	0.630	0.784	22.180	0.658	0.602	0.764	19.290
MC-Dropout, S = 20	0.633	**0.579**	0.747	16.100	0.686	**0.638**	0.782	**21.900**	0.659	0.605	0.765	**19.000**
TTA, S = 8	0.632	0.576	0.748	**16.050**	0.686	0.634	0.783	22.000	0.659	**0.609**	0.765	19.025
CEE, Ours	**0.634**	0.574	**0.752**	16.287	**0.687**	0.631	**0.788**	22.065	**0.661**	0.603	**0.770**	19.176

4 Conclusion

In this work, we introduce an uncertainty-guided coarse-to-fine framework for myocardial scar and edema segmentation in multi-sequence CMR. The approach combines a hard anatomical prior (coarse mask + ROI) with a soft prior computed as Calibrated

Ensemble Entropy (CEE). CEE is formed via transformation-marginalised, temperature-calibrated ensembling of Stage-1 probabilities, followed by normalised voxel-wise entropy; the map highlights ambiguous boundaries, while the ROI suppresses remote false positives. On the CARE 2025 MyoPS validation set, the framework achieves higher mean Dice and Precision and lower HD than baselines on average, with particularly clear gains for edema. Remaining limitations include the static ROI and the absence of end-to-end coupling between stages. Future work will explore adaptive cropping/restoration, entropy-aware joint training, and broader multi-centre validation across additional cohorts and modalities.

Acknowledgments. This work was supported in part by the National Natural Science Foundation of China under Grant 62271149, in part by the Science and Technology Project of Fujian Province under Grants 2024J01353, 2022Y4014, 2020Y9091, 2023Y9144.

References

1. Isensee, F., Jaeger, P.F., Kohl, S.A.A., Petersen, J., Maier-Hein, K.H.: NnU-Net: a self-configuring method for deep learning-based biomedical image segmentation. Nat. Methods **18**, 203–211 (2021)
2. Li, L., et al.: MyoPS: a benchmark of myocardial pathology segmentation combining three-sequence cardiac magnetic resonance images. Med. Image Anal. **87**, 102808 (2023)
3. MyoPS Challenge Organizers: *Statistical Atlases and Computational Models of the Heart. ACDC and M&Ms Challenges, and LV Full Quantification, LAScarQS, and MyoPS 2020.* In: MICCAI 2020, LNCS, vol. 12554. Springer, Cham (2020)
4. Nazzal, W., Alshehri, Y., Alduailej, M., et al.: Improving medical image segmentation using test-time augmentation. Mathematics **12**(24), 4003 (2024)
5. Tomar, D., Sengupta, S., Chandramouli, K., et al.: OptTTA: Learnable test-time augmentation for source-free domain adaptation. In: Medical Imaging with Deep Learning (MIDL) 2022, PMLR, vol. 172, pp. 1192–1217 (2022)
6. Ma, X., Tao, Y., Zhang, Y., Ji, Z., Zhang, Y., Chen, Q.: Test-Time Generative Augmentation for Medical Image Segmentation. arXiv 2406.17608 (2024)
7. Buddenkotte, T., Rieck, B., Bustreo, M., et al.: Calibrating ensembles for scalable uncertainty quantification in medical image segmentation. Comput. Biol. Med. **163**, 107096 (2023)
8. Ding, Z., Xu, J., Cordonnier, J.-B., Rosenfeld, A.: Local temperature scaling for probability calibration. In: Proceedings of the IEEE/CVF International Conference on Computer Vision (ICCV), pp. 16408–16417 (2021)
9. Kock, F.W., Ferrante, E., Rekik, I., et al.: Confidence histograms for model reliability assessment in medical image segmentation. In: Medical Imaging with Deep Learning (MIDL) 2022, PMLR, vol. 172, pp. 741–759 (2022)
10. Karimi, D., Warfield, S.K., Gholipour, A.: Improving calibration and out-of-distribution detection in medical image segmentation. IEEE Trans. Artif. Intell. **4**(2), 383–397 (2023)
11. Mody, P., Geras, K.J., Malkin, N., Azizi, S., Choi, E.: Improving uncertainty–error correspondence in deep segmentation with AvU loss. Mach. Learn. Biomed. Imaging (MELBA) **3**, e012006 (2024)
12. Luo, Z., Wei, F., Yang, Y., et al.: An uncertainty-guided tiered self-training framework for medical image segmentation. In: Linguraru, M.G., et al. (eds.) MICCAI 2024, LNCS, vol. 15009, pp. 670–680. Springer, Cham (2024)

13. Yang, B., Zhang, X., Zhang, H., Li, S., Higashita, R., Liu, J.: Structural uncertainty estimation for medical image segmentation. Med. Image Anal. **103**, 103602 (2025)
14. Sikha, O.K., et al.: Uncertainty-aware segmentation quality prediction via deep Bayesian modeling: comprehensive evaluation and interpretation on skin cancer and liver segmentation. Comput. Med. Imaging Graph. **123**, 102547 (2025)
15. Wu, S., et al.: A coarse-to-fine fusion network for small liver tumor detection and segmentation: a real-world study. Diagnostics **13**(15), 2504 (2023)
16. Isler, I.S., Mohaisen, D., Lisle, C., Turgut, D., Bagci, U.: Uncertainty-Guided Coarse-to-Fine Tumor Segmentation with Anatomy-Aware Post-Processing. arXiv 2504.12215 (2025)
17. Juwita, J., Hassan, G.M., Akhtar, N., Datta, A.: Pancreas segmentation in CT scans: a novel MOMUNet-based workflow. Comput. Biol. Med. **180**, 108932 (2025)
18. Wyburd, M.K., Dinsdale, N.K., Jenkinson, M., Namburete, A.I.L.: Anatomically plausible segmentations: explicitly preserving topology through prior deformations (TEDS-Net). Med. Image Anal. **97**, 103222 (2024)
19. Li, L., et al.: Universal topology refinement for medical image segmentation with polynomial feature synthesis. In: Linguraru, M.G., et al. (eds.) MICCAI 2024, LNCS, vol. 15009, pp. 670–680. Springer, Cham (2024)
20. Zhang, P., Cheng, Y., Tamura, S.: Shape prior-constrained deep learning network for medical image segmentation. Comput. Biol. Med. **180**, 108932 (2024)
21. Jani, V.P., Ostovaneh, M., Chamera, E., Kato, Y., Lima, J.A.C., Ambale-Venkatesh, B.: Deep learning for automatic volumetric segmentation of left ventricular myocardium and ischaemic scar from multi-slice LGE-CMR. Eur. Hear. J. – Cardiovasc. Imaging **25**(6), 829–838 (2024)
22. Ramzan, F., Chen, C., Clayton, R.H.: Improving myocardial scar segmentation with end-to-end and cascaded CNN using hybrid loss and multi-modality CMR imaging. In: Computing in Cardiology (CinC) 2024 (2024). https://doi.org/10.22489/CinC.2024.148
23. Zhuang, X.: Multivariate mixture model for myocardial segmentation combining multi-source images. IEEE Trans. Pattern Anal. Mach. Intell. **41**(12), 2933–2946 (2019)
24. Qiu, J., et al.: MyoPS-Net: myocardial pathology segmentation with flexible combination of multi-sequence CMR images. Med. Image Anal. **84**, 102694 (2023)
25. Ding, W., et al.: Aligning multi-sequence CMR towards fully automated myocardial pathology segmentation. IEEE Trans. Med. Imaging **42**(12), 3474–3486 (2023)
26. Yang et al.: Contrast-Free Myocardial Scar Segmentation in Cine MRI using Motion and Texture Fusion. ISBI (2025)
27. Ding, et al.: CineMyoPS: segmenting myocardial pathologies from cine cardiac MR. IEEE TMI (2025). https://doi.org/10.1109/TMI.2025.3586254

MA2: Unifying Modality-Agnostic Segmentation and Modality-Aware Staging for Real-World Liver Fibrosis Analysis

Derong Yu and Guoyan Zheng(✉)

Institute of Medical Robotics, School of Biomedical Engineering, Shanghai Jiao Tong University, No. 800 Dongchuan Road, Shanghai 200240, China
guoyan.zheng@sjtu.edu.cn

Abstract. Accurate liver segmentation and fibrosis staging play a pivotal role in Artificial Intelligence (AI)-assisted surgical decision-making, facilitating precise disease management, prognostic evaluation, and clinical interventions. However, existing approaches face significant limitations when applied to real-world clinical data: (1) Liver segmentation is hindered by the scarcity of annotated data, particularly for non-contrast sequences; (2) Multi-modality fibrosis staging encounters obstacles due to random modality absence and inter-sequence misalignment. To tackle these challenges, we propose MA2, a unified framework integrating two key components: **m**odality-**a**gnostic segmentation and **m**odality-**a**ware staging. For modality-agnostic liver segmentation, we develop a training pipeline that utilizes pseudo-images synthesized from supervoxels and simulated non-contrast images to enhance model generalization capability. For liver fibrosis staging, we introduce learnable modality-aware tokens that augment image patch tokens from available modalities, coupled with random modality dropout during training to enhance cross-modality information integration. Experiments on the CARE-Liver track dataset from the CARE 2025 challenge demonstrate the superior performance of our method in both validation and testing phases.

Keywords: Cross-modality and cross-center generalization · Random modality dropout · Liver segmentation · Fibrosis staging

1 Introduction

Liver fibrosis, occurring in most types of chronic liver diseases, poses a global health burden due to its potential progression to cirrhosis, liver failure, and portal hypertension [9]. Accurate liver segmentation and fibrosis staging play a vital role in computer-aided diagnosis, disease management, and prognostication for liver fibrosis. Recently, deep learning has demonstrated remarkable success in medical image segmentation and classification tasks. However, existing models often exhibit limited generalization capabilities when confronted with

X. Zhuang et al. (Eds.): CARE 2025, LNCS 16257, pp. 33–45, 2026.
https://doi.org/10.1007/978-3-032-16271-7_4

real-world clinical scenarios. This work aims to address data distribution drift caused by real-world variability in imaging scanner systems, and segmentation label scarcity for fibrosis analysis.

Generally, real-world liver segmentation and fibrosis staging face many challenges including: (1) Limited segmentation annotations with modality variations. Since manual annotation for 3D medical images is time-consuming and laborious, limited segmentation labels for contrast-enhanced hepatobiliary phase are available while annotations for non-contrast modalities are even harder to acquire; (2) Random modality absence. Due to high acquisition cost and extended acquisition time, MR modality sets may be incomplete [13]; (3) Inter-sequence misalignment. Non-rigid tissue deformation and cross-modality heterogeneity may complicate precise sequence alignment.

Prior studies have taken significant efforts to address the challenges posed by modality variations. In brain MR image analysis, convolutional neural networks (CNNs) trained exclusively on pseudo-images synthesized from brain segmentation labels have achieved robust performance across diverse domains [1,6]. However, in comparison with brain structures, abdominal organs have highly varying shapes, scales and appearance among patients, which are hard to capture. To address the challenge, we perform supervoxel-level clustering to obtain dense pseudo-labels for domain randomized image synthesis, enabling modality-agnostic segmentation using only hepatobiliary-phase annotations.

To tackle random modality absence and inter-sequence misalignment in fibrosis staging, we develop a modality-aware staging network leveraging modality-aware tokens and transformer layers. The network processes available modality images using a sliding window approach to extract overlapping patches. These image patches then undergo unified feature extraction via an encoder that is shared with the forementioned segmentation network. Subsequently, we embed learnable modality-aware tokens and integrate cross-phase information through transformer layers.

In summary, our contributions can be summarized as follows:

- We propose MA2, a unified framework for **m**odality-**a**gnostic liver segmentation and **m**odality-**a**ware fibrosis staging of real-world clinical images.
- We present a segmentation paradigm that leverages pseudo-images synthesized from supervoxel labels, complemented by simulated non-contrast images and real images as training sources, enabling modality-agnostic representation learning for liver segmentation.
- We introduce learnable modality-aware tokens that augment image patch embeddings, coupled with random modality dropout, to enhance multi-modal transformer-based information fusion for fibrosis staging.

2 Method

2.1 Problem Statement

We are aiming to develop a unified framework addressing modality-agnostic liver segmentation and modality-aware fibrosis staging. For liver segmentation,

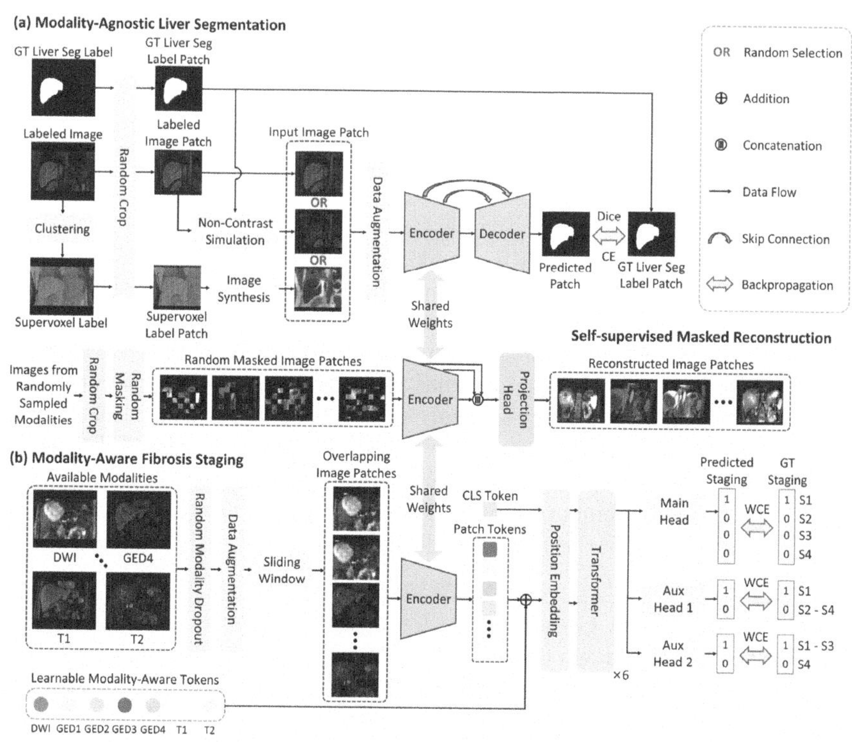

Fig. 1. Overview of the MA2 framework. (a) The modality-agnostic segmentation network is trained using pseudo-image patches synthesized from supervoxels, complemented by simulated non-contrast image patches and labeled image patches. (b) For fibrosis staging, learnable modality-aware tokens are used to augment image patch embeddings from corresponding modalities to enhance multi-modal information fusion in transformer layers. DWI: diffusion-weighted imaging. GED: Gadolinium ethoxybenzyl diethylenetriamine pentaacetic acid-enhanced. CE: cross entropy. WCE: weighted cross entropy. Seg: segmentation. CLS: classification. GT: ground truth. Aux: auxiliary.

the model needs to adapt to cross-modality variations across multiple unannotated target domains while trained on limited annotated data from a source domain. Following the setting in CARE-Liver track, our source domain comprises Gadolinium-enhanced hepatobiliary phase (GED4) MR images, while the target domains contain non-contrast diffusion-weighted (DWI), T2-weighted, and T1-weighted MR images.

For fibrosis staging, the objective is to stage liver fibrosis into four stages (S1-S4) in order to reach two clinically critical decisions: distinguishing cirrhosis (S1-S3 vs. S4) and detecting substantial fibrosis (S1 vs. S2-S4). Thus, the model requires to process multi-phase MR images despite random modality absence and inter-sequence misalignment. The CARE-Liver track defines two scenarios: non-contrast subtask using only three modalities (DWI, T2, and T1), and contrast-enhanced subtask containing seven modalities including arterial (GED1), venous (GED2), delayed (GED3), and hepatobiliary (GED4) phases alongside the non-contrast sequences.

2.2 Modality-Agnostic Liver Segmentation

As illustrated in Fig. 1 (a), the segmentation network employs an CNN-based encoder-decoder architecture with skip connections. To learn modality-agnostic representations, we train the network using three types of image patches: pseudo-image patches, simulated non-contrast image patches, and GED4 image patches. Specifically, given an GED4 image with its ground truth (GT) liver segmentation label, 3D supervoxel-level clustering [15] is applied to the image to obtain the supervoxel label. We then randomly crop spatially aligned patches of size $H \times W \times D$ from the GED4 image, the supervoxel label, and the GT liver segmentation label, yielding the GED4 image patch X_{GED4}, the supervoxel label patch S, and the GT segmentation label patch Y_s, respectively. Here H, W, and D represent respectively the height, width, and depth of each patch.

Pseudo-Image Patch Generation. Using the supervoxel label patch S, we synthesize the pseudo-image patch X_{syn} following the image generation pipeline introduced in [3]. This involves sampling intensities from Gaussian mixture models (GMMs) with randomized parameters, followed by applying Perlin noise [14]. The synthetic volume undergoes min-max normalization to standardize intensities within [0,1]. Such a synthesis pipeline generates highly unrealistic pseudo-images from randomized domains, effectively bridging the domain gaps.

Simulated Non-Contrast Image Patch Generation. From the min-max normalized GED4 image patch X_{GED4} and the GT liver segmentation label patch Y_s, we derive the simulated non-contrast image patch X_{sim} by subtracting a randomly sampled intensity value within the liver region. The non-contrast simulation can be formulated as:

$$X^i_{sim} = X^i_{GED4} - \min(\gamma, X^i_{GED4})Y^i_s, \quad \gamma \sim U(a, b) \tag{1}$$

where i indexes voxels ($1 \leq i \leq H \cdot W \cdot D$), Y^i_s indicates liver region (1 for liver, 0 for background), and γ is randomly drawn from the uniform distribution U with lower bound $a = 0$ and upper bound $b = \mu + \sigma$. Here μ and σ denote the mean intensity and the standard deviation within the liver region.

Segmentation Training. At each iteration, one image patch X_s is randomly selected with empirically determined probabilities $p_{syn} = 0.65$, $p_{sim} = 0.175$ and $p_{GED4} = 0.175$ from $\{X_{syn}, X_{sim}, X_{GED4}\}$, respectively. The selected image patch X_s is then fed to the segmentation network to get the predicted patch $\hat{Y}_s$. The GT liver segmentation label patch Y_s is used to supervise the network training with a loss function $\mathcal{L}_{seg}$ combining Dice loss and cross-entropy (CE) loss:

$$\mathcal{L}_{seg}(\hat{Y}_s, Y_s) = 1 - \text{Dice}(\hat{Y}_s, Y_s) + \text{CE}(\hat{Y}_s, Y_s) \quad (2)$$

To effectively leverage unlabeled data, we also incorporate semi-supervised learning into our segmentation training. Specifically, the training process initiates with supervised learning until achieving a validation Dice threshold $\delta = 0.85$. Then, we generate initial pseudo-labels $\{Y_u\}$ for all unlabeled samples $\{X_u\}$ across the four imaging modalities (GED4, DWI, T2, and T1) using the current trained model. These pseudo-annotations $\{Y_u\}$ undergo continuous refinement throughout subsequent training epochs. This is done by checking the validation Dice after each training epoch, keeping the model that achieves a better validation Dice than the existing one, and using the updated model to predict the pseudo-labels for the unlabeled image patches.

At each iteration, the semi-supervised learning is performed as follows. For an unlabeled image patch X_u with the corresponding pseudo liver segmentation label patch Y_u, we generate the predicted patch $\hat{Y}_u$ through the segmentation network. Simultaneously, we also sample labeled data (X_s, Y_s) and feed the sampled data into the segmentation network to obtain $\hat{Y}_s$. The semi-supervised loss $\mathcal{L}_{semi}$ combines both labeled and pseudo-labeled components:

$$\mathcal{L}_{semi}(\hat{Y}_s, Y_s, \hat{Y}_u, Y_u) = \mathcal{L}_{seg}(\hat{Y}_s, Y_s) + \lambda_{semi}\mathcal{L}_{seg}(\hat{Y}_u, Y_u) \quad (3)$$

where λ_{semi} represents the dynamically weighted contribution of the pseudo-labeled data loss. This weight follows a cosine scheduler, gradually increasing from 0.01 to 1.0 throughout the training process.

2.3 Modality-Aware Fibrosis Staging

Our fibrosis staging method leverages cross-phase complementary information from dynamic MRI sequences (see Fig. 1 (b)). During training, given the available modalities in one patient, random modality dropout [10] with probability $p_m = 0.5$ is applied to each modality, which means each modality has a 50% chance of being excluded from the input. During the modality dropout process, we ensure that at least one modality remains active. Such a strategy enhances model robustness against random modality absence.

Patch Token Extraction. We extract overlapping patches $X_c \in \mathbb{R}^{N \times H \times W \times D}$ from images of the kept modalities using a sliding window approach with 50% overlap ratio, where N represents the number of patches. These image patches are processed through an encoder that is shared with the segmentation network, to generate patch embeddings $F_{pat} \in \mathbb{R}^{N \times C \times \frac{H}{32} \times \frac{W}{32} \times \frac{D}{32}}$, with C denoting the feature dimension. The embeddings are then flattened into patch tokens of size $N \times (\frac{H}{32} \cdot \frac{W}{32} \cdot \frac{D}{32}) \times C$.

Modality-Aware Token Integration. To incorporate modality-specific information while maintaining the modality-agnostic feature extraction capability of the encoder, we introduce learnable modality-aware tokens. The complete set of modality tokens $F_{mod} \in \mathbb{R}^{N_m \times C}$ (where $N_m = 7$ equals the total number of modalities) are combined with their corresponding patch tokens by addition. Spatial information is preserved through position embeddings $F_{pos} \in \mathbb{R}^{(\frac{H}{32} \cdot \frac{W}{32} \cdot \frac{D}{32}) \times C}$ added to patch tokens based on their spatial indexes [4].

Cross-Phase Information Fusion. The patch tokens are reshaped to size $(N \cdot \frac{H}{32} \cdot \frac{W}{32} \cdot \frac{D}{32}) \times C$ and concatenated with a classification (CLS) token $F_{cls} \in \mathbb{R}^{1 \times C}$, forming the overall tokens $F_{all} \in \mathbb{R}^{(N \cdot \frac{H}{32} \cdot \frac{W}{32} \cdot \frac{D}{32} + 1) \times C}$. The CLS token also receives position embeddings $(1 \times C)$ [4]. After that, F_{all} undergoes six transformer layers [4,16], where self-attention mechanism is used to integrate information from all modalities and spatial locations, effectively fusing complementary information from cross-phase MRI sequences.

Fibrosis Stage Classification. The CLS token, after being processed through the transformer layers, serves as the final feature representation for fibrosis stage prediction. Our network incorporates a main classification head (1×4 output for stages S1-S4) supplemented by two auxiliary classification heads: one distinguishing S1 from S2-S4 (1×2 output) and the other separating S1-S3 from S4 (1×2 output). To address class imbalance, all heads are trained using weighted cross-entropy (WCE) loss functions, with class weights set inversely proportional to their respective frequencies in the training dataset. The overall classification loss $\mathcal{L}_{cls}$ integrates contributions from all prediction heads:

$$\mathcal{L}_{cls} = \mathcal{L}_{main} + \lambda_{aux1}\mathcal{L}_{aux1} + \lambda_{aux2}\mathcal{L}_{aux2} \tag{4}$$

Here, $\mathcal{L}_{main}$ represents the main classification loss, while $\mathcal{L}_{aux1}$ and $\mathcal{L}_{aux2}$ correspond to the losses from the auxiliary heads, as shown in Fig. 1 (b). Throughout our experiments, we empirically set $\lambda_{aux1} = \lambda_{aux2} = 1.0$.

2.4 Self-Supervised Masked Image Reconstruction

We additionally incorporate self-supervised masked image reconstruction [2] at each iteration before the forementioned supervised and semi-supervised learning in order to learn a generalizable feature representation. For each training sample, we randomly crop an image patch of size $H \times W \times D$ from any available modality. We then apply random masking to regions of size $h \times w \times d$, with a masking ratio r uniformly sampled between 0.5 and 0.8 ($r \sim U(0.5, 0.8)$). Here h, w, and d represent respectively the height, width, and depth of each masked region. The masked patch is processed through the shared encoder, as shown in Fig. 1, after which we upsample all hierarchical encoder features to the original patch size $H \times W \times D$ and concatenate them. A linear projection layer subsequently reconstructs the original unmasked patch, with L1 loss serving as the reconstruction loss function.

2.5 Alternative Training

The MA2 framework employs an alternative training approach to jointly learn modality-agnostic segmentation and modality-aware fibrosis staging, along with self-supervised masked image reconstruction. Such a design addresses the gradient weakening issue observed during simultaneous optimization of both tasks, which can cause confusion in weight updating [12]. Our training protocol cycles through masked image reconstruction, supervised and semi-supervised segmentation, and fibrosis staging in each iteration: first performing self-supervised masked image reconstruction, then optimizing the segmentation task, followed by the fibrosis staging task.

2.6 Inference

At inference stage, for liver segmentation, a sliding window approach with overlap ratio of 75% is adopted. The sampled image patches from each modality (DWI, T2, and T1) are fed to the trained segmentation network to get liver segmentation predictions. Post-processing involves applying a maximum connected area operation to the predicted liver masks. For fibrosis staging, the network processes: (1) all available modalities for contrast-enhanced subtask, and (2) all available DWI, T2, and T1 modalities for non-contrast subtask, without random modality dropout. The overlap ratio is the same (50%) as that in training. The final predicted probabilities are the average of the predicted probabilities from both the main and the auxiliary classification heads.

3 Experiments and Results

3.1 Datasets

In this study, we employ the LiQA data [5,11,17] from the CARE-Liver track in the CARE 2025 challenge, supplemented by the CHAOS 2019 challenge data [7] as the additional training data.

LiQA Data. LiQA data [5,11,17] comprises 610 patients diagnosed with liver fibrosis from four centers (A, B1, B2, and C) using three different MRI scanner vendors. The dataset consists of seven MRI phases (DWI, T2, T1, GED1, GED2, GED3, and GED4), with individual subjects potentially missing random phases except for the GED4 phase. The sequences lack pre-alignment through spatial registration. The data is partitioned into training, validation, and testing sets as detailed in Table 1. While all samples in the challenge training set include fibrosis staging annotations, only 10 samples per center contain GED4 liver segmentation labels. For model selection, we further divided the challenge training set into our customized training and validation subsets. Rigid spatial alignment was performed on our validation set to generate noise ground truth for DWI, T2, and T1 modalities. The challenge testing set contains both in-distribution samples (Centers A, B1, and B2) and out-of-distribution samples (Center C), enabling comprehensive evaluation of model generalization capabilities.

Table 1. Data split of LiQA data from the CARE-Liver track in the CARE 2025 challenge. #: number of. Seg: segmentation.

Challenge Training Set					Challenge Validation Set		Challenge Testing Set	
Our Training Set			Our Validation Set					
Center	#Cases	#Seg Labels	#Cases	#Seg Labels	Center	#Cases	Center	#Cases
A	117	9	13	1	A	20	A	40
B1	153	9	17	1	B1	20	B1	40
B2	54	9	6	1	B2	20	B2	40
							C	70

CHAOS 2019 Challenge Data. To improve segmentation capability, we incorporated MR scans from the CHAOS (Combined Healthy Abdominal Organ Segmentation) 2019 challenge [7] into our training set. This dataset comprises 60 MR volumes with manual segmentation labels of multiple abdominal organs. These MR volumes are acquired from 20 subjects, with each subject scanned using two different pulse sequences: T1-DUAL (with in and out phases) and T2-SPIR. For our experiments, only the provided liver masks were utilized as ground truth. During training, we processed CHAOS data through the same pipeline as described in Sect. 2.2.

3.2 Evaluation Metrics

In the CARE-Liver track, the liver segmentation task employs Dice score and Hausdorff distance (HD) as evaluation metrics, while fibrosis staging performance is assessed through the area under receiver operating characteristic curve (AUC) and accuracy (ACC).

3.3 Implementation Details

The MA2 framework was implemented using PyTorch v2.1 and MONAI v1.4, with a feature dimension of $C = 1024$ in the transformer layers. Our implementation utilized an input patch size of $H = W = D = 128$ at $2.0 \times 2.0 \times 2.0$ mm^3 spacing, with masked regions sized $h = w = d = 16$. For model training, we employed following batch sizes: 2 for segmentation and masked image reconstruction tasks, and 5 for fibrosis staging task. The encoder-decoder architecture followed the same structure as described in [3], initialized with their pre-trained weights. For segmentation training, we used the Adam [8] optimizer with a weight decay of 1.0×10^{-5} and an initial learning rate of 2.0×10^{-4}, applying cosine annealing scheduling. Similarly, both masked image reconstruction and classification training were optimized using the same optimizer but with a lower initial learning rate of 3.0×10^{-5}. To enhance model robustness, we employed data augmentation including Gaussian noise, Gibbs noise, bias field, contrast adjustment, Gaussian smoothing and sharpening, random low-resolution simulation, elastic deformation, affine transformation, flipping, and rotation operations. The training process comprised 75k iterations, taking 2 days on a single NVIDIA H100 GPU with 55GB memory consumption. During testing, MA2 achieved an average inference rate of 1.27, 0.39, and 1.25 cases per second using 5GB, 15GB, and 8GB memory for segmentation, contrast, and non-contrast staging, respectively.

Table 2. Quantitative results for non-contrast liver segmentation when our method was evaluated on the challenge validation dataset. Best results are highlighted in bold. ✓: employ the corresponding component. ✗: do not employ the corresponding component. ↑: higher value indicates better performance. ↓: lower value indicates better performance. Semi-sup: semi-supervised segmentation. FS: fibrosis staging. MIR: masked image reconstruction. HD: Hausdorff distance.

Pseudo	Alternative Training			DWI		T2		T1	
Images	Semi-sup	FS	MIR	Dice (%) ↑	HD (mm) ↓	Dice (%) ↑	HD (mm) ↓	Dice (%) ↑	HD (mm) ↓
✗	✗	✗	✗	44.41	92.37	39.72	112.49	87.06	180.77
✓	✗	✗	✗	79.42	29.92	86.91	34.64	92.05	**45.48**
✓	✓	✗	✗	82.28	37.56	87.27	55.40	92.14	72.88
✓	✓	✓	✗	82.45	30.06	**88.28**	34.12	**92.53**	49.11
✓	✓	✓	✓	**84.21**	**26.72**	87.87	**32.42**	92.30	46.06

3.4 Results from Validation Phase

To investigate the effectiveness of our proposed modality-agnostic segmentation approach, we conducted an ablation study using exclusively the LiQA data with GED4 segmentation annotations. The validation phase results, as shown in Table 2, reveal that the baseline model trained solely on GED4 images exhibited inferior performance, while incorporating pseudo-images and simulated non-contrast images yielded substantial improvements, with average Dice score gains of 35.01%/47.19%/4.99% and average HD reductions of 62.45/77.85/135.29 mm for DWI/T2/T1 modalities, respectively. These results substantiate that our domain randomization-based pseudo-image synthesis significantly improves model robustness against contrast variations. The progressive incorporation of semi-supervised segmentation, fibrosis staging, and masked image reconstruction into the training pipeline yielded further performance enhancements, ultimately achieving respectively an average Dice score of 84.21%, 87.87%, and 92.30% with an average HD of 26.72 mm, 32.42 mm, and 46.06 mm across the three target modalities. Visual results presented in Fig. 2 further validate the effectiveness of our modality-agnostic training approach.

For fibrosis staging validation, an ablation study was performed on LiQA data. Quantitative results in Table 3 show that when incrementally adding segmentation and masked image reconstruction into the training pipeline, progressive performance improvements were observed, achieving AUC/ACC values of 71.65%/70.00% for cirrhosis detection and 68.00%/70.00% for substantial fibrosis detection in contrast-enhanced cases. Similar improvement was observed in non-contrast cases, with AUC/ACC reaching 73.09%/65.00% and 67.11%/73.33% for cirrhosis and substantial fibrosis detection, respectively. These results verify the effectiveness of our MA2 framework.

3.5 Results from Testing Phase

Tables 4 and 5 present respectively the quantitative results for non-contrast liver segmentation and fibrosis staging from the testing phase. The segmentation results indicate reliable performance across both in-distribution and out-of-distribution testing data, confirming the efficacy of our model against modality variations and inter-center domain shifts. For fibrosis staging, while our method

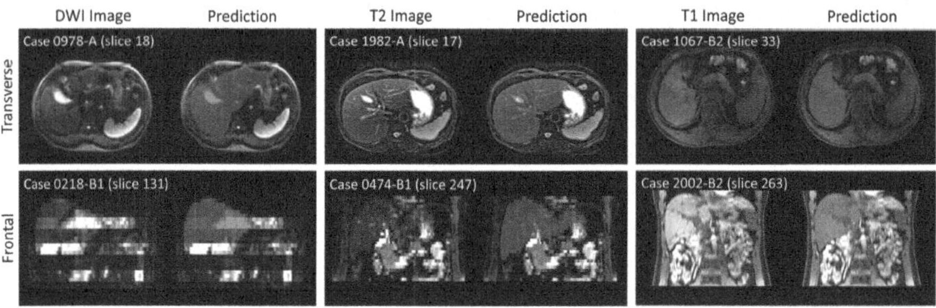

Fig. 2. Qualitative results of our MA2 framework for modality-agnostic segmentation on the challenge validation set. The first row shows examples in 2D slices of the transverse plane. The second row shows examples in 2D slices of the frontal plane.

Table 3. Quantitative results for liver fibrosis staging when our method was evaluated on the challenge validation dataset. Best results are highlighted in bold. ✓: employ the corresponding component. ✗: do not employ the corresponding component. ↑: higher value indicates better performance. MIR: masked image reconstruction. AUC: area under receiver operating characteristic curve. ACC: accuracy.

Contrast-Enhanced Liver Fibrosis Staging						
Modality-aware	Alternative Training		Cirrhosis		Substantial Fibrosis	
Tokens	Segmentation	MIR	AUC (%) ↑	ACC (%) ↑	AUC (%) ↑	ACC (%) ↑
✓	✗	✗	65.79	63.33	63.56	**73.33**
✓	✓	✗	66.99	66.67	61.33	68.33
✓	✓	✓	**71.65**	**70.00**	**68.00**	70.00
Non-Contrast Liver Fibrosis Staging						
Modality-aware	Alternative Training		Cirrhosis		Substantial Fibrosis	
Tokens	Segmentation	MIR	AUC (%) ↑	ACC (%) ↑	AUC (%) ↑	ACC (%) ↑
✓	✗	✗	67.94	60.00	**70.07**	**73.33**
✓	✓	✗	71.77	60.00	65.26	71.67
✓	✓	✓	**73.09**	**65.00**	67.11	**73.33**

achieved reasonable performance on in-distribution testing data, we observed significant performance degradation in out-of-distribution scenario. These results suggest that while our MA2 framework excels in segmentation generalization, further research is needed to enhance fibrosis staging generalization across large domain gaps.

Table 4. Quantitative results for non-contrast liver segmentation when our method was evaluated on the challenging testing data. ↑: higher value indicates better performance. ↓: lower value indicates better performance. HD: Hausdorff distance.

In-Distribution					
DWI		T2		T1	
Dice (%) ↑	HD (mm) ↓	Dice (%) ↑	HD (mm) ↓	Dice (%) ↑	HD (mm) ↓
83.74	26.96	88.90	34.60	92.62	27.80
Out-of-Distribution					
DWI		T2		T1	
Dice (%) ↑	HD (mm) ↓	Dice (%) ↑	HD (mm) ↓	Dice (%) ↑	HD (mm) ↓
88.57	11.21	88.94	24.52	94.44	25.54

Table 5. Quantitative results for liver fibrosis staging when our method was evaluated on the challenging testing dataset. ↑: higher value indicates better performance. AUC: area under receiver operating characteristic curve. ACC: accuracy.

Contrast-Enhanced Liver Fibrosis Staging							
In-Distribution				Out-of-Distribution			
Cirrhosis		Substantial Fibrosis		Cirrhosis		Substantial Fibrosis	
ACC (%) ↑	AUC (%) ↑	ACC (%) ↑	AUC (%) ↑	ACC (%) ↑	AUC (%) ↑	ACC (%) ↑	AUC (%) ↑
70.83	75.10	75.00	78.45	41.43	46.81	64.29	52.62
Non-Contrast Liver Fibrosis Staging							
In-Distribution				Out-of-Distribution			
Cirrhosis		Substantial Fibrosis		Cirrhosis		Substantial Fibrosis	
ACC (%) ↑	AUC (%) ↑	ACC (%) ↑	AUC (%) ↑	ACC (%) ↑	AUC (%) ↑	ACC (%) ↑	AUC (%) ↑
71.67	78.61	70.00	73.70	42.86	49.31	70.00	31.08

4 Conclusion

In this paper, we proposed a unified framework to achieve modality-agnostic segmentation and modality-aware fibrosis staging. Specifically, the segmentation network leveraged a novel training paradigm incorporating pseudo-image patches derived from supervoxels, combined with simulated non-contrast image patches and real image patches to ensure robustness against both modality heterogeneity and inter-center variability. For fibrosis staging, learnable modality-aware tokens were designed to augment patch embeddings from corresponding modalities, enhancing multi-modal information fusion in transformer layers.

Acknowledgments. This work was supported in part by the National Natural Science Foundation of China via project 62471293. We would like to acknowledge organizers of CARE 2025 challenge for their organization and the provision of LiQA data.

References

1. Billot, B., Greve, D.N., Puonti, O., Thielscher, A., Van Leemput, K., Fischl, B., Dalca, A.V., Iglesias, J.E., et al.: Synthseg: segmentation of brain mri scans of any contrast and resolution without retraining. Med. Image Anal. **86**, 102789 (2023)
2. Chen, Z., Agarwal, D., Aggarwal, K., Safta, W., Balan, M.M., Brown, K.: Masked image modeling advances 3d medical image analysis. In: Proceedings of the IEEE/CVF Winter Conference on Applications of Computer Vision, pp. 1970–1980 (2023)
3. Dey, N., Billot, B., Wong, H.E., Wang, C., Ren, M., Grant, E., Dalca, A.V., Golland, P.: Learning general-purpose biomedical volume representations using randomized synthesis. In: The Thirteenth International Conference on Learning Representations (2025), https://openreview.net/forum?id=xOmC5LiVuN
4. Dosovitskiy, A., Beyer, L., Kolesnikov, A., Weissenborn, D., Zhai, X., Unterthiner, T., Dehghani, M., Minderer, M., Heigold, G., Gelly, S., Uszkoreit, J., Houlsby, N.: An image is worth 16x16 words: transformers for image recognition at scale. In: International Conference on Learning Representations (2021), https://openreview.net/forum?id=YicbFdNTTy
5. Gao, Z., Liu, Y., Wu, F., Shi, N., Shi, Y., Zhuang, X.: A reliable and interpretable framework of multi-view learning for liver fibrosis staging. In: International Conference on Medical Image Computing and Computer-Assisted Intervention, pp. 178–188 (2023)
6. Gopinath, K., Greve, D.N., Magdamo, C., Arnold, S., Das, S., Puonti, O., Iglesias, J.E., Initiative, A.D.N., et al.: "recon-all-clinical": cortical surface reconstruction and analysis of heterogeneous clinical brain mri. Med. Image Anal. 103608 (2025)
7. Kavur, A.E., Gezer, N.S., Barış, M., Aslan, S., Conze, P.H., Groza, V., Pham, D.D., Chatterjee, S., Ernst, P., Özkan, S., et al.: Chaos challenge-combined (ct-mr) healthy abdominal organ segmentation. Med. Image Anal. **69**, 101950 (2021)
8. Kingma, D.P., Ba, J.: Adam: a method for stochastic optimization. arXiv preprint arXiv:1412.6980 (2014)
9. Li, Q., Chen, T., Shi, N., Ye, W., Yuan, M., Shi, Y.: Quantitative evaluation of hepatic fibrosis by fibro scan and gd-eob-dtpa-enhanced t1 mapping magnetic resonance imaging in chronic hepatitis b. Abdom. Radiol. **47**(2), 684–692 (2022)
10. Li, X., Dou, Q., Chen, H., Fu, C.W., Qi, X., Belavỳ, D.L., Armbrecht, G., Felsenberg, D., Zheng, G., Heng, P.A.: 3d multi-scale fcn with random modality voxel dropout learning for intervertebral disc localization and segmentation from multi-modality mr images. Med. Image Anal. **45**, 41–54 (2018)
11. Liu, Y., Gao, Z., Shi, N., Wu, F., Shi, Y., Chen, Q., Zhuang, X.: Merit: multi-view evidential learning for reliable and interpretable liver fibrosis staging. Med. Image Anal. **102**, 103507 (2025)

12. Ma, D., Pang, J., Gotway, M.B., Liang, J.: Foundation ark: accruing and reusing knowledge for superior and robust performance. In: International Conference on Medical Image Computing and Computer-Assisted Intervention, pp. 651–662. Springer (2023)
13. Meng, X., Sun, K., Xu, J., He, X., Shen, D.: Multi-modal modality-masked diffusion network for brain mri synthesis with random modality missing. IEEE Trans. Med. Imaging **43**(7), 2587–2598 (2024)
14. Perlin, K.: An image synthesizer. ACM Siggraph Comput. Graph. **19**(3), 287–296 (1985)
15. Stutz, D., Hermans, A., Leibe, B.: Superpixels: an evaluation of the state-of-the-art. Comput. Vis. Image Underst. **166**, 1–27 (2018)
16. Vaswani, A., Shazeer, N., Parmar, N., Uszkoreit, J., Jones, L., Gomez, A.N., Kaiser, Ł., Polosukhin, I.: Attention is all you need. Adv. Neural Inf. Process. Syst. **30** (2017)
17. Wu, F., Zhuang, X.: Minimizing estimated risks on unlabeled data: a new formulation for semi-supervised medical image segmentation. IEEE Trans. Pattern Anal. Mach. Intell. **45**(5), 6021–6036 (2023)

Transfer Learning for Multimodal Whole Heart Segmentation Supported by Intensity Transformations

Johanna Brosig[1,2,3(✉)], Lisa Bautz[1,2,3], Inna Khasyanova[2,3], Lars Walczak[1,2,3], Simon Sündermann[3,4,6], Jörg Kempfert[3,4,6], Titus Kühne[2,3,6], Anja Hennemuth[1,2,3,5,6], and Markus Hüllebrand[1,2,3,6]

[1] Fraunhofer Institute for Digital Medicine MEVIS, Berlin, Germany
{johanna.brosig,lisa.bautz}@mevis.fraunhofer.de
[2] Deutsches Herzzentrum der Charité, Institute of Computer-assisted Cardiovascular Medicine, Berlin, Germany
[3] Charité Universitätsmedizin Berlin, corporate member of Freie Universität Berlin and Humboldt-Universität zu Berlin, Berlin, Germany
[4] Department of Cardiothoracic and Vascular Surgery, Deutsches Herzzentrum der Charité (DHZC), Berlin, Germany
[5] Department of Diagnostic and Interventional Radiology and Nuclear Medicine, University Medical Center Hamburg-Eppendorf, Hamburg, Germany
[6] DZHK (German Center for Cardiovascular Research), Berlin, Germany

Abstract. The CARE-WHS challenge focuses on achieving precise whole-heart segmentations across various computed tomography (CT) and magnetic resonance (MR) images, addressing the complexities arising from anatomical variability and different scanning protocols. Previous efforts have highlighted limitations in both model-based and deep-learning-based approaches to cardiac segmentation. This study evaluates the performance of two state-of-the-art architectures, nnU-Net and SwinUNETR, in the context of the CARE-WHS challenge. We explore three training strategies: a basic configuration using only challenge data for training, a model trained on public CT data, and a transfer learning approach, where the model trained on public data is finetuned to the available challenge data. Additionally, a random smooth gray value transformation is implemented as data augmentation for nnU-Net and SwinUNETR to mitigate discrepancies between CT and MR scans. Our results indicate that while nnU-Net consistently outperforms SwinUNETR, the SwinUNTER in combination with random smooth gray value transformation (GVT) shows the highest potential for unseen intensities.

Keywords: Gray value transformation · Multi-modality · Segmentation

X. Zhuang et al. (Eds.): CARE 2025, LNCS 16257, pp. 46–56, 2026.
https://doi.org/10.1007/978-3-032-16271-7_5

1 Introduction

The CARE-WHS challenge aims to find accurate whole-heart segmentation solutions to facilitate exact quantification on both CT and MR images of different sites. However, anatomical variations, different scanning protocols, and different modalities complicate the development of a solution that generalizes well.

The task of automatic whole-heart segmentation has been approached in previous work numerous times. In 2013, Zhuang et al. [13] reviewed different model-based algorithms and found many limitations in both accuracy and computational efficiency. With the rise of machine learning, the focus shifted to deep-learning-based segmentations. Bernard et al. [1] reviewed methods for cardiac multi-structure MR segmentation in 2018 and pronounced the problem nearly solved. They concluded that state-of-the-art machine learning methods can already produce highly accurate segmentations, although they perform slightly worse near the heart's apex.

Similar to the CARE Challenge, the MM-WHS segmentation challenge [15] in 2019 strived to find whole-heart segmentation methods for CT and MR images. They reported that while the majority of submitted algorithms were deep-learning-based, hybrid models that combine prior knowledge with machine learning have good potential. Habijan et al. [5] give a more recent overview of both model and deep-learning-based methods for whole heart segmentation. They conclude that the performance of deep-learning-based methods highly depends of the amount and the quality of training data and annotations available. A general review of deep-learning based methods for cardiac image segmentations is found in [3]. They name the following challenges: Scarcity of labels, lack of model interpretability and model generalization across various imaging modalities, scanners, and pathologies.

As the nnU-Net [7] already performed best on MR images in 2018 [1], we evaluate its performance in combination with CT images in the context of the CARE-WHS challenge. Furthermore, we compare it to the SwinUNETR [6] architecture, as this architecture already outperformed the nnU-Net on the task of brain tumor segmentation. Inspired by Habijan et al.'s [5] claim, that the performance of deep-learning methods highly depends on the available training data, we test different configurations: a *basic* version trained only on the challenge data, a version *pretrained* on various public datasets, and a third version with *transfer learning*. In order to ease the differences between CT and MR data, we apply GVT [8] to the intensity values as data augmentation.

2 Methods

We compare the performance of the nnU-Net [7] to the performance of the SwinUNETR [6] using different training data and strategies. As shown in Fig. 1, we compare the performance of both architectures for the following training configurations:

- *Pretraining*: training on public CT datasets supplemented by manually corrected private data
- *Transfer*: finetuning of the pretrained model using the challenge training data
- *Basic*: training on challenge training data

In addition, the performance with and without GVT [8] is evaluated.

2.1 Data

In addition to the datasets provided by the CARE-WHS Challenge [4,14,16], we use four public and one private dataset of CT images. Figure 1 gives an overview of the data processing workflow. Table 1 specifies the dataset properties. The four public datasets include the TotalSegmentator data v1 and v2 [9]. They consist of randomly sampled CT scans from clinical routine and thereby represent a wide range of pathologies, institutions, and scanners. Version v2 contains improved annotations of the aorta and pulmonary artery (PA), but only one label for the complete heart is provided, while v1 contains annotations of the heart chambers and myocardium. Therefore, the annotations of v1 and v2 are merged. Furthermore, we use the ImageCAS [12] dataset consisting of CTs of patients with diagnosed ischemic stroke, transient ischemic attack, and/or peripheral artery disease. The dataset comprises annotations of the coronary arteries. The ImageCHD [11] dataset contains CT scans of patients with Congenital Heart Disease (CHD). Annotations of the heart chambers, myocardium, aorta (Ao), and PA are provided.

We use the merged TotalSegmentator dataset to train an nnU-Net [7]. This *CardiacAnnotationNet* is then used to produce annotations for the remaining datasets. For the ImageCHD [11] data, myocardium annotations are missing in some cases. For others, the complete myocardium is annotated. In contrast, the annotations for this challenge include only the myocardium surrounding the left ventricle left ventricle (LV). Therefore, we merge the predicted myocardium segmentation with the annotations provided. Cases in which we deemed the annotation inaccurate after merging are excluded.

As previous experiments have shown that trained models had problems segmenting the LV in late systolic phases, private data acquired at Charit–Universittsmedizin Berlin are added. The institutional review board (Ethikkommission Charit–Universittsmedizin Berlin, approval number EA1/062/19) approved the use of retrospective data for this study and waived individual informed consent. 24 cases are segmented using the *CardiacAnnotationNet* and corrected manually by domain experts. Similarly, a subset of the ImageCAS [12] dataset is corrected. This was done using a self-developed software with a threshold-based brush tool.

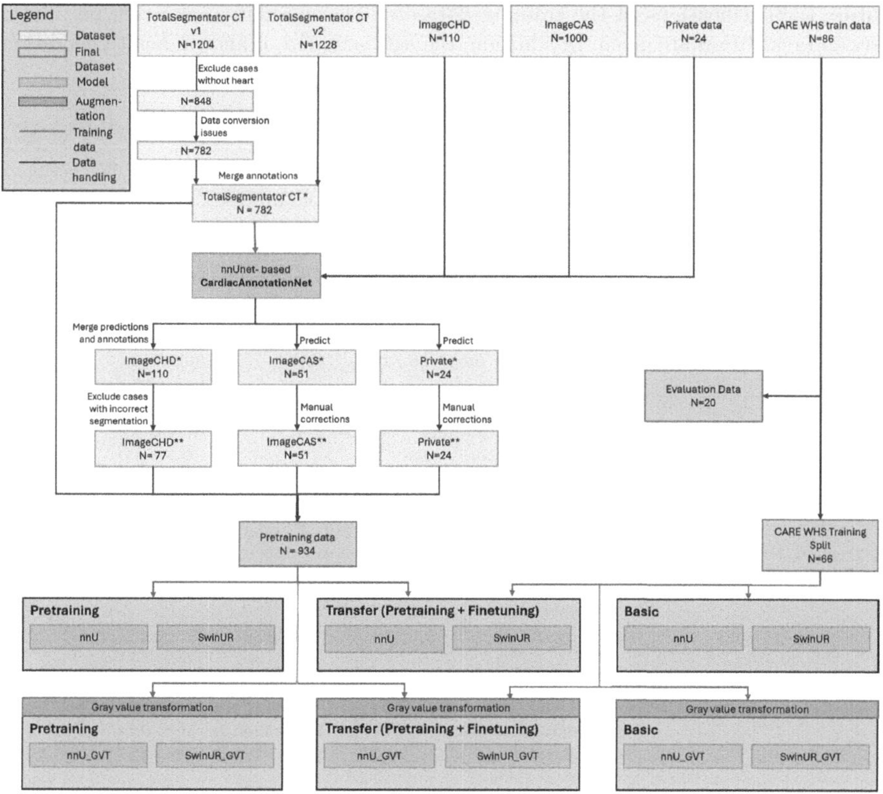

Fig. 1. Processing pipeline. An annotation model is trained using the TotalSegmentator [9] data. The annotation model is used to initialize the annotations for CT data. After manual corrections of a subset, models with nnU-Net [7] (nnU) and SwinUNETR [6] (SwinUR) architectures are trained with the corrected annotations and publicly available data. We compare the performance with and without gray value transformation (GVT).

In total, our pretraining dataset consists of 934 samples. This includes 77 samples from the ImageCHD [11] data, 51 samples from the ImageCAS [12] data, 782 TotalSegmentator [9] training samples, and 24 private samples from Charit–Universittsmedizin Berlin. The CARE challenge training data [4,14,16] is split into a training set of 66 samples and an evaluation set of 20 samples. The evaluation set comprises 10 randomly selected MR and 10 randomly selected CT scans.

Table 1. Specifications of the training datasets. The modality, scanner type, image size, and resolution are given. In addition, the age, sex, and, if known, health condition are given.

Name	Modality	Subjects	Scanner type	Resolution	Voxel size in mm^3
TotalSegmentator v1 / v2 [9]	CT	510 females, 716 males,2 unknown800 abnormality, 404 none,24 unknown 15-98 years	16 scanners (most Siemens)	(63-437) (89-430) (37-838)	1.51.51.5
ImageCHD [11]	CT	1 month to 40 years / 104 with CHD	Siemens biograph 64	512 512 (129-357)	typically 0.250.250.5
ImageCAS [12]	CT	414 females (59.98 years) 586 males (57.68 years) ischemic stroke, transient ischemic attack and/or peripheral artery disease	Siemens 128-slice dual-source	512 512 (206-275)	(0.290.43) (0.290.43) (0.250.45)
CARE-WHS [4,14,16]	CT,MR	n/a	n/a	(167-512) (148-512) (50-363)	(0.28-1.21) (0.28-1.21) (0.45-3.0)
Private	CT	5 female, 2 male (multiple timepoints) 16-74 years	Siemens	(256-512)(256-512)(122-412)	(0.30-0.74) (0.30-0.74) (0.5-1.0)

2.2 Models

We use the nnU-Net [7] and SwinUNETR [6] for multi-class segmentation. The nnU-Net is a framework proposing self-configuring segmentation networks. Hence, the network handles resampling, normalization, and hyperparameter selection by design. Dice Similarity Coefficient (DSC) and cross-entropy determine the loss function. The challenge data are used to create the fingerprint for all nnU-Net models. The 3D high-resolution configuration is selected.

The SwinUNETR is composed of a Swin transformer as encoder and a fully convolutional neural network as decoder. We use MONAI [2] to implement SwinUNETR. We select a patch token size of 2 and a feature size of 48. DSC and cross-entropy are used as the loss function. The input is resampled to the median voxel size of the challenge training data, an isotropic voxel size of 0.88 mm. The input is cropped to 224^3 voxels. The cropping window is centered around the center of mass of the heart label predicted using the TotalSegmentator [10]. The input is clipped using the 5th and 95th percentiles and normalized to intensity values between 0 and 1.

Augmentations For both architectures, we compare the performance using the default augmentations to the performance using additional gray value transformation as an augmentation. The nnU-Net default implementation comprises rotations, scaling, Gaussian noise, Gaussian blur, brightness, contrast, simulation of low resolution, gamma intensity transformation, and mirroring [7]. As suggested in [6] for the SwinUNETR, we apply random axis mirror flip along each axis, random intensity shift, and random scale shift as augmentations.

Random Smooth Gray Value Transformation As the challenge aims at an accurate segmentation for CT and MR, we integrate random smooth gray value transformations (GVT) [8] into the augmentations applied to the data before feeding it to the models. The transformation facilitates reducing cross-modality differences. Thus, we evaluate its performance at whole heart CT and MR segmentation. More specifically, the voxel values are continuosly mapped using a sum of sines with random frequencies, amplitudes, and offsets. Figure 2 shows an example of both CT and MR image with and without GVT.

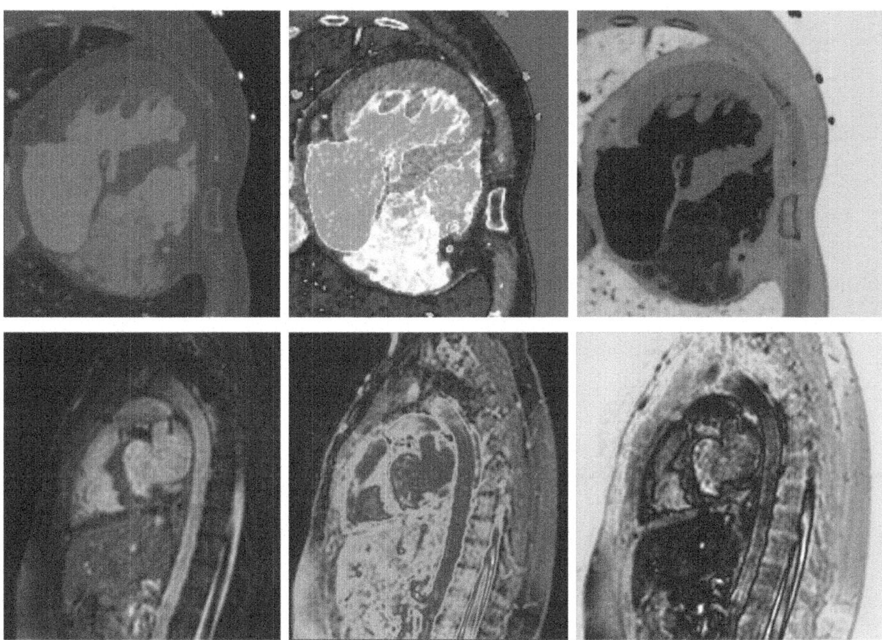

Fig. 2. Examples of GVT applied to CT (upper row) and MR (lower row). The left images are the original slices; GVT was applied to the middle and right slices.

3 Results

For evaluation, we use the metrics proposed by the CARE challenge: DSC, 95th percentile Hausdorff Distance (HD95), and Average Surface Distance (ASD). Table 2 shows results for the configurations and architectures used in this work. The performance of all models is better on CT data than on MR. Furthermore, the nnU-Net outperforms the SwinUNETR in all scenarios except the the pretraining tested on MR images. In Fig. 4, the DSC for the labels for each configuration and architecture is displayed. While the performance of all models is similar between the heart chambers, the segmentation of the arteries is more error-prone. For the submitted transfer nnU_GVT model, Fig. 3 shows exemplary slices indicating regions with differences between the reference annotation and the prediction.

Table 2. Segmentation results for nnU-Net (nnU) and SwinUNETR (SwinUR) architecture with and without gray value transformation as data augmentation. The DSC, HD95, and ASD are given as mean±standard deviation for CT and MR images. In addition, we compare three different training datasets: only publicly available data (pre), only the challenge data (basic), and publicly available data for pretraining and challenge data for finetuning (transfer).

		CT			MR		
Model		DSC	HD95 [mm]	ASD [mm]	DSC	HD95 [mm]	ASD [mm]
pre	nnU	0.89 ± 0.03	22.73 ± 10.31	1.11 ± 0.45	0.52 ± 0.22	48.83 ± 24.21	2.84 ± 2.58
	nnU_GVT	0.89 ± 0.03	20.01 ± 10.87	1.09 ± 0.44	0.54 ± 0.24	77.36 ± 120.09	3.49 ± 3.92
	SwinUR	0.88 ± 0.04	20.7 ± 11.98	4.48 ± 2.41	0.79 ± 0.11	22.54 ± 10.88	5.49 ± 2.79
	SwinUR_GVT	0.89 ± 0.03	23.4 ± 8.44	4.6 ± 1.89	0.82 ± 0.06	29.39 ± 18.83	6.98 ± 4.36
transfer	nnU	0.96 ± 0.01	2.43 ± 1.32	0.45 ± 0.14	0.91 ± 0.03	9.15 ± 7.81	1.12 ± 0.41
	nnU_GVT	0.96 ± 0.02	2.45 ± 1.27	0.47 ± 0.15	0.91 ± 0.03	8.97 ± 7.81	1.15 ± 0.43
	SwinUR	0.93 ± 0.02	6.08 ± 5.0	1.50 ± 0.64	0.87 ± 0.06	10.94 ± 5.44	2.15 ± 0.92
	SwinUR_GVT	0.93 ± 0.02	4.06 ± 2.0	0.94 ± 0.26	0.88 ± 0.04	9.58 ± 5.77	1.85 ± 0.54
basic	nnU	0.96 ± 0.02	11.15 ± 25.94	0.46 ± 0.14	0.91 ± 0.03	8.96 ± 7.88	1.15 ± 0.4
	nnU_GVT	0.96 ± 0.02	2.63 ± 1.63	0.46 ± 0.15	0.91 ± 0.03	8.77 ± 7.8	1.14 ± 0.46
	SwinUR	0.95 ± 0.02	4.23 ± 3.38	1.04 ± 0.53	0.89 ± 0.04	10.86 ± 5.94	1.85 ± 0.7
	SwinUR_GVT	0.92 ± 0.01	6.4 ± 3.18	1.53 ± 0.48	0.87 ± 0.03	10.18 ± 5.01	2.07 ± 0.44

4 Discussion

As shown in Table 2, the nnU-Net DSC achieved using the transfer learning and only challenge data is the same, while the transfer learning on the SwinUNTER architecture led to a slightly improved DSC compared to using only challenge data. For CT, HD95 and ASD are improved using transfer learning compared to only using the challenge data with both architectures. This could indicate that transfer learning to enlarge the training dataset leads to a better understanding of cardiac shapes, as neither ASD nor HD95 is part of the loss functions.

The performance is worse using only pretraining compared to transfer and only challenge data for training for both architectures. Especially, the results on the MR data are worse with pretraining only. This is most likely due to the fact that MR data was not part of the training data. Using pretraining data only, the SwinUNETR_GVT model achieves the best DSC and outperforms the nnU-Net

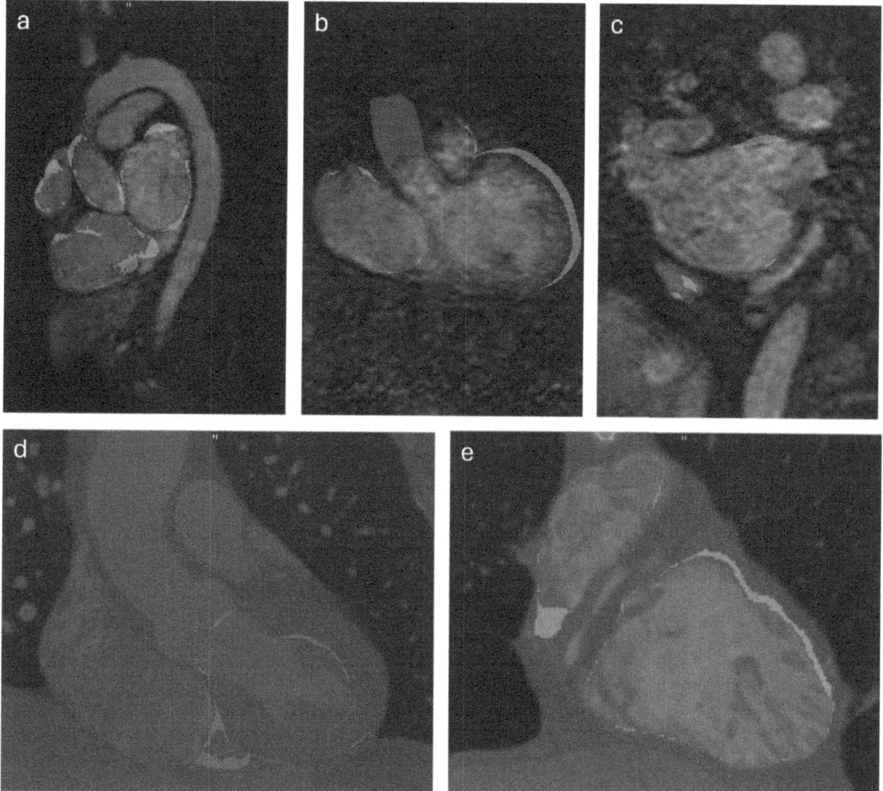

Fig. 3. Differences between reference annotation and prediction for transfer nnU_GVT for selected slices of (a-c) MR and (d-e) CT volumes. The colors highlight regions with differences to the ground truth annotations. The red color indicates under-segmented areas, while blue marks over-segmented regions.

versions on MR data. This could be explained by the SwinUNETR self-attention modules facilitating modeling long-range dependencies, making it less dependent on local intensity changes. This could indicate that the SwinUNETR_GVT has the highest potential for segmenting data with unseen intensities. Future work could investigate whether adjusting the GVT frequencies can further improve the result.

The mean DSC is equal or lower using the SwinUNETR compared to the nnU-Net for all training strategies, but for using pretraining data only. Hyperparameter optimization could potentially improve the SwinUNETR results. In [6], the performance of both architectures is compared for brain tumor segmentation. They report that the SwinUNETR outperforms the nnU-Net on average by 0.05 in terms of DSC. The DSC using SwinUNETR with GVT is higher for MR compared to SwinUNETR without GVT using pretraining data only. However, using the challenge data as part of the training results in similar DSC. This indicates that GVT is beneficial if intensity distributions are expected in the test set that were not present in the training set.

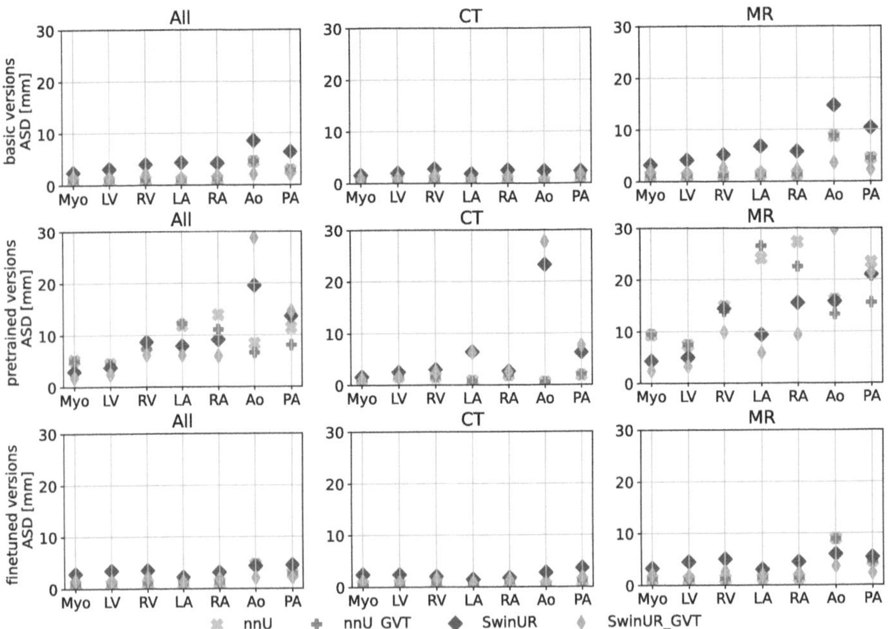

Fig. 4. Comparison of the label-specific performance in terms of ASD between all models. The evaluated segmentation labels are myocard (Myo), left ventricle (LA), right ventricle (RV), left atrium (LA), right atrium (RA), aorta (Ao), and pulmonary artery (PA). The first row shows the results of all models trained on the basic dataset. The second row shows the results of the pretrained models, and the last row shows the results of the finetuned versions. The first column shows results evaluated on the whole test data, the second column shows results evaluated on CT data, and the last column shows results for MR data.

Figure 4 shows the ASD each model scored for the different labels of the whole heart segmentation. The basic and transfer variants of nnU-Net versions outperform the SwinUNTER models in most categories. However, for the aorta and PA segmentation on MR data, the SwinUR_transfer_GVT performs best.

For CT, the ASD of the PA is comparatively high for all models. This could be explained by the reference annotations showing differences in how far the vessels are considered part of the PA. On MR the same holds true for the aorta and PA segmentation.

This is also shown in Fig. 3. The high ASD for the aorta is caused by the predictions only covering parts of the ascending aorta, while the reference annotation additionally covers parts of the descending aorta. Due to many training data annotations only covering parts of the ascending aorta the model weights are optimized towards only labeling parts of the ascending aorta. Figure 3 shows that drops in the evaluation metrics can be explained by differences along the boundary regions. In Fig. 3, differences around the pulmonary veins are displayed. Potentially, because there is no clear line of demarcation indicating the transition between left atrium (LA) and pulmonary veins, high inter-observer variance causes the differences between annotation and prediction. Hence, in some training annotations, the positions of the veins are evident, in some, they are not.

5 Conclusion

We evaluated the performance of the nnU-Net and SwinUNETR with and without GVT and different training datasets. The nnU-Net outperformed the SwinUNETR for all configurations. Our results suggest that GVT can improve the whole heart segmentation performance. However, the GVT could not account for limited diversity in the training data. For data with unseen intensities, the SwinUNETR with GVT showed the highest potential.

Acknowledgments. This work was supported by the Fraunhofer Internal Programs under Grant No. SME 40-09567 the DFG SFB 1470 and the EU-project SIMCOR.

References

1. Bernard, O., Lalande, A., Zotti, C., Cervenansky, F., Yang, X., Heng, P., et al.: Deep learning techniques for automatic MRI cardiac multi-structures segmentation and diagnosis: Is the problem solved? IEEE Trans. Med. Imaging **37**(11), 2514–2525 (2018). https://doi.org/10.1109/TMI.2018.2837502
2. Cardoso, M.J., Li, W., Brown, R., Ma, N., Kerfoot, E., Wang, Y., Murrey, B., et al.: Monai: An open-source framework for deep learning in healthcare. arXiv preprint arXiv:2211.02701 (2022)
3. Chen, C., Qin, C., Qiu, H., Tarroni, G., Duan, J., Bai, W., et al.: Deep learning for cardiac image segmentation: a review. Front. Cardiovascular Med. **7**, 25 (2020). https://doi.org/10.3389/fcvm.2020.00025

4. Gao, S., Zhou, H., Gao, Y., Zhuang, X.: Bayeseg: Bayesian modeling for medical image segmentation with interpretable generalizability. Med. Image Anal. **89**, 102889 (2023). https://doi.org/10.1016/J.MEDIA.2023.102889
5. Habijan, M., Babin, D., Galić, I., Leventić, H., Romić, K., Velicki, L., et al.: Overview of the whole heart and heart chamber segmentation methods. Cardiovasc. Eng. Technol. **11**(6), 725–747 (2020). https://doi.org/10.1007/s13239-020-00494-8
6. Hatamizadeh, A., Nath, V., Tang, Y., Yang, D., Roth, H.R., Xu, D.: Swin UNETR: swin transformers for semantic segmentation of brain tumors in MRI images. In: Crimi, A., Bakas, S. (eds.) Brainlesion: Glioma, Multiple Sclerosis, Stroke and Traumatic Brain Injuries–7th International Workshop, BrainLes 2021, Held in Conjunction with MICCAI 2021, Virtual Event, September 27, 2021, Revised Selected Papers, Part I. Lecture Notes in Computer Science, vol. 12962, pp. 272–284. Springer (2021). https://doi.org/10.1007/978-3-031-08999-2_22
7. Isensee, F., Jaeger, P.F., Kohl, S.A., Petersen, J., Maier-Hein, K.H.: nnu-net: a self-configuring method for deep learning-based biomedical image segmentation. Nat. Methods **18**(2), 203–211 (2021). https://doi.org/10.1038/s41592-020-01008-z
8. Lessmann, N., van Ginneken, B.: Random smooth gray value transformations for cross modality learning with gray value invariant networks. CoRR **abs/2003.06158** (2020), https://arxiv.org/abs/2003.06158
9. Wasserthal, J.: Dataset with segmentations of 117 important anatomical structures in 1228 ct images (Oct 2023). https://doi.org/10.5281/zenodo.10047292, https://doi.org/10.5281/zenodo.10047292
10. Wasserthal, J., Meyer, M., Breit, H., Cyriac, J., Yang, S., Segeroth, M.: Totalsegmentator: robust segmentation of 104 anatomical structures in CT images. CoRR **abs/2208.05868** (2022). https://doi.org/10.48550/ARXIV.2208.05868
11. Xu, X., Wang, T., Zhuang, J., Yuan, H., Huang, M., Cen, J., et al.: Imagechd: A 3d computed tomography image dataset for classification of congenital heart disease. In: Martel, A.L., Abolmaesumi, P., Stoyanov, D., Mateus, D., Zuluaga, M.A., Zhou, S.K., Racoceanu, D., Joskowicz, L. (eds.) Medical Image Computing and Computer Assisted Intervention–MICCAI 2020–23rd International Conference, Lima, Peru, October 4-8, 2020, Proceedings, Part IV. Lecture Notes in Computer Science, vol. 12264, pp. 77–87. Springer (2020). https://doi.org/10.1007/978-3-030-59719-1_8
12. Zeng, A., Wu, C., Lin, G., Xie, W., Hong, J., Huang, M., et al.: Imagecas: A large-scale dataset and benchmark for coronary artery segmentation based on computed tomography angiography images. Comput. Medical Imaging Graph. **109**, 102287 (2023). https://doi.org/10.1016/J.COMPMEDIMAG.2023.102287
13. Zhuang, X.: Challenges and methodologies of fully automatic whole heart segmentation: a review. J. Healthcare Eng. **4**(3), 371–407 (2013). https://doi.org/10.1260/2040-2295.4.3.371
14. Zhuang, X.: Multivariate mixture model for myocardial segmentation combining multi-source images. IEEE Trans. Pattern Anal. Mach. Intell. **41**(12), 2933–2946 (2019). https://doi.org/10.1109/TPAMI.2018.2869576
15. Zhuang, X., Li, L., Payer, C., Stern, D., Urschler, M., Heinrich, M.P., et al.: Evaluation of algorithms for multi-modality whole heart segmentation: An open-access grand challenge. Medical Image Anal. **58** (2019). https://doi.org/10.1016/J.MEDIA.2019.101537
16. Zhuang, X., Shen, J.: Multi-scale patch and multi-modality atlases for whole heart segmentation of MRI. Medical Image Anal. **31**, 77–87 (2016). https://doi.org/10.1016/J.MEDIA.2016.02.006

CoSSeg-TTA: Contrast-Aware Semi-Supervised Segmentation with Domain Generalization and Test-Time Adaptation

Jincan Lou[1], Jingkun Chen[3(✉)], Haoquan Li[1], Hang Li[1], Wenjian Huang[1], Weihua Chen[2], Fan Wang[2], and Jianguo Zhang[1(✉)]

[1] Southern University of Science and Technology, Guangdong, China
zhangjg@sustech.edu.cn
[2] DAMO Academy, Hangzhou, China
[3] Department of Engineering Science, University of Oxford, Oxford, UK
jingkun.chen@eng.ox.ac.uk

Abstract. Accurate liver segmentation from contrast-enhanced MRI is essential for diagnosis, treatment planning, and disease monitoring. However, it remains challenging due to limited annotated data, heterogeneous enhancement protocols, and significant domain shifts across scanners and institutions. Traditional image-to-image translation frameworks have made great progress in domain generalization, but their application is not straightforward. For example, Pix2Pix requires image registration, and cycle-GAN cannot be integrated seamlessly into segmentation pipelines. Meanwhile, these methods are originally used to deal with cross-modality scenarios, and often introduce structural distortions and suffer from unstable training, which may pose drawbacks in our single-modality scenario. To address these challenges, we propose CoSSeg-TTA, a compact segmentation framework for the GED4 (Gd-EOB-DTPA enhanced hepatobiliary phase MRI) modality built upon nnU-Netv2 and enhanced with a semi-supervised mean teacher scheme to exploit large amounts of unlabeled volumes. A domain adaptation module, incorporating a randomized histogram-based style appearance transfer function and a trainable contrast-aware network, enriches domain diversity and mitigates cross-center variability. Furthermore, a continual test-time adaptation strategy is employed to improve robustness during inference. Extensive experiments demonstrate that our framework consistently outperforms the nnU-Netv2 baseline, achieving superior Dice score and Hausdorff Distance while exhibiting strong generalization to unseen domains under low-annotation conditions.

Keywords: Contrast enhancement · Semi-supervised learning · Medical segmentation · Test-time adaptation · Domain generalization

X. Zhuang et al. (Eds.): CARE 2025, LNCS 16257, pp. 57–67, 2026.
https://doi.org/10.1007/978-3-032-16271-7_6

1 Introduction

Liver fibrosis, a common consequence of chronic liver injuries, can progress to cirrhosis, liver failure, or hepatocellular carcinoma, posing serious global health concerns. Accurate liver segmentation is essential in clinical workflows, including diagnosis, treatment planning, and surgical navigation. However, acquiring high-quality annotations is labor-intensive, requires expert knowledge, and is prone to inter-observer variability, which often leads to annotation scarcity [14,17].

Beyond annotation scarcity, two major technical challenges remain. First, clinical liver assessment always uses contrast-enhanced MRI, such as Gd-EOB-DTPA-enhanced imaging, but it suffers from artifacts and uneven enhancement [4,12,18]. Second, modern clinical datasets are often collected from multiple centers and scanners, leading to severe domain shifts due to variations in vendors, acquisition protocols, and noise characteristics [16,18,20].

Recent advances such as GAN-based domain transfer and image-to-image translation exhibit strong cross-domain generative capability. However, these approaches have critical limitations. Methods like Pix2Pix [10] always require image registration, and those like cycle-GAN [26] cannot be integrated seamlessly into our framework. Meanwhile, a large body of work uses GANs for cross-modality tasks, rather than for small scanner- or protocol-induced shifts within modality [24] , and will introduce artifacts and blur tissue edges. Their behavior is not ideal for our setting, which is domain shift within the same modality.

To address these issues, we propose a semi-supervised segmentation framework that integrates domain generalization and test-time adaptation. Our approach builds on nnU-Netv2 [9] under mean teacher paradigm with pseudo-labels learning to solve annotation scarcity. A pre-processing module combines domain transfer method with contrast-aware network, while continual test-time adaptation (CoTTA) [21] improves robustness to unseen domains. Finally post-processing is applied to trim the prediction mask.

Our contributions are threefold: (1) We design a semi-supervised framework based on nnU-Netv2 under mean teacher strategy with pseudo-labels learning, effectively leveraging unlabeled dataset. (2) We introduce a domain adaptation pipeline combining appearance translation via random histogram matching and a contrast-aware network, integrated with test-time adaptation to improve cross-domain generalization. (3) Our approach is validated on a real-world multi-center dataset, demonstrating superior robustness and accuracy compared to existing methods in low-label and cross-domain scenarios.

2 Method

Figure 1 illustrates the overall pipeline: during training, the model applies pre-processing techniques, including domain adaptation, contrast enhancement, and data augmentation, and is trained under the framework of mean teacher with pseudo-labels learning; during inference, continual test-time adaptation and post-processing further improve robustness.

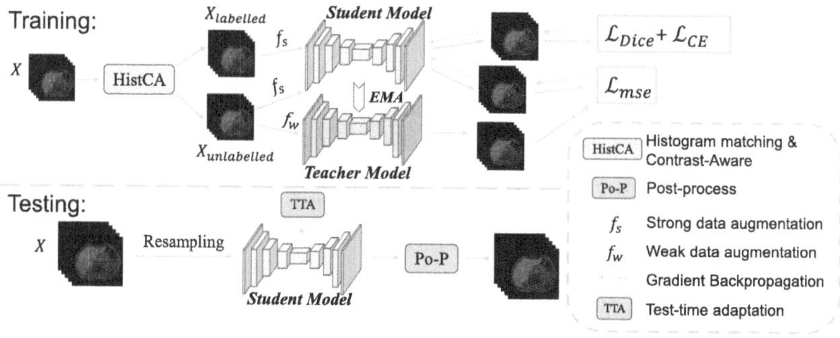

Fig. 1. An overview of the proposed semi-supervised liver segmentation framework

2.1 Semi-Supervised Learning with Mean Teacher

Since manual annotations are scarce and costly to obtain in clinical practice [2,3,25], we adopt a semi-supervised learning framework based on the mean teacher paradigm [5,19]. This approach enables the model to effectively leverage large amounts of unlabeled data alongside a limited set of labeled examples [1].

The framework consists of two models: a student network h_θ with parameters θ, and a teacher network h_ϕ with parameters ϕ. The teacher is updated as the exponential moving average (EMA) of the student parameters:

$$\phi \leftarrow \alpha\phi + (1-\alpha)\theta \tag{1}$$

where $\alpha \in [0, 1)$ is a smoothing coefficient that controls the update rate. This strategy ensures that the teacher evolves more smoothly, providing stable targets for consistency training.

Given a labeled training dataset $\mathcal{D}_l^s$ and an unlabeled training dataset $\mathcal{D}_u^s$, the overall training objective is formulated as:

$$\mathcal{L} = \mathcal{L}_{\text{sup}}(\mathcal{D}_l^s) + \lambda_{\text{mse}} \cdot \mathcal{L}_{\text{mse}}(\mathcal{D}_u^s) \tag{2}$$

$$\mathcal{L}_{\text{sup}} = \mathcal{L}_{\text{Dice}} + \mathcal{L}_{\text{ce}}(\mathcal{D}_l^s) \tag{3}$$

where $\mathcal{L}_{\text{sup}}$ is the supervised segmentation loss to learn from labeled dataset. $\mathcal{L}_{\text{mse}}$, which is mean square error loss, is used as consistency loss that enforces agreement between student and teacher predictions on unlabeled data under different perturbations.

In practice, we apply strong data augmentation (e.g., histogram matching, geometric transformations) to generate two perturbed views of each unlabeled sample, encouraging the student to produce consistent outputs with the teacher. This design effectively exploits unlabeled data, improves feature representation learning, and mitigates overfitting in low-annotation settings.

2.2 Domain Adaptation via Appearance Translation

In multi-domain medical imaging, the marginal input distribution $P(x)$ often varies significantly across centers and scanners, a phenomenon known as covariate shift. If unaddressed, this distribution discrepancy causes poor cross-domain generalization.

Instead of GAN based methods, we adapt a lightweight appearance translation strategy based on histogram matching, which can be directly embedded into data pre-processing and training. The method of random histogram matching efficiently deal with domain generalization, and avoid the generation of artifacts and blurred pattern (see Fig. 2).

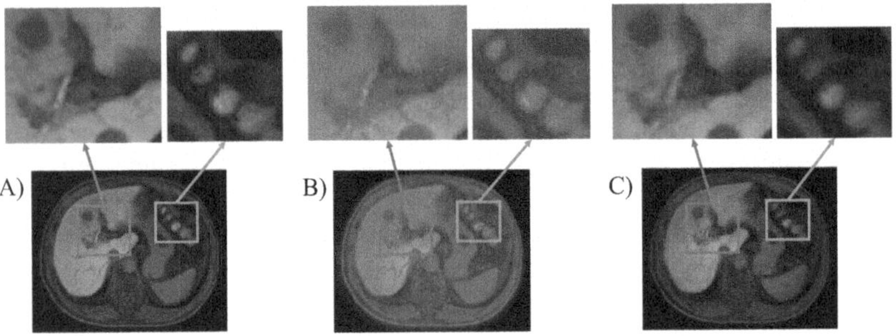

Fig. 2. A) Original GED4 modality image; B) Style transferred with random matching histogram; C) Style transferred with GAN. The red triangle areas show the comparison of artifacts, while the blue triangle areas show the comparison of blurred pattern

2.3 Contrast-Aware Module

To address the inconsistent visibility of liver structures across contrast phases, we design a learning-based contrast-aware module that exploits the contrast relationship between T1-weighted modality (T1WI) and GED4 modalities.

In contrast-enhanced medical imaging, different acquisition phases often exhibit significant differences in soft tissue visibility and organ boundary clarity. Specifically, in our dataset, T1WI corresponds to the pre-contrast phase, while the GED4 modality represents the final post-contrast enhanced phase, where liver lesions and vascular structures are more conspicuously visualized due to contrast agent accumulation. Motivated by this inherent contrast evolution, we propose a learning-based module that captures the mapping between T1WI and GED4 modalities to enhance the contrast representation in GED4 images.

We hypothesize that the contrast relationship between the T1WI and GED4 phases can be exploited using deep learning to generate contrast-enhanced representations that emphasize relevant anatomical structures. To this end, we first perform rigid registration and 3D alignment between T1WI and GED4 volumes using the FSL-Flirt toolkit [11]. Subsequently, all volumes are resampled to a unified spatial resolution of $1.0 \times 1.0 \times 2.5$ mm^3 to ensure spatial consistency and facilitate voxel-wise correspondence learning.

A 3D U-Net [6] is applied to learn the forward mapping function $G : X_{\mathrm{T1}} \rightarrow \hat{X}_{\mathrm{GED4}}$. The objective is to reconstruct a synthetic contrast-enhanced image $\hat{X}_{\mathrm{GED4}}$ that closely approximates the corresponding real X_{GED4}.

The training loss for this module combines two components:

$$\mathcal{L}_{\text{con-enh}} = \mathcal{L}_{\mathrm{MSE}} + \lambda_{\mathrm{SSIM}} \cdot \Big(1 - \mathrm{SSIM}(\hat{X}_{\mathrm{GED4}}, X_{\mathrm{GED4}})\Big) \tag{4}$$

where $\mathcal{L}_{\mathrm{MSE}}$ is the mean squared error between the synthetic and real GED4 images, and SSIM [22] is the structural similarity index that encourages perceptual and textural consistency. This combination ensures that the reconstructed images are not only pixel-wise accurate but also preserve high-frequency anatomical structures relevant to contrast uptake.

2.4 Pseudo-Labels Learning

In addition to the semi-supervised learning approach, we further enhance the model's ability to generalize by leveraging pseudo-labels. Pseudo-labeling is an effective strategy to exploit unlabeled data by using the model's own predictions as labels. In our framework, after training the mean teacher model on the training set, we apply the trained student model to segment the new unlabeled dataset, generating pseudo-labels for each new sample.

These pseudo-labels are generated under the assumption that the model has already learned meaningful features from the training set data and are then used to augment the original training set. We combine the training set $\mathcal{D}^s$ with the pseudo-labeled new set $\mathcal{D}^{new}_{\mathrm{pseudo}}$ to fine-tune the model. The fine-tuning process incorporates both the true labels and pseudo-labels, refining the model's parameters to improve its generalization to unseen data. This final fine-tuning step strengthens the model's robustness by exposing it to a larger variety of data, enhancing segmentation accuracy and generalization.

Formally, the new fine-tuning objective becomes:

$$\mathcal{L}_{\mathrm{finetune}} = \mathcal{L}_{\mathrm{sup}}(\mathcal{D}^s_l \cup \mathcal{D}^{new}_{\mathrm{pseudo}}) + \lambda_{\mathrm{mse}} \cdot \mathcal{L}_{\mathrm{mse}}(\mathcal{D}^s_u) \tag{5}$$

2.5 Test-Time Adaptation Module and Post-processing

Even with domain adaptation during training, unseen test domains may still introduce significant distribution shifts due to scanner-dependent noise patterns or different acquisition protocols. To further enhance robustness at inference time, we integrate a test-time adaptation (TTA) module with CoTTA [21] into our framework. Unlike static domain transfer methods, CoTTA adapts the model online by updating its parameters as new test samples are encountered, without requiring access to the source training data.

Specifically, given a pretrained student model h_θ, CoTTA maintains an exponential moving average (EMA) teacher model h_ϕ to provide stable pseudo-labels.

For each incoming test volume x_t, the model prediction $\hat{y}_t = h_\theta(x_t)$ is refined by consistency regularization with the teacher output $h_\phi(x_t)$. At the same time, stochastic restoration is applied to a subset of network parameters, preventing error accumulation and catastrophic forgetting during continual adaptation.

The overall objective at test time can be expressed as:

$$\mathcal{L}_{\text{TTA}} = \|h_\theta(x_t) - h_\phi(x_t)\|^2, \tag{6}$$

Allowing θ to adapt progressively to the target distribution.

However, the predicted mask may still surrounding with noise points or areas. To further address this issue, we apply 3D morphological post-processing to further trim the segmentation mask.

3 Experiment

3.1 Dataset and Metrics

The dataset utilizes the CARE-Liver track of CARE 2025, collected from multiple clinical centers using different MRI scanners [7,13,23]. It includes a training set with 330 unlabeled and 30 labeled cases, a validation set with 60 unlabeled cases, and an unseen test set with 60 labeled cases. Each case includes 7 imaging modalities, while in our framework, we only require T1WI and GED4 modalities among them.

During the training phase, the whole training set is used during the pre-train stage for semi-supervised learning, and whole the validation set is used during the finetune stage for pseudo-labels learning. For each experiment, we use five fold cross validation to split these 30 labeled cases for evaluating experiment.

To quantitatively evaluate the performance of liver segmentation, we adopt two widely used metrics in medical image analysis: Dice score (DICE) and standard Hausdorff Distance (HD). The HD is computed in the physical space with millimeters (mm) as the unit. We report the average performance of five fold cross validation on each method.

3.2 Setup

All experiments were run on a single RTX 3090 GPU. We use the same epochs of 150 and learning rate of 0.01 with the same scheduler policy for each training. During the ablation experiments, for mean teacher frame, λ_{mse} is dynamically increased from 0.0 to 1.0 with a ramp-up step of 40 epochs. During the training of contrast-aware module, we set λ_{SSIM} as 0.8.

For the training stage, we first use aligned T1WIGED4 pairs to train the contrast-aware module. Once trained, this module is applied to the input GED4 data to generate enhanced GED4 volumes. The original and enhanced GED4 images are subsequently concatenated as a two-channel input to the nnU-Netv2 model. Before feeding into the network, random histogram matching and standard data augmentation strategies are applied. The segmentation model is trained under the mean teacher framework with pseudo-labels learning to leverage both labeled and unlabeled data.

For the inference stage, the trained student model produces segmentation predictions, which are further refined by the post-processing module to remove small false positives and fragmented regions. In addition, when test samples originate from previously unseen domains, the CoTTA module is activated to dynamically adapt the model to the target distribution during deployment.

3.3 Segmentation Results Analysis

Table 1. Comparison between different baselines

Metrics	U-Net [6]	VNet [15]	nnU-Netv2 [9]	Swin UNETR [8]
DICE	95.01	94.83	**95.78**	93.63
HD	75.06	66.69	69.35	**42.64**

Baseline Comparison We first use labeled training set to evaluate the segmentation performance of different classic baseline models and select the best baseline model without TTA and post-processing strategies. As shown in Table 1, the nnU-Netv2 [9] model achieved the highest DICE score of 95.78, surpassing

Table 2. Ablation analysis of methods over cycle-GAN, random histogram matching, mean teacher framework, pseudo-labels learning, contrast-aware module, continual test-time adaptation and post-processing. The baseline model is nnU-Netv2. Mean DICE and HD are used to evaluate each method. Five fold cross validation is used to get the mean DICE and HD. A∼G are local experiments result, while the last two rows are the challenge test phase results with an unseen domain dataset. ID* refers to the source domain test dataset, and OOD* refers to an unseen domain test dataset

Exp	GAN	HIST	Mean-T	pseu-learn	Con-Aware	CoTTA	Post-P	DICE ↑	HD ↓
A								95.78	69.35
B	✓							95.94	55.67
C		✓						96.30	70.45
D		✓	✓					96.46	60.88
E		✓	✓	✓				96.52	64.29
F		✓	✓	✓	✓			96.67	55.24
G		✓	✓	✓	✓	✓		96.85	64.64
H		✓	✓	✓	✓	✓	✓	**96.88**	**49.22**
ID*								97.03	21.4
OOD*								97.65	15.17

other baselines such as U-Net [6], VNet [15], and Swin UNETR [8]. Note that the maximum HD is highly sensitive to single outliers and does not fully capture overall boundary quality. Thus, although nnU-Netv2 had a higher HD score (69.35), the primary focus of our study was on improving DICE, where nnU-Netv2 demonstrated the most promising results.

Ablation Analysis In the ablation study, various methods were incorporated into the nnU-Netv2 to assess their impact on model performance. The techniques evaluated include cycle-GAN, random histogram matching, mean teacher pseudo-labels learning, and the contrast-aware module. Table 2 summarizes the results of the ablation study. Each method was tested in combination, and the mean DICE and HD scores were used to quantify the performance.

From the results, we observe that the inclusion of both GAN and random histogram matching lead to an improvement compared to the baseline model. While in comparison, random histogram matching shows a better performance in DICE. Their different effects could have been foreseen in Fig. 2, where cycle-GAN has a poor generalization ability and image quality.

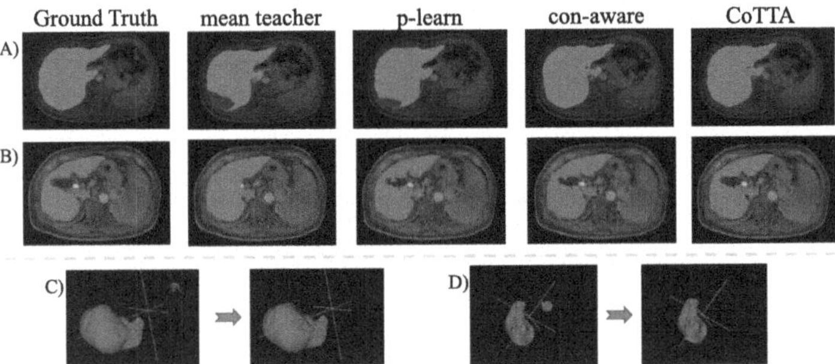

Fig. 3. Visualization of typical segmentation results comparing different methods on the CARE-Liver track dataset of CARE 2025. In A) and B), from the *2nd* to the *5th*, we add mean teacher, pseudo-labels learning, contrast-aware module and CoTTA in sequence. C) and D) show the optimization of segmentation results by post-processing module

During the training phase, we add the methods of mean teacher framework, pseudo-labels learning and contrast-aware module. The integration of mean teacher, pseudo-labels learning, and contrast-aware module resulted in a much better performance, which helps the model learn detailed knowledge about the liver region. CoTTA further improve the segmentation precision, and the model achieves the best performance with post-processing at DICE of 96.88 and HD of 49.22 in local experiments. Finally, the model achieves excellent results (ID*: 97.03 DICE, 21.4 HD; OOD*: 97.65 DICE, 15.17 HD) on the CARE 2025 challenge test phase. The visualization of some typical segmentation results by applying different methods is shown in Fig. 3.

4 Conclusion

We proposed CoSSeg-TTA, a semi-supervised framework for liver segmentation from contrast-enhanced MRI, addressing annotation scarcity and domain shifts. Built on nnU-Netv2 under the mean teacher framework with pseudo-labels learning, it leverages unlabeled data, while a domain adaptation module with histogram-based style transfer and a contrast-aware network enhances segmentation robustness. CoTTA and post-processing further improve performance, achieving excellent results on the CARE 2025 challenge test phase. CoSSeg-TTA offers a robust solution for clinical liver segmentation tasks.

However, the contrast-aware module of our framework relies on paired T1WI and GED4 modalities, which may not always be available. Extreme domain shifts and noisy pseudo-labels can affect performance, and computational demands may limit real-time use. Future work includes extending to other modalities, improving the contrast-aware module with generative models, incorporating uncertainty estimation, and validating on larger datasets. Federated learning could address multi-center privacy concerns, enhancing clinical applicability.

Acknowledgments. This work is supported in part by National Natural Science Foundation of China (Grant No. 62276121), the TianYuan funds for Mathematics of the National Science Foundation of China (Grant No. 12326604).

References

1. Chen, J., Chen, C., Huang, W., Zhang, J., Debattista, K., Han, J.: Dynamic contrastive learning guided by class confidence and confusion degree for medical image segmentation. Pattern Recogn. **145**, 109881 (2024)
2. Chen, J., Duan, H., Zhang, X., Gao, B., Tan, T., Grau, V., Han, J.: From gaze to insight: Bridging human visual attention and vision language model explanation for weakly-supervised medical image segmentation. arXiv preprint arXiv:2504.11368 (2025)
3. Chen, J., Huang, W., Zhang, J., Debattista, K., Han, J.: Addressing inconsistent labeling with cross image matching for scribble-based medical image segmentation. IEEE Trans, Image Process (2025)
4. Chen, J., Li, W., Li, H., Zhang, J.: Deep class-specific affinity-guided convolutional network for multimodal unpaired image segmentation. In: International Conference on Medical Image Computing and Computer-Assisted Intervention. pp. 187–196. Springer (2020)
5. Chen, J., Zhang, J., Debattista, K., Han, J.: Semi-supervised unpaired medical image segmentation through task-affinity consistency. IEEE Trans. Med. Imaging **42**(3), 594–605 (2023)
6. Çiçek, Ö., Abdulkadir, A., Lienkamp, S.S., Brox, T., Ronneberger, O.: 3d u-net: learning dense volumetric segmentation from sparse annotation. In: International conference on medical image computing and computer-assisted intervention. pp. 424–432. Springer (2016)

7. Gao, Z., Liu, Y., Wu, F., Shi, N., Shi, Y., Zhuang, X.: A reliable and interpretable framework of multi-view learning for liver fibrosis staging. In: International Conference on Medical Image Computing and Computer-Assisted Intervention. pp. 178–188 (2023)
8. Hatamizadeh, A., Nath, V., Tang, Y., Yang, D., Roth, H.R., Xu, D.: Swin unetr: Swin transformers for semantic segmentation of brain tumors in mri images. In: International MICCAI brainlesion workshop. pp. 272–284. Springer (2021)
9. Isensee, F., Jaeger, P.F., Kohl, S.A., Petersen, J., Maier-Hein, K.H.: nnu-net: a self-configuring method for deep learning-based biomedical image segmentation. Nat. Methods **18**(2), 203–211 (2021)
10. Isola, P., Zhu, J.Y., Zhou, T., Efros, A.A.: Image-to-image translation with conditional adversarial networks. In: Proceedings of the IEEE conference on computer vision and pattern recognition. pp. 1125–1134 (2017)
11. Jenkinson, M., Bannister, P., Brady, M., Smith, S.: Improved optimization for the robust and accurate linear registration and motion correction of brain images. Neuroimage **17**(2), 825–841 (2002)
12. Li, C., Lin, X., Mao, Y., Lin, W., Qi, Q., Ding, X., Huang, Y., Liang, D., Yu, Y.: Domain generalization on medical imaging classification using episodic training with task augmentation. Comput. Biol. Med. **141**, 105144 (2022)
13. Liu, Y., Gao, Z., Shi, N., Wu, F., Shi, Y., Chen, Q., Zhuang, X.: Merit: Multi-view evidential learning for reliable and interpretable liver fibrosis staging. Med. Image Anal. **102**, 103507 (2025)
14. Marinov, Z., Jäger, P.F., Egger, J., Kleesiek, J., Stiefelhagen, R.: Deep interactive segmentation of medical images: A systematic review and taxonomy. IEEE transactions on pattern analysis and machine intelligence (2024)
15. Milletari, F., Navab, N., Ahmadi, S.A.: V-net: Fully convolutional neural networks for volumetric medical image segmentation. In: 2016 fourth international conference on 3D vision (3DV). pp. 565–571. Ieee (2016)
16. Nichyporuk, B., Cardinell, J., Szeto, J., Mehta, R., Falet, J.P.R., Arnold, D.L., Tsaftaris, S.A., Arbel, T.: Rethinking generalization: The impact of annotation style on medical image segmentation. arXiv preprint arXiv:2210.17398 (2022)
17. Rajchl, M., Koch, L.M., Ledig, C., Passerat-Palmbach, J., Misawa, K., Mori, K., Rueckert, D.: Employing weak annotations for medical image analysis problems. arXiv preprint arXiv:1708.06297 (2017)
18. Sendra-Balcells, C., Campello, V.M., Martín-Isla, C., Viladés, D., Descalzo, M.L., Guala, A., Rodriguez-Palomares, J.F., Lekadir, K.: Domain generalization in deep learning for contrast-enhanced imaging. Comput. Biol. Med. **149**, 106052 (2022)
19. Tarvainen, A., Valpola, H.: Mean teachers are better role models: Weight-averaged consistency targets improve semi-supervised deep learning results. Adv. Neural Inf. Process. Syst. **30** (2017)
20. Vorontsov, E., Molchanov, P., Gazda, M., Beckham, C., Kautz, J., Kadoury, S.: Towards annotation-efficient segmentation via image-to-image translation. Med. Image Anal. **82**, 102624 (2022)
21. Wang, Q., Fink, O., Van Gool, L., Dai, D.: Continual test-time domain adaptation. In: Proceedings of the IEEE/CVF Conference on Computer Vision and Pattern Recognition. pp. 7201–7211 (2022)
22. Wang, Z., Bovik, A.C., Sheikh, H.R., Simoncelli, E.P.: Image quality assessment: from error visibility to structural similarity. IEEE Trans. Image Process. **13**(4), 600–612 (2004)

23. Wu, F., Zhuang, X.: Minimizing estimated risks on unlabeled data: A new formulation for semi-supervised medical image segmentation. IEEE Trans. Pattern Anal. Mach. Intell. **45**(5), 6021–6036 (2023)
24. Zhang, H., Li, H., Dillman, J.R., Parikh, N.A., He, L.: Multi-contrast mri image synthesis using switchable cycle-consistent generative adversarial networks. Diagnostics **12**(4), 816 (2022)
25. Zhang, X., Wu, S., Zhang, P., Jin, Z., Xiong, X., Bu, Q., Chen, J., Feng, J.: Helpnet: Hierarchical perturbations consistency and entropy-guided ensemble for scribble supervised medical image segmentation. Medical Image Analysis p. 103719 (2025)
26. Zhu, J.Y., Park, T., Isola, P., Efros, A.A.: Unpaired image-to-image translation using cycle-consistent adversarial networks. In: Proceedings of the IEEE international conference on computer vision. pp. 2223–2232 (2017)

CardioSeqM: A Scalable and Context-Aware Model for Unified Heart Segmentation from Volumetric Cardiac Data

Abdul Qayyum[1(✉)], Moona Mazher[2], and Steven A Niederer[1]

[1] Faculty of Medicine, National Heart and Lung Institute, Imperial College London, London, UK
a.qayyum@imperial.ac.uk

[2] Department of Computer Science, UCL Hawkes Institute, University College London, London, UK

Abstract. Cardiovascular diseases (CVDs) are the leading cause of death worldwide, highlighting the need for accurate diagnostic and therapeutic strategies. Unified cardiac segmentation from medical images, including single structures, whole heart anatomy, and myocardial pathology, is critical for understanding cardiac morphology, assessing disease progression, and guiding treatment planning. This task is challenging due to dynamic cardiac motion, motion artifacts, low contrast-to-noise ratio, and variability across multi-center datasets, with CT and MRI each presenting unique difficulties. To address these challenges, we propose a two-stage unified segmentation framework using 3D CardioNet. In the first stage, a Masked Autoencoder (MAE)-based self-supervised learning approach pretrains 3D CardioNet on all available unlabeled cardiac data, enabling robust volumetric feature representation without extensive manual annotation. In the second stage, the CardioNet encoder and decoder are combined with the CardioSeq module, which models 3D cardiac volumes as sequences to capture long-range spatial dependencies, improving segmentation of both local structures and global anatomy. The pretrained encoder is frozen while the decoder is fine-tuned for unified segmentation. Evaluated across left atrial segmentation from LGE MRI, whole heart segmentation from CT and MRI, and myocardial pathology segmentation, our approach demonstrates superior performance, highlighting the effectiveness of MAE pretraining and CardioSeq within 3D CardioNet for robust, generalizable automated cardiac segmentation.

Keywords: 3D MAE SSL · CardioSeq · Self-supervised · CardioNet · Whole heart segmentation · Pathology segmentation · Left atrial segmentation

X. Zhuang et al. (Eds.): CARE 2025, LNCS 16257, pp. 68–78, 2026.
https://doi.org/10.1007/978-3-032-16271-7_7

1 Introduction

Cardiovascular diseases (CVDs) remain the leading cause of mortality worldwide, accounting for millions of deaths each year [19]. This underscores the urgent need for precise diagnostic and therapeutic strategies, where accurate quantification of cardiac structures and pathological regions is critical [18]. Segmentation of these regions from medical images enables detailed morphological analysis, assessment of disease progression, and informed clinical decision-making. Traditional approaches often rely on separate models for individual structures or pathologies, such as left atrial delineation, myocardial scar detection, or whole heart segmentation. However, such task-specific models lead to fragmented workflows, limited knowledge transfer, and reduced robustness to heterogeneous or incomplete data.

Medical image segmentation has significantly benefited from advances in deep learning, particularly convolutional neural networks (CNNs) and their variants [4,6,9,14–16]. Deep learning-based approaches can automatically learn hierarchical feature representations from large-scale datasets, capturing complex anatomical structures and subtle pathological variations that traditional hand-crafted methods struggle to modulate. Models such as U-Net and its 3D extensions have become standard for volumetric segmentation, enabling accurate delineation of organs and tissues across multiple modalities, including MRI, CT, and ultrasound. These methods have demonstrated state-of-the-art performance in diverse tasks in segmentation [8,11–13], highlighting the potential of data-driven approaches for robust and reproducible medical image analysis.

Developing a unified cardiac segmentation framework addresses the limitations of task-specific approaches by jointly handling multiple tasks, including segmentation of single structures (e.g., left atrium), whole heart anatomy, and myocardial pathologies (left ventricle, myocardium, and scar) across diverse imaging modalities such as LGE MRI, CT, and MRI. Accurate delineation of these structures is inherently challenging due to several factors: the heart exhibits dynamic motion throughout the cardiac cycle, imaging artifacts such as motion blur and low contrast-to-noise ratio complicate visual interpretation, and the significant variability in multi-center, multi-modality data creates domain shifts that hinder generalization. Furthermore, pathological regions such as myocardial scars are often small, irregularly shaped, and visually subtle, making their segmentation particularly difficult even for advanced algorithms.

To overcome these challenges, we leverage self-supervised learning (SSL) with a Masked Autoencoder (MAE) [7] to pretrain a robust encoder on all available unlabeled cardiac data. This enables the model to learn rich volumetric representations that capture both local anatomical details and global contextual dependencies, reducing dependence on extensive manual annotation. In addition, we propose the CardioSeq module, which models 3D cardiac volumes as sequences to capture long-range spatial dependencies and integrates these with convolutional features. This approach improves segmentation performance across all structures and pathologies by effectively encoding both fine-grained details and global spatial context.

In this work, we present a unified cardiac segmentation model, trained and tested on a large, multi-center, multi-modality dataset, capable of simultaneously segmenting single structures, whole heart anatomy, and myocardial pathology. Our approach demonstrates strong generalization across in-distribution and out-of-distribution data, establishing a robust framework for comprehensive automated cardiac analysis and addressing the challenges of limited annotations, anatomical variability, and pathological heterogeneity.

2 Proposed Method

2.1 Dataset

The challenge dataset is a large-scale, multicenter, and multimodal data set designed for unified cardiac segmentation across three tasks: (1) left atrial segmentation from LGE MRI, (2) whole heart segmentation from both CT and MRI, and (3) myocardial pathology segmentation (left ventricle, myocardium, and scar) from LGE MRI. Training data are sourced from multiple institutions, comprising over 400 cases with diverse imaging protocols, while separate validation and test sets cover both in-distribution (seen centers) and out-of-distribution (unseen centers) scenarios. This heterogeneous dataset provides a robust foundation for developing generalizable models that can adapt to anatomical variability, imaging modality differences, and clinical heterogeneity [1,17]. We leveraged all available unlabeled cardiac imaging data for self-supervised pretraining.

2.2 Proposed CardioNet for Unified Heart Segmentation

Accurate segmentation of cardiac structures is vital for quantitative analysis in clinical practice and research. The proposed model is shown in Fig. 1. Existing convolutional neural network architectures, such as UNet, have achieved strong performance in medical image segmentation tasks by capturing local features through hierarchical encoderdecoder structures. we present CardioNet, an encoderdecoder architecture for unified heart segmentation. Our approach leverages a 3D Masked Autoencoder (3D-MAE) for unsupervised pretraining, enabling the model to learn rich volumetric representations from unlabeled data. These pretrained weights initialize the encoder of CardioNet, providing a strong feature extraction backbone. The decoder is then fine-tuned in a supervised manner on labeled datasets to generate accurate segmentation maps. Additionally, we integrate a CardioSeq block at the bottleneck of the network to capture global spatial dependencies through bidirectional quasiseparable mixing. This combination of 3D-MAE pretraining, convolutional local feature extraction, and global sequence-based mixing results in a robust and generalizable cardiac segmentation model.

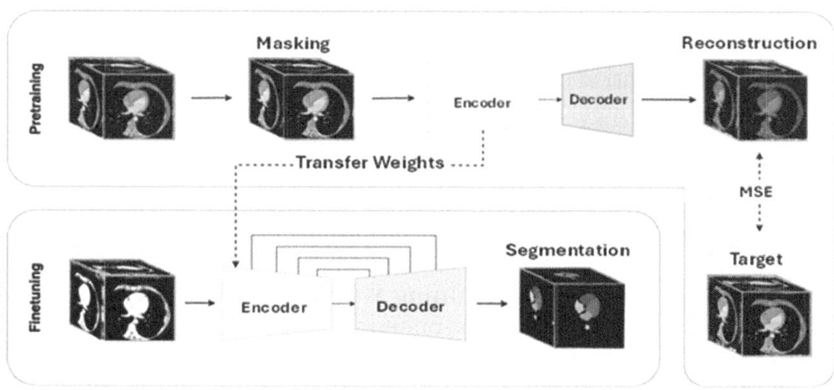

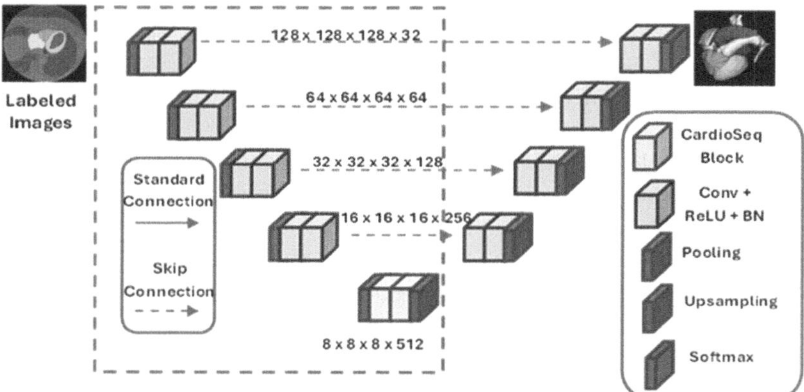

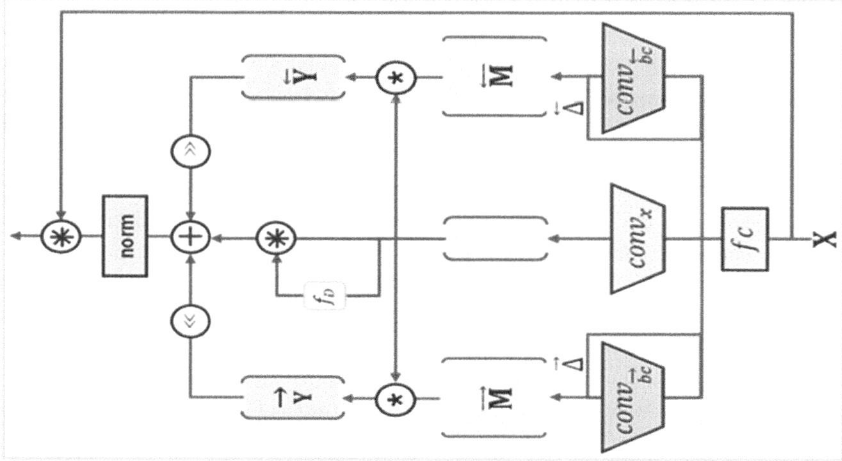

Fig. 1. The proposed CardioNet for unified cardiac segmentation

EncoderDecoder Framework CardioNet follows a classical encoderdecoder design:

- **Encoder:** Convolutional layers extract rich local features while progressively downsampling the input volume to capture hierarchical context. The encoder is initialized with weights from the 3D-MAE pretraining.
- **Decoder:** Symmetric upsampling layers reconstruct spatial resolution and integrate skip connections from the encoder, preserving fine anatomical details for precise segmentation.

3D Masked Autoencoder Pretraining We adopt a 3D Masked Autoencoder (3D-MAE) as the self-supervised pretraining strategy. During pretraining, random patches of the input 3D medical volumes are masked, and the model learns to reconstruct the missing patches. This forces the encoder to develop robust volumetric feature representations, capturing both local structure and global spatial context. The pretrained encoder is then transferred to CardioNet and fine-tuned with labeled data for segmentation. This approach allows the model to effectively leverage large-scale unlabeled cardiac imaging datasets, significantly reducing the dependency on annotated data while improving generalization.

CardioSeq Block for Global Context In our proposed CardioNet, an encoder–decoder architecture for unified heart segmentation, the encoder employs convolutional layers to extract rich local spatial features while progressively reducing spatial resolution. The decoder uses upsampling layers to restore spatial details and generate the final segmentation output. At the network's bottleneck, we integrate the CardioSeq layer, which implements bidirectional quasiseparable mixing. This layer flattens the 3D spatial feature map into a one-dimensional sequence, enabling the modeling of long-range dependencies across the entire spatial context. By treating spatial locations as sequential positions, CardioSeq efficiently captures global contextual information in both forward (causal) and backward (anti-causal) directions using semiseparable state-space models (SSMs). This combination of local convolutional feature extraction and global sequence-based context modeling enhances the representational capacity at the bottleneck, improving segmentation accuracy through richer spatial feature integration.

The CardioSeg block takes an input sequence X (features or embeddings) and processes it in two parallel streams: a fully connected (fc) channel-mixing layer for feature-wise interactions, and a block/bottleneck convolution (`conv_bc`) along the sequence to capture local temporal context. These streams run in both forward and backward directions, controlled by directional masks ($\rightarrow M, \leftarrow M$) that enforce causal flow. An additional convolution (`conv_x`) provides further local mixing. The forward and backward outputs are then fused using a feature-wise gate f_D, with elementwise addition ($\oplus$), concatenation ($\ll, \gg$), and multiplicative gating ($*$) used to combine pathways. Overall, it produces a bidirectional representation that mixes local context and channel features for segmentation.

Bidirectional quasiseparable mixing is specifically designed for sequences derived from volumetric data. Given an input volume of shape (B, C, H, W, D), the spatial dimensions (H, W, D) are flattened into a sequence length $S = H \times W \times D$. This transformation allows the model to process the volume as a sequence of spatial positions, facilitating the application of sequential mixing operations that aggregate information across the entire spatial domain. The quasiseparable structure implies a low-rank representation that enables efficient computation without explicitly forming a large dense matrix [3]. Together, this bidirectional quasiseparable mixing yields a powerful context-aware feature representation that integrates global spatial relationships effectively.

The equation describes below how the output at each sequence position i is computed by combining three components: contributions from all past positions $j < i$, contributions from all future positions $j > i$, and direct self-connection at position i. The matrix M organizing these parameters is structured so that its diagonal elements δ_i represent self-connections preserving local features. The lower triangle contains parameters $A_i b_j$ that govern how information flows causally from past positions to the current one, while the upper triangle contains parameters $A_i' b_j'$ for anti-causal mixing, aggregating information from future positions. This quasiseparable structure enables efficient modeling of bidirectional dependencies without explicitly storing a full dense matrix.

For each batch b, position i:

$$Y_{(b,i)} = \sum_{j<i} A_i b_j X_{(b,j)} + \sum_{j>i} A_i' b_j' X_{(b,j)} + \delta_i X_{(b,i)} \quad (1)$$

where A_i, b_j: causal parameters, A_i', b_j': anti-causal parameters, and δ_i: diagonal/self-connection.

The matrix M shown for sequence length 16 illustrates how the bidirectional mixing operates. Its diagonal elements δ_i represent self-connection weights that preserve local information at each position i. The lower triangular part (below the diagonal) contains parameters $A_i b_j$ that mix information causally from past positions $j < i$ to the current position i. Conversely, the upper triangular part (above the diagonal) holds parameters $A_i' b_j'$ responsible for mixing information anti-causally from future positions $j > i$ back to position i. This structured matrix efficiently captures dependencies in both directions while maintaining a sparse, low-rank form for fast computation.

$$M = \begin{bmatrix} \delta_1 & A_1' b_2' & A_1' b_3' & \cdots & A_1' b_{16}' \\ A_2 b_1 & \delta_2 & A_2' b_3' & \cdots & A_2' b_{16}' \\ A_3 b_1 & A_3 b_2 & \delta_3 & \cdots & A_3' b_{16}' \\ \vdots & \vdots & \vdots & \ddots & \vdots \\ A_{16} b_1 & A_{16} b_2 & A_{16} b_3 & \cdots & \delta_{16} \end{bmatrix} \quad (2)$$

Where:

- **Diagonal:** δ_i for $i = 1, \ldots, 16$
- **Lower triangle:** $A_i b_j$ for $i > j$

- **Upper triangle:** $A_i' b_j'$ for $i < j$
- **Lower triangle (below diagonal):** Each entry M_{ij} for $i > j$ mixes information from past positions using parameters A_i and b_j (causal direction)
- **Upper triangle (above diagonal):** Each entry M_{ij} for $i < j$ mixes information from future positions using parameters A_i' and b_j' (anti-causal direction)
- **Diagonal:** Each M_{ii} is a self-connection parameter δ_i

3 Results

Our proposed CardioNet model achieved strong performance across all three cardiac segmentation tasks: single cardiac structure (left atrium), whole heart structures, and myocardial pathology (left ventricle, myocardium, and scar demonstrating the effectiveness of the unified framework and SSL pretraining. Tables 1 and 2 summarize the validation and test performance of our proposed CardioNet(SSL) model on the CARE Cardiac dataset.

The validation and test leaderboard results demonstrate the effectiveness of our Car-dioNet (SSL) model on the CARE-Cardiac dataset. On the validation set, CardioNet (SSL) outperforms both the standard CardioNet and 3D ResUNet [10], achieving the highest Dice scores across structure and pathology (0.7329), whole heart structures (0.8634), and single cardiac structures (0.8671), with lower or comparable Hausdorff distances, indicating improved segmentation accuracy and boundary delineation. Transformer-CNN [2] and nnUNet [5] achieve slightly lower Dice scores and higher Hausdorff distances, highlighting the advantage of our CardioNet with SSL pretraining.

On the test set, the model shows strong performance for whole heart structures (average DICE 0.8721, HD 29.80) across in-distribution and out-of-distribution data, while single cardiac structures perform well on in-distribution data (DICE 0.923) but decrease on out-of-distribution data (DICE 0.4442), highlighting domain sensitivity. Structure and pathology segmentation achieves moderate overall performance (average DICE 0.6545, HD 40.36), reflecting the challenge of pathological region segmentation. Overall, these results confirm that CardioNet (SSL) provides robust and generalizable automated cardiac segmentation across multi-center, multi-modality datasets.

The self-supervised Masked Autoencoder (MAE) pretraining on all available unlabeled cardiac images allowed the encoder to learn rich volumetric representations capturing both local and global dependencies. This strong initialization reduced reliance on labeled data and enhanced model generalization across diverse modalities, improving segmentation accuracy for complex structures such as atria, ventricles, and myocardial scars. A central contribution of our approach is the CardioSeq module, integrated at the bottleneck of the encoder-decoder architecture. By flattening the 3D spatial volume into sequences, the bidirectional quasiseparable mixing of CardioSeq captures long-range dependencies both forward and backward across the spatial domain. This allows the model to combine local convolutional features with global contextual information efficiently. In practice, this is particularly beneficial for whole heart segmentation,

Table 1. Validation Leaderboard Score for CARE-Cardiac: Quantitative comparison of segmentation algorithms on structure and pathology, whole heart structures, and single cardiac structure.

	Structure and pathology		Whole heart		Single structure	
Algorithm	**DICE**	**HD**	**DICE**	**HD**	**DICE**	**HD**
CardioNet (SSL)	**0.732**	**11.24**	**0.863**	**27.72**	**0.867**	**28.59**
CardioNet (without SSL)	0.728	11.89	0.860	27.81	0.856	25.91
Base_3DResUNet	0.709	12.05	0.854	35.98	0.855	26.21
Transformer-CNN	0.693	13.07	0.823	38.20	0.829	30.18
nnUNet	0.717	11.98	0.859	29.09	0.859	27.76

Table 2. Test Leaderboard Score for CARE-Cardiac test task.

	ID		OOD		AVG	
	DSC	HD	DSC	HD	DSC	HD
Single Cardiac Structure	0.923	73.773	0.444	69.728	0.596	71.015
Whole Heart Structures	0.850	38.270	0.903	17.091	0.872	29.798
Structure and Pathology	0.539	83.773	0.723	14.319	0.654	40.364
Average	**0.771**	**65.272**	**0.690**	**33.7132**	**0.707**	**47.059**

where capturing relationships among multiple chambers and vessels is critical. The module enhances feature representation, improves boundary delineation, and contributes significantly to the high Dice scores and reduced Hausdorff distances observed in both validation and test sets. Overall, the combination of unified dataset training, MAE-based SSL pretraining, and the CardioSeq module enabled our model to achieve robust and accurate segmentation across all tasks, demonstrating its practical applicability for comprehensive cardiac image analysis.

Figure 2 presents a qualitative comparison of segmentation performance across three tasks: Structure and Pathology, Whole Heart Structures, and Single Cardiac Structures. The second column shows results from the proposed CardioNet with self-supervised learning (SSL), the third column shows its baseline variant without SSL, and the fourth column displays results from the 3D ResNet model.

In all tasks, the proposed CardioNet with SSL demonstrates the most accurate and visually coherent segmentations, closely aligning with the ground truth (GT) annotations shown in the first column. Notably, fine anatomical details, such as thin myocardial walls and subtle pathological regions, are better preserved and delineated in the SSL-enhanced model compared to the baselines. While all models are capable of identifying the major cardiac structures, the baseline CardioNet (without SSL) occasionally produces minor boundary deviations, and the 3D ResNet exhibits slight over- or under-segmentation in more complex regions. These visual differences highlight the benefit of incorporating SSL, which appears to enhance feature representation and structural consistency, allowing the model to capture intricate spatial relationships. Overall, the proposed approach not only maintains global shape fidelity but also preserves local structural details, resulting in superior qualitative segmentation performance.

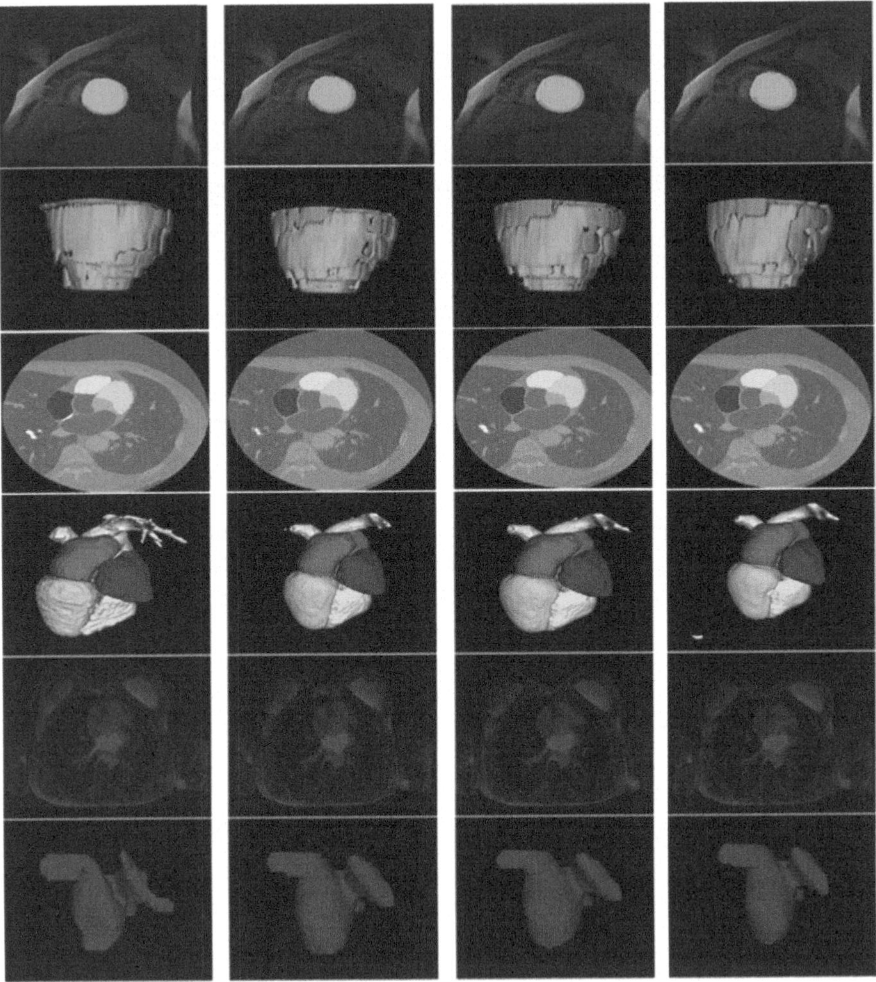

Fig. 2. Segmentation maps generated by our proposed method and baseline methods.

4 Conclusion

We propose a two-stage unified cardiac segmentation framework that combines self-supervised pretraining with advanced 3D modeling for robust automated analysis. In the first stage, a Masked Autoencoder (MAE) is employed to pretrain 3D CardioNet on all available unlabeled cardiac data, enabling rich volumetric feature learning without relying on extensive manual annotations. In the second stage, the pretrained encoder, integrated with the CardioSeq module, is fine-tuned for unified segmentation. This design captures long-range spatial dependencies, enhancing performance across both local structures and global anatomical context. We evaluated our approach on multi-center, multi-modality datasets, including left atrial segmentation from LGE MRI, whole heart segmentation from CT and MRI, and myocardial pathology segmentation. The results demonstrate superior performance, highlighting the effectiveness of MAE pretraining and the CardioSeq module in achieving robust, generalizable cardiac segmentation.

Future work will focus on multimodal fusion strategies and task-adaptive modeling to further improve segmentation accuracy across diverse imaging conditions and complex anatomical variations, ultimately advancing precision cardiac care and personalized treatment planning.

.

Disclosure of Interests. All authors declare no competing financial or non-financial interests.

Acknowledgments. The authors would like to thank the organizers of the CARE-2025 MICCAI Challenge for providing the dataset, evaluation framework, and support that made this work possible.

References

1. Gao, S., Zhou, H., Gao, Y., Zhuang, X.: Bayeseg: Bayesian modeling for medical image segmentation with interpretable generalizability. Med. Image Anal. **89**, 102889 (2023)
2. Hatamizadeh, A., Nath, V., Tang, Y., Yang, D., Roth, H.R., Xu, D.: Swin unetr: Swin transformers for semantic segmentation of brain tumors in mri images. In: International MICCAI brainlesion workshop. pp. 272–284. Springer (2021)
3. Hwang, S., Lahoti, A., Puduppully, R., Dao, T., Gu, A.: Hydra: Bidirectional state space models through generalized matrix mixers. Adv. Neural. Inf. Process. Syst. **37**, 110876–110908 (2024)
4. Imran, M., Krebs, J.R., Sivaraman, V.B., Zhang, T., Kumar, A., Ueland, W.R., Fassler, M.J., Huang, J., Sun, X., Wang, L., et al.: Multi-class segmentation of aortic branches and zones in computed tomography angiography: The aortaseg24 challenge. arXiv preprint arXiv:2502.05330 (2025)
5. Isensee, F., Jaeger, P.F., Kohl, S.A., Petersen, J., Maier-Hein, K.H.: nnu-net: a self-configuring method for deep learning-based biomedical image segmentation. Nat. Methods **18**(2), 203–211 (2021)

6. Mazher, M., Razzak, I., Qayyum, A., Tanveer, M., Beier, S., Khan, T., Niederer, S.A.: Self-supervised spatial-temporal transformer fusion based federated framework for 4d cardiovascular image segmentation. Inf. Fusion **106**, 102256 (2024)
7. Munk, A., Ambsdorf, J., Llambias, S., Nielsen, M.: Amaes: Augmented masked autoencoder pretraining on public brain mri data for 3d-native segmentation. arXiv preprint arXiv:2408.00640 (2024)
8. Nan, Y., Xing, X., Wang, S., Tang, Z., Felder, F.N., Zhang, S., Ledda, R.E., Ding, X., Yu, R., Liu, W., et al.: Hunting imaging biomarkers in pulmonary fibrosis: benchmarks of the aiib23 challenge. Med. Image Anal. **97**, 103253 (2024)
9. Payette, K., Steger, C., Licandro, R., De Dumast, P., Li, H.B., Barkovich, M., Li, L., Dannecker, M., Chen, C., Ouyang, C., et al.: Multi-center fetal brain tissue annotation (feta) challenge 2022 results. IEEE transactions on medical imaging (2024)
10. Qayyum, A., Ang, C.K., Sridevi, S., Khan, M.A., Hong, L.W., Mazher, M., Chung, T.D.: Hybrid 3d-resnet deep learning model for automatic segmentation of thoracic organs at risk in ct images. In: 2020 International Conference on Industrial Engineering, Applications and Manufacturing (ICIEAM). pp. 1–5. IEEE (2020)
11. Qayyum, A., Razzak, I., Mazher, M., Lu, X., Niederer, S.A.: Unsupervised unpaired multiple fusion adaptation aided with self-attention generative adversarial network for scar tissues segmentation framework. Inf. Fusion **106**, 102226 (2024)
12. Qayyum, A., Xu, H., Halliday, B.P., Rodero, C., Lanyon, C.W., Wilkinson, R.D., Niederer, S.A.: Transforming heart chamber imaging: Self-supervised learning for whole heart reconstruction and segmentation. arXiv preprint arXiv:2406.06643 (2024)
13. de la Rosa, E., Reyes, M., Liew, S.L., Hutton, A., Wiest, R., Kaesmacher, J., Hanning, U., Hakim, A., Zubal, R., Valenzuela, W., et al.: A robust ensemble algorithm for ischemic stroke lesion segmentation: Generalizability and clinical utility beyond the isles challenge. arXiv preprint arXiv:2403.19425 (2024)
14. de la Rosa, E., Su, R., Reyes, M., Wiest, R., Riedel, E.O., Kofler, F., Yang, K., Baazaoui, H., Robben, D., Wegener, S., et al.: Isles'24: Improving final infarct prediction in ischemic stroke using multimodal imaging and clinical data. arXiv preprint arXiv:2408.10966 (2024)
15. Wang, K., Qin, C., Shi, Z., Wang, H., Zhang, X., Chen, C., Ouyang, C., Dai, C., Mo, Y., Dai, C., et al.: Extreme cardiac mri analysis under respiratory motion: Results of the cmrxmotion challenge. arXiv preprint arXiv:2507.19165 (2025)
16. Yang, K., Musio, F., Ma, Y., Juchler, N., Paetzold, J.C., Al-Maskari, R., Höher, L., Li, H.B., Hamamci, I.E., Sekuboyina, A., et al.: Benchmarking the cow with the topcow challenge: Topology-aware anatomical segmentation of the circle of willis for cta and mra. ArXiv pp. arXiv–2312 (2025)
17. Zhuang, X.: Multivariate mixture model for myocardial segmentation combining multi-source images. IEEE Trans. Pattern Anal. Mach. Intell. **41**(12), 2933–2946 (2018)
18. Zhuang, X., Li, L., Payer, C., Štern, D., Urschler, M., Heinrich, M.P., Oster, J., Wang, C., Smedby, Ö., Bian, C., et al.: Evaluation of algorithms for multi-modality whole heart segmentation: an open-access grand challenge. Med. Image Anal. **58**, 101537 (2019)
19. Zhuang, X., Shen, J.: Multi-scale patch and multi-modality atlases for whole heart segmentation of mri. Med. Image Anal. **31**, 77–87 (2016)

A Latent-Guided Hybrid Architecture for Liver Segmentation in Contrast-Enhanced MRI

Ting Yu Tsai, An Yu, Wenqi Li, and Ming-Ching Chang(✉)

University at Albany, State University of New York, Albany, NY 12222, USA
{ttsai2,ayu,wli31,mchang2}@albany.edu

Abstract. Liver segmentation in hepatobiliary-phase (GED4) MRI is crucial for fibrosis assessment but remains challenging due to the scarcity of annotated data. Recent advances in large language models (LLMs), such as LLaMA, have demonstrated remarkable generalization capabilities in learning transferable latent representations across domains. In this work, we introduce LLaMba-Seg, a framework that integrates frozen LLaMA into a selective state-space U-Mamba, forming a hybrid architecture for robust liver segmentation. Our model consists of a trainable U-Mamba encoder-decoder, with a frozen LLaMA module at the bottleneck, which distills high-level semantic context and guides representation alignment. U-Mamba captures spatial details at multiple resolutions for precise boundary delineation in low-contrast settings, while LLaMA's contextual embeddings enable the creation of high-confidence pseudo-labels from unannotated GED4 scans. Focusing on the contrast-enhanced subtask of segmenting the GED4 sequence, we train the model on a combined dataset that includes the challenge's GED4 data along with external AMOS and ATLAS data to enhance domain robustness. On the Liver Fibrosis Quantification and Analysis Task 2 (LiSeg) validation benchmark, our model achieves a Dice score of 0.97 and a Hausdorff Distance of 21.34 mm, demonstrating its effectiveness under limited supervision.

Keywords: Liver Segmentation · Hepatobiliary-Phase MRI · Contrast-Enhanced MRI · Latent Representation Transfer · State-Space Models · U-Mamba · Domain Robustness · Limited Supervision

1 Introduction

The accurate segmentation of the liver from hepatobiliary-phase magnetic resonance imaging (MRI) is a critical prerequisite for assessing liver function and diagnosing hepatic fibrosis [24]. This task is hindered by a confluence of challenges: low-contrast boundaries, high anatomical variability, scarcity of annotated data [2,13,23], and the inherent difficulty of learning discriminative latent representations from such limited and complex information [4,17].

X. Zhuang et al. (Eds.): CARE 2025, LNCS 16257, pp. 79–89, 2026.
https://doi.org/10.1007/978-3-032-16271-7_8

To address these challenges, previous research [20,31] has primarily focused on refining deep learning architectures and data augmentation strategies. Aggressive augmentation methods such as elastic deformations and contrast adjustments have been employed to artificially expand limited datasets and improve robustness to anatomical variability. Many other approaches have similarly relied on the U-Net/U-Mamba [20,25] architecture, leveraging its powerful encoder-decoder structure to capture both contextual information and precise spatial details [25]. These methods still struggled to learn fine-grained latent space representations, often capturing only coarse, high-level features of the anatomy.

Recent advancements in large language models (LLMs), such as LLaMA [32], have showcased remarkable capabilities in learning transferable, high-level latent representations that generalize effectively across various domains [26]. Inspired by this, we propose a novel hybrid architecture that synergistically combines the strengths of vision-specific models with the powerful semantic understanding of LLMs for medical image segmentation.

In this work, we introduce LLaMba-Seg (LLaMA-enhanced Mamba for Segmentation), a framework that integrates a frozen LLaMA model [5,32] into a selective state-space U-Mamba [20] architecture. Our model leverages a trainable U-Mamba encoder-decoder to capture fine-grained spatial details at multiple resolutions, enabling precise boundary delineation in challenging low-contrast settings. A frozen LLaMA layer is strategically placed between the encoder and decoder to distill high-level semantic features from the image embeddings. This allows the model to leverage LLaMA's rich contextual understanding to guide representation alignment and, crucially, to generate high-confidence pseudo-labels from unannotated scans.

We validated our approach on the Liver Fibrosis Quantification and Analysis (LiQA) Task 2 Liver Segmentation (LiSeg) challenge's contrast-enhanced sub-task of segmenting the GED4 sequence. To improve the model's domain robustness, we employed a multi-source training strategy, utilizing a composite dataset that combines the challenge's dataset [6,18,29] with external scans from the AMOS [13] and ATLAS [23] datasets. Strong performance is obtained on the LiQA Task 2 validation benchmark, where our model achieved a Dice score of 0.97 and a Hausdorff Distance of 21.34 mm. These results underscore the effectiveness of our hybrid architecture under limited supervision and cross-domain variability.

2 Related Work

Backbone of medical image segmentation. U-Net popularized the symmetric encoder–decoder with skip connections for precise localization under limited supervision [25]. Building on this idea, nnU-Net standardized preprocessing, architecture, training and postprocessing into a self-configuring pipeline that generalizes across datasets [12]. To overcome the locality of convolutions and better capture long-range dependencies, hybrid and pure-Transformer designs were introduced: TransUNet couples a CNN with a ViT encoder [3], and UNETR adopts a pure Transformer encoder for 3D volumes with U-Net style decoding [9]. The quadratic complexity of self-attention, however, is costly for high-resolution 3D inputs. State-space models (SSMs) address this with linear-time sequence modeling. Mamba provides selective SSM blocks with high throughput and linear scaling [8]. Its visual adaptation, VMamba, implements visual state-space blocks that efficiently aggregate global context [19]. In medical imaging, U-Mamba integrates convolutional and Mamba blocks within a U-shaped hierarchy, reporting strong accuracy with favorable memory/speed trade-offs [20]. Concurrent 3D variants such as SegMamba further validate SSMs for volumetric segmentation [30].

LLM/LLaMA layers for medical vision. A complementary line of work leverages large language models (LLMs) as frozen global priors via lightweight adapters. BLIP-2 bridges frozen image encoders and frozen LLMs using a small querying transformer, reducing trainable parameters for vision–language pre-training [16]. LLaMA-Adapter and its V2 variant efficiently inject instructional or visual tokens into a frozen LLaMA through prompts/adapters and early-fusion strategies [5,32]. In biomedicine, LLaVA-Med adapts a conversational VLM to biomedical imagery for open-ended VQA [15], and Med-Flamingo enables few-shot medical VQA via continued multimodal pretraining [22]. Beyond VQA, a frozen LLM transformer block can be inserted directly as an encoder layer for purely visual biomedical tasks, acting as a plug-and-play global regularizer without prompts [14]. Our method follows this parameter-efficient philosophy: we place a frozen LLaMA adapter at the bottleneck of a U-Mamba and use its output as the deepest skip connection, injecting a globally consistent prior at the coarsest scale while preserving linear-time long-range modeling in the encoder.

3 Method

3.1 Data and Preprocessing

We train on Liver Fibrosis Quantification and Analysis (LiQA) dataset [6,18,29] hepatobiliary-phase (GED4) annotations (30 cases) and incorporate two external MRI sources for supervision: the ATLAS [23] training subset (60 MRI cases; liver label retained) and the AMOS [13] Task-2 MRI training split (60 MRI cases; liver label extracted from the multi-organ masks). All images and labels are harmonized with SimpleITK by resampling to 1.5 mm isotropic spacing (BSpline for images, nearest-neighbor for labels) while preserving the original origin and direction. We subsequently standardize intensities per volume and apply foreground cropping to reduce empty background.

3.2 Network Architecture: UNet + Mamba + LLaMA

Our model, named LLaMba-Seg, is a 3D U-Mamba encoder–decoder augmented with a frozen LLaMA-2 (7B) [27] adapter at the bottleneck (Fig. 1). Each

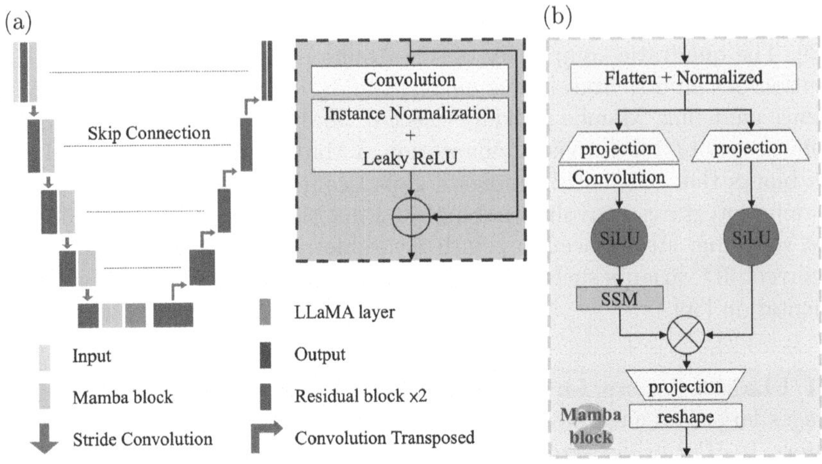

Fig. 1. Overview of LLaMba-Seg architecture: **a** Overall: The encoder stacks residual conv blocks with Mamba to couple local detail and linear-time global context. A frozen LLaMA-2 adapter at the bottleneck projects deepest features to LLaMA space, processes them, and projects back, thereby replacing the deepest skip. The decoder upsamples with residual blocks, fusing this LLaMA-conditioned bottleneck with shallower skips; freezing LLaMA keeps parameters low while injecting strong priors. **b** Mamba block: The 3D feature map is flattened and layer-normalized, then split into a sequence path and a gating path. The two branches are combined via a Hadamard product, projected back to the feature width, reshaped to 3D, and added with a residual connection.

encoder stage stacks two residual blocks [10] (Convolution + InstanceNorm [28] + LeakyReLU [21]) followed by a Mamba block [8], which provides linear-time long-range dependency modeling. In the Mamba block, the 3D feature map is first flattened and layer-normalized [1], then processed along two parallel paths: (i) a sequence path that applies a linear projection, depthwise 1D convolution, SiLU [11], and a selective state-space (SSM) update [7]; and (ii) a gating path with a linear projection and SiLU. The two outputs are fused via an element-wise (Hadamard) product, projected back to the original feature width, reshaped to 3D, and added through a residual skip connection. Compared with self-attention, this design aggregates global context with linear time and memory complexity, making it well suited for high-resolution volumes.

At the bottleneck, we insert a frozen LLaMA adapter. The encoder's deepest features are linearly projected to LLaMA's hidden width, passed through the frozen transformer stack, and projected back to the encoder width. The resulting LLaMA-conditioned feature serves as deepest connection into the decoder, which then concatenates it with the upsampled decoder features as in U-Net. This design injects globally regularized context while keeping LLaMA frozen and adding only lightweight trainable projection layers.

We follow a 3D full-resolution training plan at 1.5 mm isotropic spacing with patch size of $96 \times 128 \times 192$, batch size 2, and per-volume z-score normalization.

Optimization uses SGD with an initial learning rate of 1×10^{-3}, weight decay 3×10^{-5}, and a polynomial learning-rate schedule over 1000 epochs. We report Dice and HD95 on the LiQA validation set.

4 Experiement

4.1 Experimental Settings and Datasets

We evaluate our approach on the LiQA GED4 validation split and the blinded test set. All experiments are implemented in PyTorch and run on a DGX cluster using a single NVIDIA A100 (80 GB) GPU per job.

LiQA Dataset We use the LiQA liver-fibrosis cohort comprising 610 patients collected across multiple centers and three MRI platforms: Philips Ingenia 3.0 T, Siemens Skyra 3.0 T, and Siemens Aera 1.5 T [6,18,29]. Each case includes T2-weighted imaging, diffusion-weighted imaging, and Gadolinium ethoxybenzyl diethylenetriamine pentaacetic acid (Gd-EOB-DTPA) to cover the non-contrast, arterial, portal, delayed, and hepatobiliary phases. Data are provided in the Neuroimaging Informatics Technology Initiative (NIfTI) file format; phases other than the hepatobiliary phase may be absent, and no inter-phase or inter-subject pre-alignment is applied. Table 1 summarizes the splits across vendors and centers.

In this study, we train, validate, and test exclusively on hepatobiliary-phase (GED4) images. The training set contains 30 annotated cases in total (10 per center). The validation set includes 60 cases (20 per center), all with liver annotations. The held-out test split comprises 190 GED4 cases drawn from four vendor/center pairs; ground-truth liver annotations are withheld and used only for blinded evaluation. Notably, Vendor C is unseen during training/validation, providing an opportunity to assess cross-vendor generalization. This multi-vendor, multi-center design, combined with the lack of pre-registration, introduces substantial appearance and geometric variability, offering a realistic and challenging testbed for robust segmentation.

ATLAS Dataset The ATLAS (A Tumour and Liver Automatic Segmentation) dataset [23] was introduced in the MICCAI 2023 ATLAS Challenge to benchmark automated liver and tumor delineation on contrast-enhanced MRI and is used in this study as an external training dataset. It comprises 90 hepatocellular carcinoma (HCC) cases with liver and tumor annotations, released as a public CE-MRI resource with a 60/30 train–test split. Metadata (sequence/phase, resolution, scanner vendor) allow studies of domain variability and robustness. As one of the first openly available, fully annotated CE-MRI datasets for HCC segmentation, ATLAS supports evaluation under realistic clinical heterogeneity. In this study, we use only the training subset as external training data; no test data or labels are used.

Table 1. LiQA dataset [6,18,29] composition across training, validation, and test splits. Test annotations are withheld by the challenge organizers for blinded evaluation.

Split	Vendor	Center	#Cases	#Annotations
Training	A	A	130	10
	B	B1	170	10
	B	B2	60	10
Validation	A	A	20	20
	B	B1	20	20
	B	B2	20	20
Testing	A	A	40	–
	B	B1	40	–
	B	B2	40	–
	C	C	70	–

Table 2. Network comparison on LiQA GED4 validation dataset (higher Dice is better; lower HD is better). Best in bold.

Network	Dice ↑	HD (mm) ↓
U-MambaBot	0.9603	26.53
U-MambaEnc	0.9684	22.63
U-MambaBot + LLaMA	0.9686	22.03
LLaMba-Seg (U-MambaEnc + LLaMA)	**0.9700**	**21.34**

Table 3. LiQA GED4 blind-test results using our LLaMba-Seg model. Higher Dice is better; lower HD is better.

Split	Dice ↑	HD (mm) ↓
in-distribution cases (ID)	0.9630	25.75
out-of-distribution cases (OOD)	0.9716	16.41

AMOS Dataset We incorporate external supervision from the MICCAI 2022 AMOS (Multi-Modality Abdominal Multi-Organ Segmentation) dataset [13], which contains 600 3D abdominal scans (500 CT, 100 MRI) with voxelwise annotations for 15 organs. Following the official Task 2 partitioning (300 CT + 60 MRI for training), we use the 60 MRI training cases as external training data to match our MRI target domain; all CT scans and the AMOS validation/test splits are excluded. Volumes are provided in NIfTI format, and from the multi-organ labels, we retain only the liver mask for supervision.

4.2 Evaluation Metrics

We evaluate liver segmentation with two standard metrics: the Dice coefficient and the Hausdorff Distance (HD). Dice measures volumetric overlap between the prediction $\hat{Y}$ and reference Y, Dice $= \frac{2|\hat{Y} \cap Y|}{|\hat{Y}|+|Y|}$, with higher values indicating better agreement. HD (reported in millimeters) quantifies the worst-case boundary discrepancy as the maximum surface-to-surface distance between the predicted and reference masks; lower values indicate more precise boundary alignment.

Table 4. Per-case liver segmentation performance on five LiQA GED4 validation cases (the same cases shown in Fig. 2). Metrics are Dice (↑) and symmetric Hausdorff distance in millimetres, HD (↓).

	Case 1	Case 2	Case 3	Case 4	Case 5
Dice ↑	0.98285	0.98305	0.98067	0.97959	0.98020
HD (mm) ↓	22.299	24.047	41.024	162.651	17.685

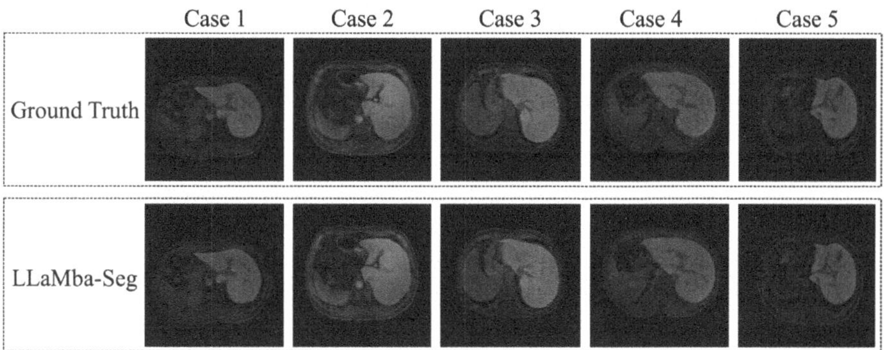

Fig. 2. Qualitative liver segmentation on five LiQA GED4 cases. Columns correspond to Cases 1–5 in Table 4. Top row: ground-truth masks; bottom row: LLaMba-Seg predictions. Red overlays denote the liver on the hepatobiliary-phase MR slices.

4.3 Results

Table 2 compares four configurations on LiQA dataset: U-Mamba with Mamba blocks in all encoder (U-MambaEnc) or only at the bottleneck (U-MambaBot), each with and without a frozen LLaMA-2 (7B) bottleneck adapter. Adding LLaMA improves both variants: for U-MambaEnc, Dice increases from 0.9684 to 0.9700 and HD drops from 22.63 to 21.34 mm. For U-MambaBot, Dice rises from 0.9603 to 0.9686 and HD decreases from 26.53 to 22.03 mm. While the LLaMA adapter yields larger relative gains on the bottleneck-only design, LLaMba-Seg remains the top performer overall on both metrics.

We also conduct a comprehensive evaluation of the challenge testing set, explicitly separating in-distribution (ID) cases, which are sourced from vendors and imaging centers included during training (Vendors A, B1, and B2), and out-of-distribution (OOD) cases that were collected from a completely held-out site (Vendor C). This setup enables us to rigorously assess the model's robustness to variations in imaging protocols, scanner hardware, and acquisition environments. As summarized in Table 3, the model maintains strong overall performance on the ID subset while demonstrating even better results on the OOD subset, highlighting its ability to generalize across clinical sites.

Specifically, the OOD cases exhibit a higher Dice score (+0.0086) compared to ID cases, indicating more accurate volumetric overlap between predicted and ground-truth segmentation, despite differences in acquisition settings. Furthermore, the OOD set achieves a substantially lower HD by −9.34 mm, reflecting more precise boundary delineation and fewer extreme segmentation errors on unseen sites. This is particularly noteworthy given that OOD data typically present additional challenges, such as shifts in image intensity distributions, heterogeneous contrast properties, and center-specific acquisition artifacts.

Figure 2 presents overlays for five cases (Cases 1–5 in Table 4). In each column, the top row displays the expert-annotated ground truth segmentations, while the bottom row shows the predicted masks generated from the proposed LLaMba-Seg model. Regions marked in red denote the segmented liver boundaries. Overall, the predicted contours visually align well with the true hepatic boundaries, demonstrating the model's ability to adapt to diverse liver morphologies, varying contrast levels, and challenging anatomical contexts. Importantly, while the model achieves consistently high overlap across cases, subtle differences highlight the complementary insights provided by different evaluation metrics. For instance, Case 4 attains a high Dice (0.9796) yet a large HD (162.65 mm) due to a tiny distant false positive. This illustrates HD's heightened sensitivity to even small, isolated false-positive regions, which may be clinically less significant but still strongly influence the boundary-based metric. Such observations emphasize the importance of jointly evaluating volumetric similarity and boundary accuracy for a comprehensive assessment of segmentation quality.

5 Conclusion

We introduced LLaMba-Seg, a U-Mamba encoder–decoder with a frozen LLaMA adapter at the bottleneck. By projecting the encoder features into LLaMA's hidden space and back, the model injects contextual priors with minimal additional trainable parameters, complementing U-Net–style skips and improving boundary fidelity. On the LiQA hepatobiliary-phase cohort, our best configuration achieved a Dice of 0.9700 and HD95 of 21.34 mm, surpassing the original U-Mamba and both bottleneck variants, with robust generalization across multiple vendors/centers, including an unseen site. **Limitations of our method** include the use of a frozen, non-medically pretrained LLM, sequence-length overhead from bottleneck tokenization, and reliance on a single phase at 1.5 mm isotropic resolution. **Future work** will explore lightweight adapter tuning with clinical corpora, self-supervised pretraining for the Mamba encoder, multi-phase fusion, domain and test-time adaptation, uncertainty estimation for quality control, and efficiency improvements via tokenization or distillation to remove the LLaMA adapter at inference.

Acknowledgments. We also thank the organizers of the CARE 2025 Challenge for their excellent organization and for providing the Liver Fibrosis Quantification and Analysis (CARE-Liver/LiQA) dataset.

References

1. Ba, J.L., Kiros, J.R., Hinton, G.E.: Layer normalization (2016). arXiv:1607.06450
2. Bilic, P., Christ, P., Li, H.B., et al.: The liver tumor segmentation benchmark (LiTS). Med. Image Anal. **84**, 102680 (2023). https://doi.org/10.1016/j.media.2022.102680
3. Chen, J., Lu, Y., Yu, Q., et al.: Transunet: transformers make strong encoders for medical image segmentation (2021). arXiv:2102.04306
4. Cheplygina, V., de Bruijne, M., Pluim, J.P.: Not-so-supervised: a survey of semi-supervised, multi-instance, and transfer learning in medical image analysis. Med. Image Anal. **54**, 280–296 (2019). https://doi.org/10.1016/j.media.2019.03.009
5. Gao, P., Han, J., Zhang, R., et al.: LLaMA-adapter V2: parameter-efficient visual instruction model (2023). arXiv:2304.15010
6. Gao, Z., Liu, Y., Wu, F., Shi, N., Shi, Y., Zhuang, X.: A reliable and interpretable framework of multi-view learning for liver fibrosis staging. In: International Conference on Medical Image Computing and Computer-Assisted Intervention, pp. 178–188 (2023)
7. Gu, A.: Modeling Sequences with Structured State Spaces. Stanford University (2023)
8. Gu, A., Dao, T.: Mamba: linear-time sequence modeling with selective state spaces (2024). arXiv:2312.00752
9. Hatamizadeh, A., Yang, D., Roth, H.R., Xu, D.: UNETR: transformers for 3D medical image segmentation. In: 2022 IEEE/CVF Winter Conference on Applications of Computer Vision (WACV), pp. 1748–1758 (2021). https://api.semanticscholar.org/CorpusID:232290634
10. He, K., Zhang, X., Ren, S., Sun, J.: Deep residual learning for image recognition. In: 2016 IEEE Conference on Computer Vision and Pattern Recognition (CVPR), pp. 770–778 (2016)
11. Hendrycks, D., Gimpel, K.: Gaussian error linear units (GELUs) (2023). arXiv:1606.08415
12. Isensee, F., Jaeger, P.F., Kohl, S.A.A., Petersen, J., Maier-Hein, K.H.: nnU-Net: a self-configuring method for deep learning-based biomedical image segmentation. Nat. Methods **18**, 203–211 (2020). https://api.semanticscholar.org/CorpusID:227947847

13. Ji, Y., Bai, H., Yang, J., Ge, C., Zhu, Y., Zhang, R., Li, Z., Zhang, L., Ma, W., Wan, X., Luo, P.: AMOS: a large-scale abdominal multi-organ benchmark for versatile medical image segmentation (2022). arXiv:2206.08023
14. Lai, Z., Wu, J., Chen, S., Zhou, Y., Hovakimyan, N.: Residual-based language models are free boosters for biomedical imaging tasks. In: 2024 IEEE/CVF Conference on Computer Vision and Pattern Recognition Workshops (CVPRW), pp. 5086–5096 (2024). https://api.semanticscholar.org/CorpusID:268692032
15. Li, C., Wong, C., Zhang, S., Usuyama, N., Liu, H., Yang, J., Naumann, T., Poon, H., Gao, J.: LLaVA-med: training a large language-and-vision assistant for biomedicine in one day. In: Proceedings of the 37th International Conference on Neural Information Processing Systems, NIPS '23. Curran Associates Inc., Red Hook, NY, USA (2023)
16. Li, J., Li, D., Savarese, S., Hoi, S.: BLIP-2: bootstrapping language-image pre-training with frozen image encoders and large language models. In: Proceedings of the 40th International Conference on Machine Learning, ICML'23, JMLR.org (2023)
17. Litjens, G., Kooi, T., Bejnordi, B.E., Setio, A.A.A., Ciompi, F., Ghafoorian, M., van der Laak, J.A., van Ginneken, B., Sánchez, C.I.: A survey on deep learning in medical image analysis. Med. Image Anal. **42**, 60–88 (2017). https://doi.org/10.1016/j.media.2017.07.005
18. Liu, Y., Gao, Z., Shi, N., Wu, F., Shi, Y., Chen, Q., Zhuang, X.: Merit: multi-view evidential learning for reliable and interpretable liver fibrosis staging. Med. Image Anal. **102**, 103507 (2025)
19. Liu, Y., Tian, Y., Zhao, Y., Yu, H., Xie, L., Wang, Y., Ye, Q., Jiao, J., Liu, Y.: VMamba: visual state space model. In: Advances in Neural Information Processing Systems, vol. 37, pp. 103031–103063. Curran Associates, Inc. (2024)
20. Ma, J., Li, F., Wang, B.: U-Mamba: enhancing long-range dependency for biomedical image segmentation (2024). arXiv:2401.04722
21. Maas, A.L., Hannun, A.Y., Ng, A.Y., et al.: Rectifier nonlinearities improve neural network acoustic models. In: Proceedings of the International Conference on Machine Learning(ICML), vol. 30, p. 3. Atlanta, GA (2013)
22. Moor, M., Huang, Q., Wu, S., Yasunaga, M., Dalmia, Y., Leskovec, J., Zakka, C., Reis, E.P., Rajpurkar, P.: Med-flamingo: a multimodal medical few-shot learner. In: Proceedings of the 3rd Machine Learning for Health Symposium. Proceedings of Machine Learning Research, vol. 225, pp. 353–367. PMLR (2023)
23. Quinton, F., Popoff, R., Presles, B., et al.: A tumour and liver automatic segmentation (ATLAS) dataset on contrast-enhanced magnetic resonance imaging for hepatocellular carcinoma. Data **8**(5), 79 (2023)
24. Reeder, S.B., Cruite, I., Hamilton, G., Sirlin, C.B.: Quantitative assessment of liver fat with magnetic resonance imaging and spectroscopy. J. Magn. Reson. Imaging **34**(4), 729–749 (2011)
25. Ronneberger, O., Fischer, P., Brox, T.: U-Net: convolutional networks for biomedical image segmentation. In: Medical Image Computing and Computer-Assisted Intervention–MICCAI 2015. pp. 234–241. Springer International Publishing, Cham (2015)
26. Tang, F., Ma, W., He, Z., Tao, X., Jiang, Z., Zhou, S.K.: Pre-trained LLM is a semantic-aware and generalizable segmentation booster (2025). arXiv:2506.18034
27. Touvron, H., Martin, L., Stone, K., et al.: Llama 2: open foundation and fine-tuned chat models (2023). arXiv:2307.09288
28. Ulyanov, D., Vedaldi, A., Lempitsky, V.: Instance normalization: the missing ingredient for fast stylization (2017). arXiv:1607.08022

29. Wu, F., Zhuang, X.: Minimizing estimated risks on unlabeled data: a new formulation for semi-supervised medical image segmentation. IEEE Trans. Pattern Anal. Mach. Intell. **45**(5), 6021–6036 (2023)
30. Xing, Z., Ye, T., Yang, Y., Liu, G., Zhu, L.: SegMamba: long-range sequential modeling mamba For 3D medical image segmentation. In: proceedings of Medical Image Computing and Computer Assisted Intervention–MICCAI 2024. LNCS, vol. 15008. Springer Nature Switzerland (2024)
31. Zhang, H., Zhang, M., You, X., Gu, Y., Yang, G.Z.: Computing assessment for Liver fibrosis staging using real-world MR images. In: Comprehensive Analysis and Computing of Real-World Medical Images, pp. 87–95. Springer Nature Switzerland, Cham (2025)
32. Zhang, R., Han, J., et al.: LLaMA-adapter: efficient fine-tuning of language models with zero-init attention (2023). arXiv:2303.16199

IE-UNet: Implicit Neural Representation-Driven Whole Heart Segmentation

Heng Zheng and Mingjing Yang(✉)

College of Physics and Information Engineering, Fuzhou University, Xueyuan Road, Fuzhou 350116, Fujian, China
yangmj5@fzu.edu.cn

Abstract. Automatic and accurate segmentation of the whole heart structure from 3D cardiac images plays a crucial role in assisting physicians with the diagnosis and treatment of cardiovascular diseases. However, the manual annotation of cardiac images is time-consuming and labor-intensive, making it difficult to efficiently utilize existing CT or MRI images for training deep learning networks, which restricts the improvement of whole heart segmentation accuracy. Multi-modality data contains multi-level cardiac image information due to differences in imaging mechanisms, contributing to enhanced segmentation precision. Therefore, this paper proposes a novel segmentation framework called Implicitly Enhanced UNet(IE-UNet) capable of mining 3D implicit features, which is specifically designed to mine and leverage 3D implicit features that are often overlooked in conventional approaches, primarily consisting of an Implicit Enhance (IE) module and a UNet module. The IE module extracts implicit features from 3D images and integrates them into the original image features to improve the segmentation accuracy of UNet. A notable advantage of the proposed Implicitly Enhanced module is its plug-and-play nature, allowing for seamless integration into various existing network architectures without the need for comprehensive redesign or additional complex training strategies. Experimental results on the CARE2025-WHS dataset demonstrate that IE-UNet achieves a Dice score of 90.69% on the valid set, proving the effectiveness of the proposed method.

Keywords: Whole heart segmentation · Implicit neural representation

1 Introduction

Over the past two decades, cardiovascular diseases (CVDs) have emerged as a significant public health challenge and remain a leading cause of global morbidity and mortality [1], necessitating advanced approaches for precise diagnosis and timely intervention. In modern clinical practice, non-invasive imaging techniques such as three-dimensional computed tomography (CT) and magnetic

X. Zhuang et al. (Eds.): CARE 2025, LNCS 16257, pp. 90–99, 2026.
https://doi.org/10.1007/978-3-032-16271-7_9

resonance imaging (MR) play an indispensable role in the detailed visualization and comprehensive evaluation of cardiac structures. The accurate segmentation of cardiac anatomy from these 3D images is fundamentally important for facilitating tailored treatment planning, objectively monitoring disease progression, and effectively guiding complex surgical procedures [2].

A complete 3D cardiac volume is typically composed of over three hundred serially reconstructed two-dimensional slices, each requiring meticulous annotation. The inherent complexity of cardiac anatomy–characterized by substantial morphological variability across patients and frequently ambiguous boundaries between adjacent substructures–makes manual segmentation not only exceptionally time-consuming but also highly susceptible to inter-observer variability. Given the escalating demand for large-scale, high-quality training data in data-intensive deep learning approaches, dataset distillation techniques have consequently gained prominence as a pragmatic strategy to mitigate annotation bottlenecks [3]. Certain advanced methods now facilitate the extraction of compact, synthetically generated datasets from existing larger synthetic collections, effectively preserving critical feature information while drastically reducing computational and labeling burdens [4]. This severe scarcity of reliably annotated medical imaging data, compounded by the inherent challenges of cardiac anatomy, consequently amplifies the difficulties associated with achieving robust and generalizable whole heart segmentation, presenting a significant obstacle in clinical translation and research advancement.

Cardiac segmentation primarily employs convolutional neural networks (CNNs) in deep learning to efficiently extract image features. Yang et al. [5] trained a deeply supervised 3D fully convolutional network (FCN) with an encoder-decoder architecture to achieve automated cardiac segmentation. Yan et al. [6] attained promising results in 3D medical image segmentation by integrating efficient Transformer modules to process multi-resolution data streams in parallel. Building upon the U-Net architecture, researchers have developed various improved models. Chen et al. [7] realized accurate and efficient medical image segmentation using U-Nets of different depths with shared weights. Additionally, Attention U-Net [8] and CFUN+ [9] were proposed to further enhance the accuracy and efficiency of medical image segmentation. MWG-UNet [10] employs attention mechanisms to bolster the segmentation ac-curacy of the generator, thereby enhancing the overall performance of the model in cardiac segmentation tasks.

Despite advances in fully automatic cardiac segmentation technology, several challenges persist: the high cost of manual annotation and patient privacy concerns make it difficult to acquire sufficient training data–particularly for 3D imaging and specific pathological subtypes–thereby complicating the training of robust whole-heart segmentation models. Furthermore, the blurred boundaries between adjacent substructures in 3D cardiac images often lead to mis-segmentation.

To address these issues, this paper proposes an Implicitly Enhanced UNet (IE-UNet), whose core is an implicit feature enhancement module designed to handle boundary ambiguity by mining implicitly continuous features in medical images. Integrating the Implicitly Enhanced module into the U-Net architecture enables the network to learn more discriminative and robust features. The proposed method achieved a Dice similarity coefficient of 90.69% on the test set of the CARE-WHS 2025 challenge.

2 Method

The IE-UNet framework is implemented by inserting the Implicitly Enhanced (IE) module prior to the U-Net architecture–as depicted in Fig. 1–leveraging U-Net as its backbone due to its established excellence in semantic segmentation tasks. During training, the IE module continuously infuses implicit structural and contextual features into the hierarchical feature maps, thereby not only improving segmentation accuracy through enhanced boundary sensitivity and structural consistency, but also substantially increasing the model's robustness to noise and anatomical variability across different imaging protocols and patient populations.

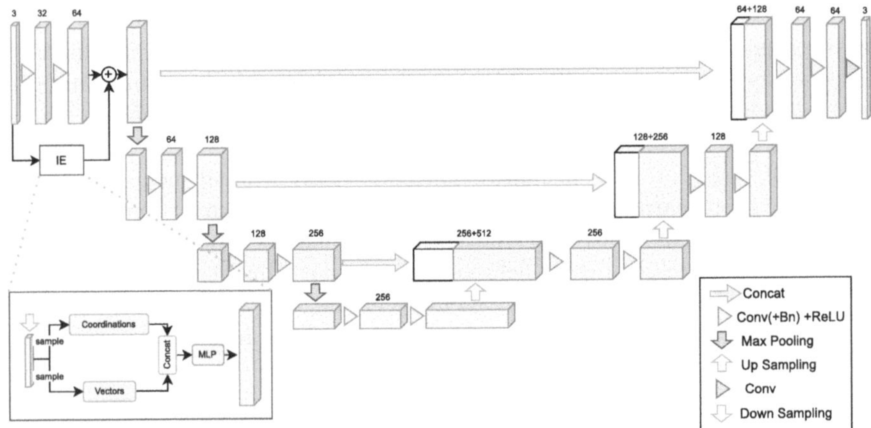

Fig. 1. IE-UNet Network Architecture for Whole Heart Segmentation.The key component of this architecture is the Implicitly Enhanced Module (IEM), which is integrated at the initial stage of the U-Net backbone. The IE module excavates implicitly continuous features from the input image and controls the incorporation of such features to enhance the model's robustness, generalization capability, and segmentation performance. Based on implicit neural representation, the IE module utilizes a multilayer perceptron (MLP) to extract continuous implicit features corresponding to spatial coordinates. For further details, refer to the main text.

2.1 Network Backbone

U-Net is characterized by its distinctive U-shaped encoder-decoder architecture, which consists of a contracting path that progressively captures multi-scale contextual information through a series of convolutional and max-pooling layers–effectively reducing spatial dimensions–and a symmetric expanding path that enables precise localization and detailed reconstruction via up-convolutional operations. Central to its design is the use of skip connections that fuse high-resolution, low-level feature maps from the encoder with the semantically rich, up-sampled features in the decoder, thereby preserving fine-grained spatial information while integrating abstract representations, which significantly enhances segmentation accuracy, particularly in regions with ambiguous or complex boundaries. Notably, U-Net demonstrates remarkable performance even when trained on limited annotated datasets, a trait attributable to its efficient feature reuse and structural elegance, making it especially suitable for medical image analysis where annotated data are scarce and precision is critical.

2.2 Implicitly Enhanced Module

The IE module is designed to address the critical challenge of boundary ambiguity in medical image segmentation by leveraging and mining continuous implicit features embedded within the imaging data. The core idea is rooted in the framework of implicit neural representations [11], which learn a continuous mapping from spatial coordinates to feature values, thereby enabling sub-voxel accuracy and smooth feature transitions essential for delineating subtle anatomical boundaries.

Preprocessing To maintain computational efficiency while preserving essential structural information, we first downsample the original 3D image and concurrently perform shallow feature extraction.This yields a compact low-resolution feature map $\mathbf{R}^{C\times D/2\times H/2\times W/2}$ that retains salient image attributes. This step significantly reduces memory footprint and processing time in subsequent operations.

$$F_{low} = Conv(Downsample(R_{origin})) \tag{1}$$

Coordination Normalization and Vector Concatenation For each voxel point p_i in the target output feature map, we obtain its spatial coordinates $x_i = (d_i, h_i, w_i)$ normalized to the range [-1, 1]. Simultaneously, the corresponding feature vector v_i is sampled via trilinear interpolation from the low-resolution feature map F_{low}. The two are concatenated to form an enriched input vector that encodes both geometric and appearance information.

$$z_i = Concat(x_i, v_i) \tag{2}$$

Here, z_i represents a fused input vector combining spatial location and local image context, providing a foundation for learning spatially-aware continuous features.

Extract Continuous Features The concatenated vector z_i is fed into an MLP to obtain the continuous implicit features f_i of that coordinate point.

$$f_i = f_\theta(z_i) \tag{3}$$

which f_θ denotes a multilayer perceptron parameterized by theta, is used to learn a continuous implicit neural representation.

Feature Map Reconstruction The predicted implicit features $f_1, f_2, ..., f_N$ are reassembled according to their original spatial coordinates into a full-resolution implicit feature map $F_{imp} \in \mathbf{R}^{C \times D \times H \times W}$, which has the same spatial dimensions as the input image. A convolutional layer is applied to refine and smooth the reconstructed feature map.

$$F_{imp} = Conv(Reshape([f_1, f_2, ..., f_N])) \tag{4}$$

Fusion Finally, the generated implicit feature map F_{imp} is fused with the shallow features $F_{shallow}$ extracted from the original image by the U-Net and fed into the subsequent backbone network of the U-Net.

$$F_{out} = F_{imp} + F_{shallow} \tag{5}$$

The fusion operation integrates both high-frequency structural details from shallow features and continuous implicit representations, thereby enhancing the network's ability to resolve ambiguities in organ or tissue boundaries.

2.3 Training Methods

To optimize the IE-UNet model, we adopt a combined loss function consisting of Dice loss and cross-entropy (CE) loss to guide the model training. The Dice loss is particularly effective in addressing class imbalance issues in medical image segmentation and significantly improves boundary prediction accuracy, while the cross-entropy loss helps minimize pixel-wise classification errors. The combined loss function is defined as follows:

$$L_{total} = \lambda_1 L_{Dice} + \lambda_2 L_{CE} \tag{6}$$

where λ_1 and λ_2 are the balance parameters. This combination fully leverages the synergistic advantages of both loss functions, thereby yielding more robust and reliable segmentation results.

3 Experiments

3.1 Dataset and Preprocessing

For the experiments and evaluations of the proposed method, we used the CARE2025-WHS for whole heart segmentation challenge dataset [12–14], which contains 86 images with ground truth for training, 50 images for validation and 80 images for testing. The complete dataset comprises CT and MR images from six independent centers, with ground truth annotations encompassing seven cardiac substructures: the left ventricle blood cavity (LV), right ventricle blood cavity (RV), left atrium blood cavity (LA), right atrium blood cavity (RA), myocardium of the left ventricle (Myo), ascending aorta (AA), and pulmonary artery (PA).

3.2 Implementation and Evaluation Details

All networks, including IE-UNet, were trained with a batch size of 2 and loss weights λ_1 and λ_2 set to 1.0 and 1.0 respectively. The training process was accelerated using an NVIDIA GeForce RTX 4090 GPU, with an initial learning rate of 0.001 and optimized using the Adam optimizer with $\beta_1 = 0.9$ and $\beta_2 = 0.999$.

Model performance was evaluated by calculating the Dice Similarity Coefficient (DSC), Average Symmetric Surface Distance (ASSD), and Hausdorff Distance (HD) between the segmentation predictions and the ground truth annotations.

4 Result

In this section, we will present both quantitative and qualitative comparison results between our proposed method and other approaches, including UNet-3D [15], UNETR [16], and SwinUNETR [17]. Additionally, we have conducted a series of ablation studies, which will be reported in the subsequent sections.

4.1 Comparison Study

Table 1. Comparison of segmentation performance metrics for different methods and heart substructures. The best DSC results are labeld in **bold**.

Methods	Metrics	Substructure of Heart							WH
		LV	RV	LA	RA	MYO	AO	PA	
Unet-3D	HD	7.15	13.56	15.72	17.31	14.03	14.35	25.86	15.42
	ASSD	4.58	5.13	4.66	6.7	5.58	3.62	6.93	5.31
	DSC	0.889	0.87	0.892	0.858	0.858	0.858	0.814	0.862
UNETR	HD	9.52	13.58	13.91	16.28	16.88	18.54	28.59	16.75
	ASSD	4.52	4.83	3.21	5.96	4.52	2.48	7.08	4.65
	DSC	0.903	0.878	0.896	0.877	0.862	0.857	0.835	0.872
SwinUNETR	HD	9.12	16.58	12.31	15.92	16.27	11.03	23.89	15.02
	ASSD	3.91	4.56	2.92	6.07	4.59	2.39	7.1	4.5
	DSC	0.914	0.889	0.929	0.889	0.856	**0.92**	0.831	0.889
Ours	HD	8.24	15.68	10.17	13.71	13.83	19.06	22.68	14.76
	ASSD	1.28	1.5	1.19	1.55	1.3	3.75	2.81	1.91
	DSC	**0.931**	**0.897**	**0.936**	**0.921**	**0.867**	0.86	**0.847**	**0.895**

We conducted comparative experiments on the CARE2025-WHS training dataset, and the experimental results are presented in Table 1. Our proposed method demonstrates competitive performance across multiple evaluation metrics when compared to existing approaches. In terms of overall performance on whole heart segmentation, our method achieves the highest DSC score of 0.895, along with the lowest Hausdorff Distance (HD) of 14.76 mm and Average Symmetric Surface Distance (ASSD) of 1.91 mm, indicating superior segmentation accuracy and boundary delineation.

Notably, our approach excels in segmenting specific cardiac substructures, achieving the best DSC scores for the left ventricle (LV, 0.931), right ventricle (RV, 0.897), left atrium (LA, 0.936), right atrium (RA, 0.921), myocardium (MYO, 0.867), and pulmonary artery (PA, 0.847). The significantly lower ASSD values across most substructures (e.g., LV: 1.28 mm, RV: 1.5 mm, LA: 1.19 mm) further confirm its enhanced boundary precision. While SwinUNETR performs best on the aorta (AO) with a DSC of 0.92, our method maintains competitive results across other metrics. These findings validate the effectiveness of our approach in handling complex cardiac anatomical structures.

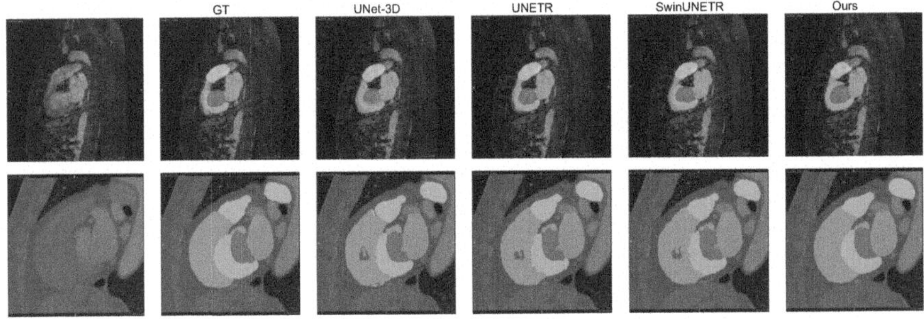

Fig. 2. A qualitative comparison of different methods, visually presenting the segmentation results of each approach, with the first column displaying CT or MR images.

As shown in Fig. 2, the qualitative comparison clearly demonstrates the superior continuity and precision of our method's segmentation results. Other methods exhibit issues such as segmentation holes and ambiguous boundaries, whereas our approach successfully captures structures that other methods fail to segment and produces clearly defined boundaries. Evidently, our IE-UNet method demonstrates greater robustness and superior performance.

4.2 Ablation Study

In this section, we conduct a series of ablation studies to demonstrate the effectiveness of our proposed IE module. The ablation study results in Table 2 provide compelling evidence for the critical role of the IE module within the overall model architecture. The incorporation of this module leads to a significant enhancement in segmentation performance: the Dice Similarity Coefficient (DSC) for whole heart segmentation increases from 0.857 to 0.895, while the Average Symmetric

Surface Distance (ASSD) boundary error is substantially reduced from 5.54 mm to 1.91 mm, signifying a breakthrough in boundary adherence accuracy. It is particularly noteworthy that the module achieves optimal DSC metrics across all cardiac substructures, with especially remarkable improvements observed in the left ventricle (0.931 vs. 0.861) and right atrium (0.921 vs. 0.859). Furthermore, boundary errors in structures such as the left atrium and pulmonary artery demonstrate an order-of-magnitude reduction. These systematic improvements conclusively prove that the IE module significantly enhances the model's capability to characterize complex anatomical structures, providing an effective solution for improving the accuracy and robustness of cardiac image segmentation.

Table 2. Results of the ablation study on the IE module. The best DSC results are labeld in **bold**.

Methods	Metrics	Substructure of Heart							WH
		LV	RV	LA	RA	MYO	AO	PA	
No-IE	HD	8.15	14.51	15.72	17.53	15.08	18.35	25.75	16.44
	ASSD	5.86	5.12	4.66	6.79	5.81	3.62	6.93	5.54
	DSC	0.861	0.87	0.891	0.859	0.858	0.851	0.814	0.857
With IE	HD	8.24	15.68	10.17	13.71	13.83	19.06	22.68	14.76
	ASSD	1.28	1.5	1.19	1.55	1.3	3.75	2.81	1.91
	DSC	**0.931**	**0.897**	**0.936**	**0.921**	**0.867**	**0.86**	**0.847**	**0.895**

4.3 Official Challenge Results

In this section, we present the results of our method on the official test dataset of CARE2025-WHS, achieving the best Dice scores on HWS CT (ID and OOD) and HWS MR (ID), and the third-best Dice score on HWS MR (OOD). The specific metrics are shown in Table 3.

5 Conclusion

In this paper, we propose IE-UNet, a novel segmentation framework that integrates an Implicitly Enhanced (IE) module with a standard U-Net backbone to tackle the persistent challenge of boundary ambiguity in whole heart segmentation from 3D cardiac images. By leveraging implicit neural representations, the IE module effectively captures and encodes continuous spatial and contextual features that are often neglected by conventional methods, thereby significantly improving the model's ability to delineate subtle anatomical boundaries and handle structural variability. Extensive experiments conducted on the multi-modality CARE2025-WHS dataset demonstrate the superiority of IE-UNet over

Table 3. Official results of our method, including WHS CT(ID and OOD) and WHS MR(ID and OOD). The metrics for different cardiac regions are all Dice scores.

Datasets	LV(↑)	Myo(↑)	RV(↑)	LA(↑)	RA(↑)	AO(↑)	PA(↑)
CT(ID)	0.9426	0.9300	0.9284	0.9653	0.9240	0.9604	0.8483
CT(OOD)	0.9754	0.9742	0.9617	0.9839	0.9695	0.9805	0.9561
MR(ID)	0.9354	0.8496	0.9148	0.8959	0.8892	0.8966	0.8148
MR(OOD)	0.9426	0.8235	0.8735	0.9116	0.8897	0.9106	0.8848
Datasets	WHS_Dice(↑)		WHS_HD(mm)(↓)		WHS_ASD(mm)(↓)		
CT(ID)	0.9410		12.5151		0.7237		
CT(OOD)	0.9740		11.6691		0.3616		
MR(ID)	0.8922		24.7081		1.1629		
MR(OOD)	0.8959		20.6044		1.5678		

state-of-the-art methods such as UNet-3D, UNETR, and SwinUNETR. Our approach achieves a Dice score of 89.5% on whole heart segmentation, with particularly notable performance across key cardiac substructures. Ablation studies further confirm the indispensable role of the IE module, showing marked improvements in both segmentation accuracy and boundary precision when the module is incorporated. The plug-and-play design of the IE module enables easy integration into existing architectures without necessitating extensive structural modifications, highlighting its versatility and potential for broader application in medical image analysis. Future work will focus on extending the framework to other anatomies and imaging modalities, as well as exploring self-supervised strategies to further reduce dependency on large annotated datasets.

Acknowledgments. This work was supported in part by the National Natural Science Foundation of China under Grant 62271149, in part by the Science and Technology Project of Fujian Province under Grants 2024J01353, 2022Y4014, 2020Y9091, 2023Y9144.

References

1. Vaduganathan, M., Mensah, G.A., Turco, J.V., Fuster, V., Roth, G.A.: The global burden of cardiovascular diseases and risk: a compass for future health. American College of Cardiology Foundation Washington DC (2022)
2. Habijan, M., Babin, D., Galić, I., Leventić, H., Romić, K., Velicki, L., Pižurica, A.: Overview of the whole heart and heart chamber segmentation methods. Cardiovasc. Eng. Technol. **11**(6), 725–747 (2020)
3. Liu, S., Wang, K., Yang, X., Ye, J., Wang, X.: Dataset distillation via factorization. Adv. Neural. Inf. Process. Syst. **35**, 1100–1113 (2022)
4. Liu, S., Ye, J., Yu, R., Wang, X.: Slimmable dataset condensation. In: Proceedings of the IEEE/CVF Conference on Computer Vision and Pattern Recognition, pp. 3759–3768 (2023)

5. Yang, X., Bian, C., Yu, L., Ni, D., Heng, P.-A.: 3D convolutional networks for fully automatic fine-grained whole heart partition. In: International Workshop on Statistical Atlases and Computational Models of the Heart, pp. 181–189. Springer (2017)
6. Yan, Q., Liu, S., Xu, S., Dong, C., Li, Z., Shi, J.Q., Zhang, Y., Dai, D.: 3d medical image segmentation using parallel transformers. Pattern Recogn. **138**, 109432 (2023)
7. Chen, G., Li, L., Zhang, J., Dai, Y.: Rethinking the unpretentious u-net for medical ultrasound image segmentation. Pattern Recogn. **142**, 109728 (2023)
8. Oktay, O., Schlemper, J., Folgoc, L.L., Lee, M., Heinrich, M., Misawa, K., Mori, K., McDonagh, S., Hammerla, N.Y., Kainz, B., et al.: Attention u-net: Learning where to look for the pancreas (2018). arXiv:1804.03999
9. Cui, H., Wang, Y., Li, Y., Xu, D., Jiang, L., Xia, Y., Zhang, Y.: An improved combination of faster r-cnn and u-net network for accurate multi-modality whole heart segmentation. IEEE J. Biomed. Health Inform. **27**(7), 3408–3419 (2023)
10. Lyu, Y., Tian, X.: Mwg-unet: hybrid deep learning framework for lung fields and heart segmentation in chest x-ray images. Bioengineering **10**(9), 1091 (2023)
11. Mildenhall, B., Srinivasan, P.P., Tancik, M., et al.: Nerf: Representing scenes as neural radiance fields for view synthesis. Commun. ACM **65**(1), 99–106 (2021)
12. Zhuang, X., Shen, J.: Multi-scale patch and multi-modality atlases for whole heart segmentation of mri. Med. Image Anal. **31**, 77–87 (2016)
13. Zhuang, X.: Multivariate mixture model for myocardial segmentation combin-ing multi-source images. IEEE Trans. Pattern Anal. Mach. Intell. **41**(12), 2933–2946 (2019)
14. Gao, S., Zhou, H., Gao, Y., Zhuang, X.: Bayeseg: Bayesian modeling for medical image segmentation with interpretable generalizability. Med. Image Anal. **89**, 102889 (2023)
15. Çiçek, Ö., Abdulkadir, A., Lienkamp, S.S., Brox, T., Ronneberger, O.: 3d u-net: Learning dense volumetric segmentation from sparse annotation. In: International Conference on Medical Image Computing and Computer-assisted Intervention, pp. 424–432. Springer (2016)
16. Hatamizadeh, A., Tang, Y., Nath, V., Yang, D., Myronenko, A., Landman, B., Roth, H.R., Xu, D.: Unetr: Transformers for 3d medical image segmentation. In: Proceedings of the IEEE/CVF Winter Conference on Applications of Computer Vision, pp. 574–584 (2022)
17. Hatamizadeh, A., Nath, V., Tang, Y., Yang, D., Roth, H.R., Xu, D.: Swin unetr: Swin transformers for semantic segmentation of brain tumors in mri images. In: International MICCAI Brainlesion Workshop, pp. 272–284. Springer (2021)

Multi-Modal MRI Fusion for Liver Fibrosis Staging and Semi-Supervised Pipeline for Liver Segmentation

Lida Yang[1], Minlu Cao[1], Yuan Cao[1], Xuecheng Fang[1], Wei Chen[2], Jax Luo[3], and Xu Qiao[1(✉)]

[1] School of Control Science and Engineering, Shandong University, Jinan, China
yanglida412@163.com, wapcml@163.com, 15829133115@163.com, pearsonfxc@163.com, qiaoxu@sdu.edu.cn

[2] School of Radiology, Shandong First Medical University and Shandong Academy of Medical Sciences, Jinan, China
chenwei9320@sdfmu.edu.cn

[3] Neurological Institute, Cleveland Clinic, Cleveland, OH, USA
jluo5@mgh.harvard.edu

Abstract. Liver fibrosis, a critical pathological feature of chronic liver diseases, requires accurate staging and segmentation to guide clinical decision-making. However, analyzing multi-center, multi-phase MRI data is challenged by cross-center imaging variability and limited annotations. To address these issues, this study proposes task-specific solutions for liver fibrosis staging (LiFS) and liver segmentation (LiSeg). For LiFS, we developed a 3D ResNet-based multi-modal deep learning framework integrating T1WI, T2WI, DWI, and GED (1–4) sequences, with an LSTM-based feature fusion module to capture inter-modal correlations. The framework targets four fibrosis stages (S1–S4) and two binary subtasks–cirrhosis detection (S1–S3 vs. S4) and substantial fibrosis detection (S1 vs. S2–S4)–and achieved an accuracy of 0.7 for cirrhosis detection and 0.7333 for substantial fibrosis detection on the validation set, demonstrating robust performance despite class imbalance. For LiSeg, to address annotation scarcity (no labels for non-contrast sequences T1WI/T2WI/DWI, limited labels for GED4), we proposed a semi-supervised pipeline integrating nnU-Net, pseudo-label technology, and deformable registration. Validation results showed excellent performance for GED4 (Dice = 0.9672) and promising outcomes for non-contrast sequences, all exceeding clinically acceptable thresholds and confirming the pipeline's clinical feasibility. Together, these methods improve the reliability of deep learning-based liver disease assessment in clinical imaging scenarios, solving key problems in multi-modal data integration and label efficiency.

Keywords: Liver fibrosis staging · Liver segmentation · Deep learning

X. Zhuang et al. (Eds.): CARE 2025, LNCS 16257, pp. 100–111, 2026.
https://doi.org/10.1007/978-3-032-16271-7_10

1 Introduction

Liver fibrosis, a critical stage in the progression of chronic liver disease to cirrhosis, can develop into liver cancer and liver failure if left untreated [1], posing a significant global public health challenge. Consequently, early and accurate assessment of liver fibrosis is crucial for monitoring and preventing disease progression, formulating personalized treatment plans, and evaluating prognosis [2], with staging (S1 for mild, S2 for moderate, S3 for severe, and S4 for cirrhosis [3]) serving as the core indicator of disease progression. Chronic liver disease affects hundreds of millions of people worldwide, and the degree of hepatic fibrosis is a decisive factor for prognosis, treatment selection, and follow-up [4]. Accurate liver segmentation on multi-phase MRI is a prerequisite for any downstream quantitative analysis, yet current solutions struggle with real-world clinical data that are both vendor-heterogeneous and annotation-scarce.

Currently, liver biopsy, the clinical gold standard for diagnosing and staging liver fibrosis, has limitations such as invasive procedures, sampling errors, and risks of complications [5,6], which severely restrict its clinical application. With the advancement of medical imaging technology, magnetic resonance imaging (MRI) has gradually become an important tool for non-invasive assessment of liver fibrosis due to its radiation-free nature and high tissue resolution [7–9]. Among its sequences, T1-weighted imaging (T1WI) clearly displays liver anatomy, T2-weighted imaging (T2WI) is sensitive to tissue edema, and diffusion-weighted imaging (DWI) reflects water molecule diffusion characteristics. The CARE-Liver 2025 challenge targets this area by releasing a large, multi-center cohort covering four complementary sequences: non-contrast T1WI, T2WI, DWI, and hepatobiliary phase (GED4) images acquired after Gd-EOB-DTPA administration. While GED4 offers superb liver–lesion contrast, only a handful of masks are provided; the remaining three sequences arrive with no annotations at all, presenting a scenario of "extremely weak supervision". Multi-sequence fusion complements information gaps between different modalities, providing multi-dimensional pathological information of liver tissue to improve the accuracy and reliability of liver fibrosis assessment, while addressing challenges like inter-scanner intensity drift and inconsistent slice orientations that amplify domain shift.

For liver fibrosis staging, this study proposes a 3D ResNet-based multi-modal fusion classification method [10]. Using data from T1WI, T2WI, DWI and GED (1–4) sequences on multi-center datasets, the method extracts and fuses features through a multi-stream network structure to achieve two binary subtasks: cirrhosis detection (S4 vs S1-S3) and substantial fibrosis detection (S1 vs S2-S4), enabling multi-stage fibrosis staging. For liver segmentation, our contribution is a concise yet effective pipeline that couples accurate registration with one-round pseudo-labelling to transform a dataset with scarce GED4 annotations and no T1WI/T2WI/DWI labels into a fully-segmented resource, yielding robust performance across all four sequences.

2 Related Work

2.1 Related Work on Liver Fibrosis Staging

Traditional radiomics methods rely on manually extracted features combined with machine learning algorithms such as support vector machines and random forests for staging. For example, Xiao et al. [6] constructed and compared radiomics models based on multiple MR parameters and fusion models using logistic regression to stage liver fibrosis in patients with chronic liver disease.

With the development of deep learning, CNN-based methods are increasingly applied to liver fibrosis assessment. Hectors et al. [11] developed a fully automated deep learning algorithm based on gadoxetate-enhanced hepatobiliary phase MRI, achieving a maximum AUC of 0.91 on the test set with good diagnostic performance. Multi-modal fusion strategies are key to improving staging performance. Xin et al. [10] developed an artificial intelligence-based liver metastasis screening system using a multi-stream feature fusion architecture, where features from each modality are extracted through independent backbone networks before fusion for prediction–an approach that informs multi-modal fusion designs in liver fibrosis staging.

2.2 Related Work on Liver Segmentation

Liver segmentation on MRI has traditionally relied on hand-crafted or atlas-driven approaches. Early atlas-based pipelines [12] and active contour methods (implemented via level sets) [13] require intensive manual tuning and degrade when confronted with inter-subject anatomical variability.

The rise of deep learning shifted the paradigm toward fully convolutional networks. Ronneberger et al. introduced U-Net [14], whose encoder–decoder design with skip connections remains the backbone for most medical-segmentation tasks. Isensee et al. later proposed nnU-Net [15], an automatically self-configuring framework that has dominated MICCAI benchmarks without manual hyper-parameter tuning.

Yet, these advances all rest on the assumption of abundant annotated volumes, which often does not hold in real-world clinical scenarios. Medical image annotation is frequently plagued by the scarcity of labeled data: some modalities may have only limited annotations, while others may lack annotations entirely. Consequently, researchers have turned to exploring semi-supervised learning and label-efficient strategies. Chen et al. popularised cross pseudo supervision, in which predictions on unlabeled data are iteratively refined and re-used as supervision [16]. Han et al. demonstrated that a single round of high-confidence pseudo-label generation, combined with entropy minimisation, can reach near-supervised accuracy on liver CT [17]. Registration-based propagation offers another route: Jansen et al. showed that deformable algorithms achieving top-ranks on public benchmarks [18] can propagate sparse labels across dynamic phases, effectively converting "no labels" into "weak labels" [19].

3 Method

3.1 Method for Liver Fibrosis Staging

Data Preprocessing Firstly, perform grayscale normalization on the image, limiting the pixel value range to [−55, 145] to remove extreme value interference, and map it to the [-1, 1] interval through linear transformation. Then standardize all images to a uniform size ($32 \times 160 \times 192$) to ensure the fusion of depth features and the spatial proportion of liver anatomical structures. For missing modalities, zero matrices matching the standardized size of the corresponding modality are used for filling, ensuring data structure integrity and stability of subsequent analyses. It is worth noting that for GED4 samples that provide a mask, corresponding regions are extracted from the original image based on the mask shape.

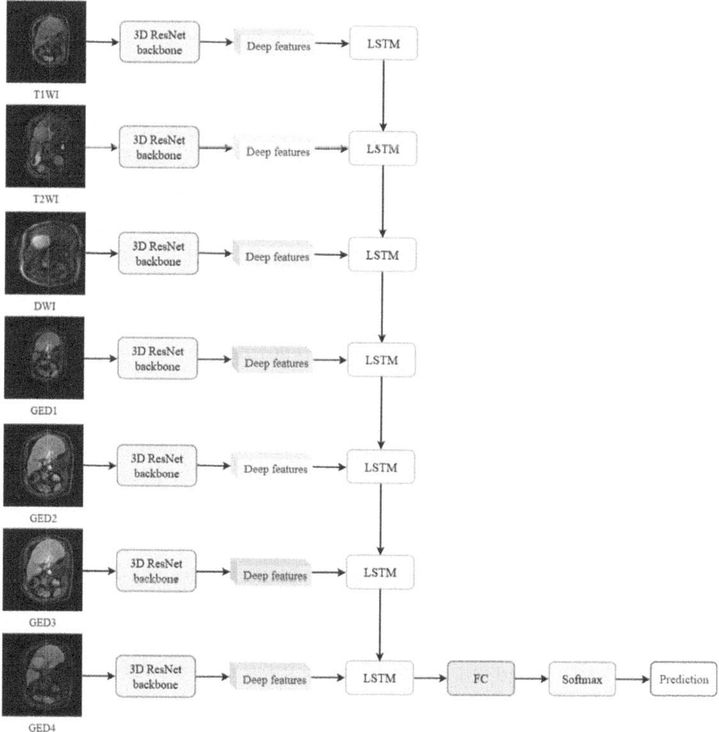

Fig. 1. Overview of the 3D ResNet-based multi-modal fusion classification model (adjusting the number of input modalities according to task requirements). MRI images from seven sequences are input into the 3D ResNet backbone of the classification module to generate image features at each stage. An LSTM model is then used to fuse information from the seven stages, which is input into a fully connected layer with a softmax function to obtain prediction probabilities.

Model Architecture The architecture of the proposed multi-modal fusion classification model is shown in Fig. 1. It consists of three basic components: a feature extraction module, a feature fusion module, and a classifier.

In the contrast-enhanced task, seven parallel 3D ResNet18 subnetworks are first used to extract their respective features from T1WI, T2WI, DWI, and GED (1–4) modalities, where each subnetwork contains conv1, bn1, relu, maxpool, and four residual blocks. Next, following the workflow of clinical radiology, the LSTM network first inputs non-contrast-enhanced images to reduce contrast agent interference and obtain baseline liver features; then multimodal images with enhanced contrast are input in physiological time sequence, capturing temporal correlations and fusing the features of seven modalities. Finally, a fully connected layer and Softmax function generate prediction probabilities for the corresponding tasks to obtain classification results. In the non-contrast task, only MRI images of T1WI, T2WI, and DWI sequences are used according to requirements, and the above operations are also performed.

3.2 Method for Liver Segmentation

nnU-Net and Pseudo-Label Technology nnU-Net is a state-of-the-art 3D U-Net variant specifically tailored for biomedical image segmentation, characterized by its self-configuring mechanism [15]. It automatically optimizes core components such as network architecture, patch size, batch size, and data augmentation strategies based on the intrinsic properties of the input dataset. This adaptability eliminates the need for manual hyperparameter tuning, enabling robust performance across diverse medical imaging tasks. Moreover, by retaining the classic encoder-decoder structure with skip connections of U-Net, it can effectively fuse high-level semantic features and low-level spatial details to enhance the segmentation accuracy of anatomical boundaries.

Pseudo-label technology, a key semi-supervised learning strategy, involves using a pre-trained model to generate "pseudo" labels for unlabeled data, which are then used as yyy supervision signals to expand the training set [20]. This approach leverages the model's own predictive power to mitigate the scarcity of labeled data, enabling the nnU-Net to learn more generalized features from the expanded data. By integrating the self-optimization capability of nnU-Net with the data expansion advantage of pseudo-label technology, the framework achieves effective segmentation performance even under conditions of limited annotations.

Inter-Sequence Deformable Registration We use the SyN framework [18] for deformable registration, with non-contrast sequences as fixed images and GED4 as moving images. SyN adopts a multi-scale optimization strategy to handle anatomical variations and cross-modal intensity differences, and ensures diffeomorphic deformation (preserving topological integrity) via symmetric normalization. This enables the physically plausible propagation of GED4 liver masks to T1WI, T2WI, and DWI sequences.

4 Experiments

4.1 Experimental Setup

The experiments were conducted on the liver dataset from the CARE-Liver 2025 challenge [21–23], which includes MRI data from 7 phases (each sample may randomly lack phases except the hepatobiliary phase). The training set comprises 360 patients, with only 30 patients having manual liver masks on the hepatobiliary-phase GED4, while all remaining GED4 volumes and all T1WI, T2WI, and DWI volumes are completely unlabeled; the validation set contains 60 patients. The two tasks were evaluated on the validation set, with specific experimental settings as follows.

Liver Fibrosis Staging Experiments The experiment is divided into non-contrast task and contrast-enhanced task: in the non-contrast task, only three sequences (T1WI, T2WI, and DWI) were used for training, while in the contrast-enhanced task, all seven sequences were used for model training. Implemented using PyTorch, the training was set to 200 epochs with the SGD optimizer, and data augmentation techniques such as random image flipping, elastic deformation, and Gaussian noise addition were applied.

Liver Segmentation Experiments For the GED4 sequence, we train a dedicated nnU-Net in two stages. Specifically, stage 1 is trained for 500 epochs using 30 manually annotated masked samples. For stage 2, training is conducted for 300 epochs on a combined dataset, which includes the original masked samples and pseudo-labels generated by the stage 1 model on unlabeled GED4 images. For the three non-contrast sequences (T1WI, T2WI, and DWI), the training process follows these steps. First, the GED4 images after stage 1 training are registered to each of these three sequences via SyN deformable registration. For each patient, a deformation field is estimated to achieve spatial alignment, enabling the propagation of GED4 liver masks to these sequences for label generation. Subsequently, a separate nnU-Net model is trained for each modality for 300 epochs, with the corresponding registered masks used as training supervision. Notably, these nnU-Net models adopt randomly initialized weights and do not leverage pre-trained weights from the stage 1 training of the GED4 sequence. All other hyperparameters for all nnU-Net models–including those designed for the GED4 sequence and the non-contrast sequences–remain consistent with the default settings of the nnU-Net framework. Finally, the trained models are applied to the validation set to perform liver segmentation.

4.2 Evaluation Metrics

For liver fibrosis staging, Accuracy (ACC) and AUC were used as evaluation metrics. ACC refers to the proportion of correctly classified results among all samples. AUC represents the area under the ROC curve, where values closer to 1 indicate better classifier performance.

To evaluate the performance of our liver segmentation results, we used Dice Similarity Coefficient (DSC) and Hausdorff Distance (HD) as evaluation metrics. DSC is mainly used to measure the overlap between the predicted results and the ground truth, while HD is used to measure the boundary error. These evaluation metrics are widely used in medical image segmentation. The Dice Similarity Coefficient is defined as:

$$\mathrm{DSC}(S_p, S_g) = \frac{2|S_p \cap S_g|}{|S_p| + |S_g|} \tag{1}$$

where S_p is the prediction result and S_g is the ground truth. The Hausdorff Distance is defined as:

$$\mathrm{HD}(S_p, S_g) = \max\left\{\sup_{x\in X}\inf_{y\in Y} d(x,y), \sup_{y\in Y}\inf_{x\in X} d(x,y)\right\} \tag{2}$$

where $\sup_{x\in X}\inf_{y\subset Y}$ represents the maximum of the minimum distances of all points in X to Y, and vice versa; $d(x, y)$ represents the distance between point x and point y.

4.3 Main Results

Liver Fibrosis Staging Results The classification results of the non-contrast task and contrast-enhanced task are presented in Tables 1 and 2, respectively; additionally, the heatmap for liver fibrosis staging is shown in Fig. 2.

Table 1. Classification results on the validation set for non-contrast tasks

Non-contrast subtask	AUC	ACC
Cirrhosis detection (S1–S3 vs. S4)	0.6818	0.6833
Substantial fibrosis detection (S1 vs. S2–S4)	0.5644	0.6833

Table 2. Classification results on the validation set for contrast-enhanced task.

Contrast-enhanced subtask	AUC	ACC
Cirrhosis Detection (S1–S3 vs. S4)	0.7512	0.7
Substantial Fibrosis Detection (S1 vs. S2–S4)	0.5585	0.7333

For liver cirrhosis detection, the AUC and ACC of the non-contrast task were 0.6818 and 0.6833, respectively, while the AUC and ACC of the contrast-enhanced task reached 0.7512 and 0.7, respectively. This indicates the model's effectiveness in identifying cirrhosis cases–since the sequences used in the contrast-enhanced task are complete and contain more complementary information, leading to better classification results. For substantial fibrosis detection,

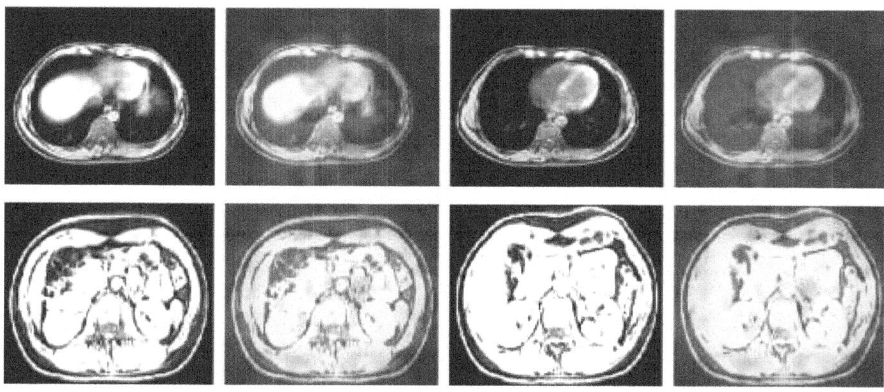

Fig. 2. Heat map

the ACC of the non-contrast task was 0.6833, while the ACC of the contrast-enhanced task was 0.7333, achieving differentiation between mild and moderate-to-severe fibrosis. However, its performance was lower compared to the cirrhosis task. This may be attributed to class imbalance: in the training set, there were 167 cases of S4 (cirrhosis) and 193 cases of S1–S3 (non-cirrhosis), which were relatively balanced; in contrast, S1 (mild fibrosis) only had 96 cases, while S2–S4 (moderate-to-severe fibrosis) had 263 cases. The smaller number of S1 samples may lead to insufficient model learning. Meanwhile, due to the threshold setting being biased toward the majority category, although ACC is improved, the model's generalization ability across different thresholds is reduced, resulting in a lower AUC.

Liver Segmentation Results Table 3 summarises the quantitative performance achieved on the 60-case validation set. GED4, benefiting from the highest contrast and limited ground truth, attains a Dice of 0.9672 and an HD95 of 20.66 mm–these values reflect strong performance compared to recent liver-MRI segmentation benchmarks. T1WI, which suffers from lower vessel-to-parenchyma contrast, still reaches a Dice of 0.9451 (with an HD95 of 54 mm), indicating that the generated masks retain sufficient quality for nnU-Net to learn robust representations. T2WI and DWI exhibit progressively lower Dice (0.8579 and 0.772, respectively) and varying HD95 (30.47 mm and 28.02 mm, respectively). Notably, label generation for non-contrast sequences depends entirely on GED4-to-sequence registration, and subtle alignment errors may marginally reduce label fidelity–this in turn restricts the upper limit of segmentation performance for T2WI and DWI. Nevertheless, all Dice values still exceed the 70% threshold commonly recognized as clinically acceptable for liver volumetry, and the HD95 values remain comparable to those reported in cirrhotic liver segmentation studies.

To further validate the generalizability of the proposed pipeline, we introduced the CirrMRI600+ dataset [24], which is the first dataset dedicated to cir-

Table 3. Liver segmentation results on the validation set.

Sequence	Dice	HD95 (mm)
GED4	0.9672	20.66
T1WI	0.9451	54
T2WI	0.8579	30.47
DWI	0.772	28.02

rhotic liver research. This dataset comprises 628 high-resolution abdominal MRI scans from 339 cirrhotic patients, including 310 T1-weighted (T1W) sequences and 318 T2-weighted (T2W) sequences. To generate labels for T1WI and T2WI in the CARE-Liver training set, we first performed deformable registration on the T1WI and T2WI sequences of annotated GED4 training cases using the deeds framework [25,26], registering each sequence to its corresponding GED4 sequence respectively. This registration process yielded labels for the T1WI and T2WI of these cases. Following label generation, we adopted the same two-stage training strategy as that used for GED4, and incorporated the CirrMRI600+ dataset as part of the training set in both stages. Table 4 presents the segmentation performance on the original CARE-Liver validation set before and after integrating the CirrMRI600+ dataset.

Table 4. Segmentation performance comparison before and after incorporating CirrMRI600+ dataset.

Dataset	T1WI (Dice/HD95 mm)	T2WI (Dice/HD95 mm)
CARE-Liver	0.946/56.81	0.8392/58.77
CARE-Liver and CirrMRI600+	0.9488/49.1	0.8553/65.15

The additional MRI data from CirrMRI600+ improves the overall liver segmentation performance. For T1WI: the Dice coefficient increases by 0.0028 (from 0.946 to 0.9488) and HD95 decreases by 7.71 mm (from 56.81 mm to 49.1 mm), indicating better accuracy and boundary alignment–this benefits from consistent imaging protocols and tissue contrast between CirrMRI600+'s T1W sequences and CARE-Liver, helping the model learn robust anatomical features. For T2WI, the Dice coefficient rises by 0.0161 (from 0.8392 to 0.8553) while HD95 increases by 6.38 mm (from 58.77 mm to 65.15 mm); the slight HD95 elevation may result from domain shifts between the two datasets' T2W sequences and T2WI's inherent susceptibility to artifacts, though overall T2WI accuracy still improves.

5 Conclusion

This study addresses two key challenges in multi-sequence MRI-based liver disease assessment: accurate liver fibrosis staging and robust liver segmentation under extremely weak supervision. For staging, we proposed a 3D ResNet-based multi-modal fusion method, which achieved effective performance in cirrhosis and substantial fibrosis detection, showing potential for non-invasive staging despite mild fibrosis sample imbalance. For segmentation, we developed a pipeline integrating registration, pseudo-labeling, and nnU-Net, propagating scarce GED4 labels to other sequences and turning weakly supervised data into fully segmented resources. Results showed robust performance across all sequences, all exceeding clinically acceptable thresholds, confirming reliable segmentation via the synergy between registration and pseudo-labeling with limited annotations.

The core components employed in this study are rooted in prior medical imaging literature, and the contribution lies more in their task-specific integration rather than standalone methodological innovation. Together, these integrated methods contribute to advancing non-invasive liver disease assessment by addressing key limitations in data availability and multi-modal information integration.

Disclosure of Interests The authors have no competing interests to declare that are relevant to the content of this article.

Acknowledgments. The authors thank the organizers of the CARE-Liver 2025 challenge for providing the dataset.

References

1. Friedman, S.L.: Liver fibrosis-from bench to bedside. J. Hepatol. **38**, 38–53 (2003). https://doi.org/10.1016/S0168-8278(02)00429-4
2. Anteby, R., Klang, E., Horesh, N., Nachmany, I., Shimon, O., Barash, Y., Kopylov, U., Soffer, S.: Deep learning for noninvasive liver fibrosis classification: a systematic review. Liver Int. **41**(10), 2269–2278 (2021). https://doi.org/10.1111/liv.14966
3. Goodman, Z.D.: Grading and staging systems for inflammation and fibrosis in chronic liver diseases. J. Hepatol. **47**(4), 598–607 (2007). https://doi.org/10.1016/j.jhep.2007.07.006
4. Tsochatzis, E.A., Bosch, J., Burroughs, A.K.: Liver cirrhosis. Lancet **383**(9930), 1749–1761 (2014). https://doi.org/10.1016/S0140-6736(14)60121-5
5. Regev, A., Berho, M., Jeffers, L.J., Milikowski, C., Molina, E.G., Pyrsopoulos, N.T., Feng, Z.Z., Reddy, K.R., Schiff, E.R.: Sampling error and intraobserver variation in liver biopsy in patients with chronic HCV infection. Am. J. Gastroenterol. **97**(10), 2614–2618 (2002). https://doi.org/10.1016/S0002-9270(02)04396-4
6. Xiao, L., Zhao, H., Liu, S., Dong, W., Gao, Y., Wang, L., Huang, B., Li, Z.: Staging liver fibrosis: comparison of radiomics model and fusion model based on multiparametric MRI in patients with chronic liver disease. Abdom. Radiol. **49**(4), 1165–1174 (2024). https://doi.org/10.1007/s00261-023-04142-2
7. Catania, R., Furlan, A., Smith, A.D., Behari, J., Tublin, M.E., Borhani, A.A.: Diagnostic value of MRI-derived liver surface nodularity score for the non-invasive quantification of hepatic fibrosis in non-alcoholic fatty liver disease. Eur. Radiol. **31**(1), 256–263 (2021). https://doi.org/10.1007/s00330-020-07114-y

8. Reiter, R., Tzschätzsch, H., Schwahofer, F., Haas, M., Bayerl, C., Muche, M., Klatt, D., Majumdar, S., Uyanik, M., Hamm, B., Braun, J., Sack, I., Asbach, P.: Diagnostic performance of tomoelastography of the liver and spleen for staging hepatic fibrosis. Eur. Radiol. **30**(3), 1719–1729 (2020). https://doi.org/10.1007/s00330-019-06471-7
9. Huang, W., Peng, Y., Kang, L.: Advancements of non-invasive imaging technologies for the diagnosis and staging of liver fibrosis: Present and future. View **5**(4), 20240010 (2024). https://doi.org/10.1002/VIW.20240010
10. Xin, H., Zhang, Y., Lai, Q., Liao, N., Zhang, J., Liu, Y., Chen, Z., He, P., He, J., Liu, J., Zhou, Y.: Automatic origin prediction of liver metastases via hierarchical artificial-intelligence system trained on multiphasic CT data: a retrospective, multicentre study. EClinicalMedicine **69**, (2024). https://doi.org/10.1016/j.eclinm.2024.102464
11. Hectors, S.J., Kennedy, P., Huang, K.H., Stocker, D., Carbonell, G., Greenspan, H., Friedman, S., Taouli, B.: Fully automated prediction of liver fibrosis using deep learning analysis of gadoxetic acid-enhanced MRI. Eur. Radiol. **31**(6), 3805–3814 (2021). https://doi.org/10.1007/s00330-020-07475-4
12. Cabezas, M., Oliver, A., Lladó, X., Freixenet, J., Cuadra, M.B.: A review of atlas-based segmentation for magnetic resonance brain images. Comput. Methods Programs Biomed. **104**(3), e158–e177 (2011). https://doi.org/10.1016/j.cmpb.2011.07.015
13. Kass, M., Witkin, A., Terzopoulos, D.: Snakes: active contour models. Int. J. Comput. Vision **1**(4), 321–331 (1988). https://doi.org/10.1007/BF00133570
14. Ronneberger, O., Fischer, P., Brox, T.: U-net: convolutional networks for biomedical image segmentation. In: Navab, N., Hornegger, J., Wells, W., Frangi, A. (eds.) Medical Image Computing and Computer-Assisted Intervention–MICCAI 2015. LNCS, vol. 9351, pp. 234–241. Springer, Cham (2015). https://doi.org/10.1007/978-3-319-24574-4_28
15. Isensee, F., Jaeger, P.F., Kohl, S.A., Petersen, J., Maier-Hein, K.H.: nnU-Net: a self-configuring method for deep learning-based biomedical image segmentation. Nat. Methods **18**(2), 203–211 (2021). https://doi.org/10.1038/s41592-020-01008-z
16. Chen, X., Yuan, Y., Zeng, G., Wang, J.: Semi-supervised semantic segmentation with cross pseudo supervision. In: Proceedings of the IEEE/CVF Conference on Computer Vision and Pattern Recognition, pp. 2613–2622. IEEE, Los Alamitos (2021). https://doi.org/10.48550/arXiv.2106.01226
17. Han, K., Liu, L., Song, Y., Liu, Y., Qiu, C., Tang, Y., Teng, Q., Liu, Z.: An effective semi-supervised approach for liver CT image segmentation. IEEE J. Biomed. Health Inform. **26**(8), 3999–4007 (2022). https://doi.org/10.1109/JBHI.2022.3167384
18. Avants, B.B., Tustison, N.J., Song, G., Cook, P.A., Klein, A., Gee, J.C.: A reproducible evaluation of ANTs similarity metric performance in brain image registration. Neuroimage **54**(3), 2033–2044 (2011). https://doi.org/10.1016/j.neuroimage.2010.09.025
19. Jansen, M.J., Kuijf, H.J., Niekel, M., Veldhuis, W.B., Wessels, F.J., Viergever, M.A., Pluim, J.P.: Liver segmentation and metastases detection in MR images using convolutional neural networks. J. Med. Imaging **6**(4), 044003–044003 (2019). https://doi.org/10.1117/1.JMI.6.4.044003
20. Arazo, E., Ortego, D., Albert, P., O'Connor, N.E., McGuinness, K.: Pseudo-labeling and confirmation bias in deep semi-supervised learning. In: 2020 Inter-

national Joint Conference on Neural Networks (IJCNN), Glasgow, UK, pp. 1–8. IEEE, Piscataway (2020). https://doi.org/10.1109/IJCNN48605.2020.9207304

21. Liu, Y., Gao, Z., Shi, N., Wu, F., Shi, Y., Chen, Q., Zhuang, X.: MERIT: multi-view evidential learning for reliable and interpretable liver fibrosis staging. Med. Image Anal. **102**, 103507 (2025). https://doi.org/10.1016/j.media.2025.103507
22. Gao, Z., Liu, Y., Wu, F., Shi, N., Shi, Y., Zhuang, X.: A reliable and interpretable framework of multi-view learning for liver fibrosis staging. In: Greenspan, H., et al. (eds.) Medical Image Computing and Computer-Assisted Intervention–MICCAI 2023. LNCS, vol. 14224, pp. 178–188. Springer, Cham (2023). https://doi.org/10.1007/978-3-031-43904-9_18
23. Wu, F., Zhuang, X.: Minimizing estimated risks on unlabeled data: a new formulation for semi-supervised medical image segmentation. IEEE Trans. Pattern Anal. Mach. Intell. **45**(5), 6021–6036 (2022). https://doi.org/10.1109/TPAMI.2022.3215186
24. Jha, D., Susladkar, O.K., Gorade, V., Keles, E., Antalek, M., Seyithanoglu, D., Velichko, Y., Ladner, D.P., Borhani, A.A., Medetalibeyoglu, A., Durak, G., Bagci, U.: Large scale MRI collection and segmentation of cirrhotic liver. Sci. Data **12**(1), 896 (2025). https://doi.org/10.1038/s41597-025-05201-7
25. Heinrich, M.P., Jenkinson, M., Brady, M., Schnabel, J.A.: MRF-based deformable registration and ventilation estimation of lung CT. IEEE Trans. Med. Imaging **32**(7), 1239–1248 (2013). https://doi.org/10.1109/TMI.2013.2246577
26. Heinrich, M.P., Maier, O., Handels, H.: Multi-modal multi-atlas segmentation using discrete optimisation and self-similarities. Visceral Challenge@ ISBI **1390**, 27. Zenodo, Geneva (2015). https://doi.org/10.5281/zenodo.32546

Two-Stage Approach for Myocardial Scar and Edema Segmentation Using Synthetic Multi-sequence MRI and Auxiliary Scar Prediction

Isabel Margolis(✉), Stefano Buoso, and Sebastian Kozerke

Institute for Biomedical Engineering, University and ETH Zurich, Zurich, Switzerland
margolis@biomed.ee.ethz.ch

Abstract. We present a two-stage deep learning framework for automated segmentation of left ventricular scar and edema from multi-sequence cardiac MRI. The method leverages late-gadolinium enhancement (LGE), T2-weighted, and balanced steady-state free precession (bSSFP) images provided by the CARE-MyoPS challenge hosted at MICCAI 2025. In the first stage, a set of 2D nnU-Nets is trained to segment the myocardium using 1–3 input channels (LGE only, LGE + bSSFP, and LGE + bSSFP + T2-weighted sequences). The resulting binary myocardium mask is then used to define a bounding box that spatially selects the input for the second stage. The second stage employs two independent 2D nnU-Net models. The primary network receives all three modalities along with the binary myocardium mask to jointly segment both scar and edema. In parallel, an auxiliary network is trained exclusively on LGE and the myocardium mask dedicated to scar segmentation. To address missing modalities in the training set, we synthetically generate bSSFP and T2-weighted images from LGE using two separate SPADE-GAN generative models. This synthetic augmentation expands the training set fivefold (n = 1954). During inference, the final prediction is assembled by replacing the scar output of the primary model with the prediction from the auxiliary network. Test-time augmentation is also applied to improve robustness. The proposed method achieves test Dice scores of 0.6097 for scar, 0.6419 for edema, and 0.6258 for scar + edema.

Keywords: Deep Learning · Myocardial pathology · Segmentation · Cardiac MRI

1 Introduction

Coronary artery disease, the underlying cause of most myocardial infarctions, is the third leading cause of death globally [1]. Accurate imaging of infarcted myocardial regions plays a critical role in clinical decision-making by enabling differentiation of cardiac pathologies, identifying patients who may benefit from revascularization, and supporting patient prognosis [2].

X. Zhuang et al. (Eds.): CARE 2025, LNCS 16257, pp. 112–123, 2026.
https://doi.org/10.1007/978-3-032-16271-7_11

Cardiovascular magnetic resonance (CMR) imaging with late gadolinium enhancement (LGE) is widely regarded as the gold standard for visualizing and delineating infarcted tissue in the left ventricle (LV) [3, 4]. In LGE CMR, gadolinium contrast shortens the T1 relaxation time, leading to increased signal intensity in regions of myocardial scarring where the washout of the contrast agent is slower.

The release of the multi-sequence MyoPS 2020 challenge dataset has accelerated research on automated segmentation methods using LGE, T2-weighted (T2), and steady-state free precession (bSSFP) CMR sequences [5–8]. bSSFP images allow for precise assessment of LV volumes and wall thickness, while T2 sequences offer complementary information by highlighting areas of myocardial edema.

Despite these imaging advances, manual scar segmentation remains common in clinical workflows, typically relying on thresholding techniques. While effective, these methods are time-consuming, require expert input, and are subject to inter- and intra-observer variability. This highlights the crucial need for automated, precise, and reproducible methodologies for segmenting myocardial scars [9].

In recent years, numerous deep learning approaches have been introduced to address the challenges of ventricular scar segmentation [10]. A common strategy is the use of fully automated cascaded architectures, in which multiple networks are trained sequentially. The output generated by one model serves as the input for the subsequent stage of the process [11–14]. The majority of existing methods rely on the U-Net architecture [15] or minor variants of it. Among these, the nnU-Net has emerged as particularly influential [16]. It processes the input images by dividing them into overlapping patches and aggregating them to generate the final segmentation. Notably, nnU-Net automates most of the design of critical pipeline components, including network architecture configuration, preprocessing, and hyperparameter tuning, making it highly adaptable to new datasets with minimal manual intervention.

Recent studies suggest that, in certain cases, separating tasks such as scar, edema, and combined pathology segmentation into distinct models can improve accuracy [17, 18]. Rather than relying on a single multitask network, this approach enables models to specialize in learning task-specific features, which can lead to improved segmentation performance in some settings.

Medical imaging datasets frequently suffer from limitations, particularly due to missing imaging sequences, which can substantially reduce the effective size of the training dataset. A solution to the problem proposed in [19] addresses the issue by leveraging Generative Adversarial Networks (GANs) to synthesize missing contrasts. While their full pipeline demonstrated improvements in precision and specificity, it revealed minimal to no enhancement in the Dice score when compared to a baseline nnU-Net trained without the additional synthetic data. Nonetheless, the approach offers a straightforward and practical means to mitigate the limitations of incomplete clinical datasets.

In this work, we address the problem of scar and edema segmentation using LGE, bSSFP, and T2 images as input. Our approach consists of two stages, incorporating an auxiliary network dedicated to scar segmentation, addressing missing modalities by generating synthetic bSSFP and T2 images from the available LGE, and applying test-time augmentation to enhance prediction robustness. Our approach was trained and validated on the Comprehensive Analysis & Computing of Real-world Medical

Images (CARE2025) Myocardial Pathology Segmentation (MyoPS) challenge dataset, organized as part of MICCAI 2025.

2 Methods

2.1 Dataset

We trained and evaluated our method using the multi-sequence CMR CARE-MyoPS dataset, excluding center H due to the absence of a myocardium reference. This dataset consists of 265 patients from seven centers located in China, France, and the United Kingdom. An overview of the dataset is presented in Table 1. The number of slices in each exam ranges from 1 to 36, with a median of 7. The average resolution is 1.3 mm $\times$ 1.3 mm $\times$ 10.6 mm. LGE and T2 images were obtained from the end-diastolic phase of the cardiac cycle. For the time-resolved bSSFP, the corresponding end-diastolic frame was identified and selected as input to the method. LGE is present in all patients; however, bSSFP sequences are absent in 31% of patients, and T2 sequences are missing in 40% of patients.

Table 1. Overview of the dataset provided by the Myocardial Pathology Segmentation (CARE-MyoPS) challenge 2025.

Center	Patients	Sequences	Labels
A	81	LGE	Scar, left ventricle and myocardium
B	65	LGE, T2, bSSFP	Scar, edema, left and right ventricles, myocardium
C	45	LGE, T2, bSSFP	Scar, edema, left and right ventricles, myocardium
D	50	LGE, T2, bSSFP	Scar, edema, left and right ventricles, myocardium
E	07	LGE, bSSFP	Scar, left and right ventricles, myocardium
F	09	LGE, bSSFP	Scar, left and right ventricles, myocardium
G	08	LGE, bSSFP	Scar, left and right ventricles, myocardium

Data from center D was withheld and used exclusively for challenge validation and testing, representing the out-of-distribution evaluation set. Additionally, 15 patients from center B were included in the challenge test set to assess in-distribution performance. For internal validation, we randomly selected a separate set of 9 patients from centers B and C, as these were the only centers that contained all three imaging modalities. The results presented in this paper are based on both the challenge validation set and our holdout validation set.

2.2 Preprocessing

The available dataset consists of images with varying spatial dimensions, with widths ranging from 158 to 518 pixels. To standardize the inputs, we resized them to 256 $\times$ 256 pixels following the steps outlined in Fig. 1.

First, we applied a center crop based on the smallest dimension of the original image. Next, we rescaled the images to 300 × 300 pixels using cubic interpolation for the three sequences and nearest-neighbor interpolation for the ground truth masks. Finally, to remove any remaining borders, a second center crop was applied to obtain a final size of 256 × 256 pixels. To complete the process, the images were normalized using the histogram-based Nyul normalization method [20].

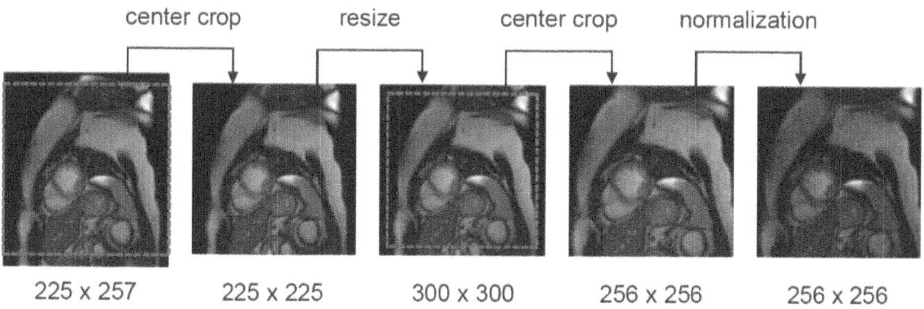

Fig. 1. Pipeline of the preprocessing steps on an example bSSFP image.

2.3 Models

An overview of our proposed two-stage approach using synthetic data is presented in Fig. 2.

First Stage. In the initial step, we trained a set of 2D nnU-Net models to predict the myocardium mask from input images of size 256 × 256 pixels. Each network was trained with a different input channel configuration: LGE only, LGE + bSSFP, and LGE + bSSFP + T2. Based on the available modalities, the corresponding model was used to generate the binary mask. Using this output mask, we calculated its center of mass and cropped both the input images and binary mask to 128 × 128 pixels. The cropped images and mask were then used in the second stage.

Second Stage. In the second stage, bSSFP and T2 images were synthetically generated for cases where these modalities were missing. Segmentation was performed by integrating predictions from two distinct 2D nnU-Nets: a primary network and an auxiliary network.

For image synthesis, we trained two independent image-to-image translation models based on the SPADE-GAN framework [21] to generate synthetic bSSFP and T2 images from preprocessed in vivo LGE images and corresponding ground truth masks. Input images and conditional masks were cropped using the bounding box defined in the first stage. The LGE-to-bSSFP model was trained using data from centers B, C, E, F, and G (n = 549), while the LGE-to-T2 model was trained on data from centers B and C (n = 381). The discriminator architecture followed a three-layer PatchGAN [22] design. Training was conducted over 1000 epochs using the Wasserstein loss [23], with learning rates of 1 × 10–5 for the Generator and 3 × 10–5 for the Discriminator. The generator loss also incorporated a weighted absolute error, assigning greater weight to the myocardium compared to the background, and a perceptual VGG loss [24] to encourage realistic structural details.

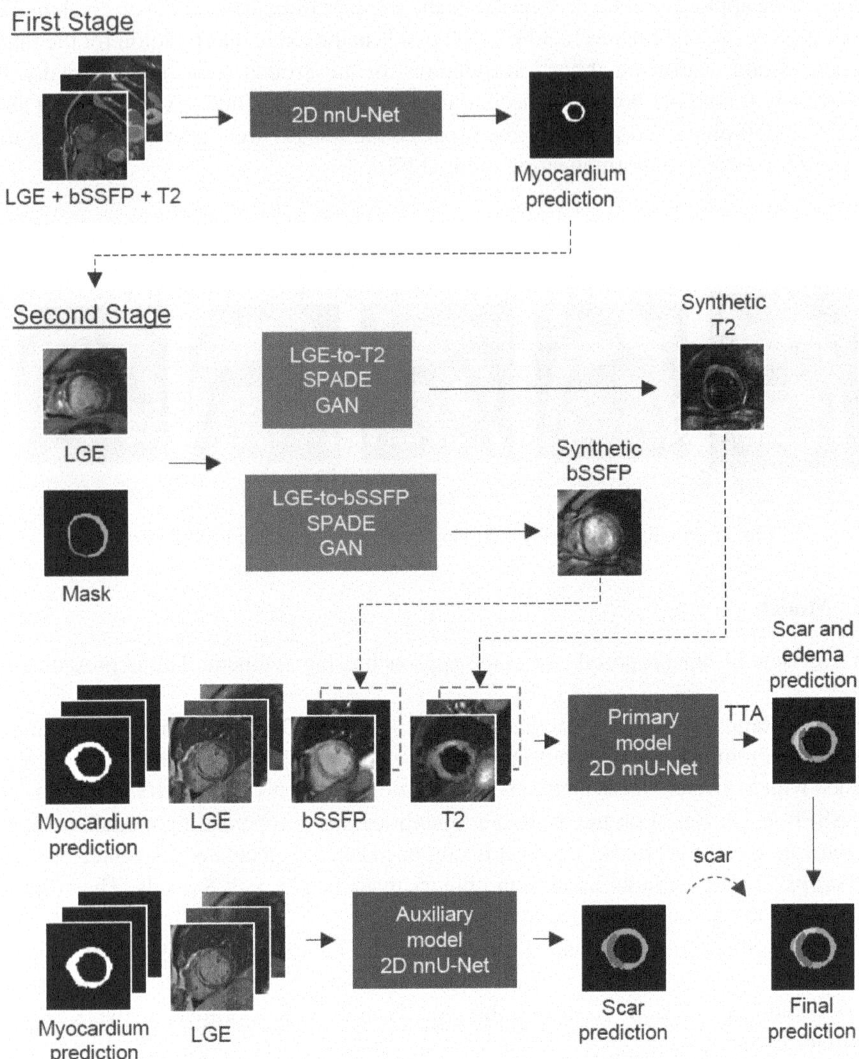

Fig. 2. Overview of the proposed two-stage framework. First Stage: A set of 2D nnU-Net models was trained with 1–3 input channels (LGE only, LGE + bSSFP, and LGE + bSSFP + T2) to segment the myocardium. A bounding box from the binary mask was used for cropping and passed to the next stage. Second Stage: Two SPADE-GANs (LGE-to-bSSFP and LGE-to-T2) synthesized missing modalities, conditioned on LGE and the corresponding reference mask. Two 2D nnU-Nets were used for pathology segmentation. The primary model segmented scar and edema using all inputs and exploiting TTA, and the auxiliary model segmented scar using LGE and myocardium only. Scar predictions from the primary network were replaced by the predictions from the auxiliary network to produce the final results. Segmented results display healthy myocardium in green, scar in red, and edema in pink.

The primary segmentation network was trained on 4-channel inputs (n = 1954), consisting of LGE, bSSFP, T2, and binary myocardium masks. It was designed to segment healthy myocardium, scar, and edema. As only 381 cases had in vivo bSSFP and T2 sequences, the remaining cases were supplemented with synthetically generated modalities using trained image-to-image translation models. To improve robustness, test-time augmentation (TTA) was applied at inference using flips, rotations (90°, 180°, 270°), Gaussian noise, and Gaussian blur. Final predictions were obtained by averaging outputs across all augmented inputs.

The auxiliary network, trained on 2-channel images (n = 1954) consisting of LGE and binary myocardium masks, was focused on segmenting healthy myocardium and scar. Since LGE was consistently available across centers and effectively highlights scar, this network was used to refine scar boundary delineation.

All nnU-Net models were trained for 200 epochs. In the final step, predictions from the auxiliary network were used to overwrite the scar regions from the primary network. Edema labels from the primary network were preserved in regions where the auxiliary network did not predict scar. In all other regions, the final label followed the output of the auxiliary network. The final masks were then rescaled to the original image dimensions.

2.4 Loss Function and Evaluation Metric

All segmentation networks were trained to minimize both the Dice loss (DICE) and the cross-entropy loss (CE):

$$l(y, \hat{y}) = l_{DICE}(y, \hat{y}) + l_{CE}(y, \hat{y})$$

The segmentation accuracy was evaluated using the metrics specified by the CARE-MyoPS challenge organizers: Dice score (DSC), Sensitivity (SEN), Precision (PRE), and Hausdorff Distance (HD).

2.5 Implementation Details

We trained all models using Python 3.8 and the PyTorch library on an NVIDIA TITAN RTX GPU. Most hyperparameters, including the learning rate and optimizer, were predefined by the nnU-Net framework, with the specific configuration detailed in [16]. Additionally, other hyperparameters, such as batch size, were optimized automatically. All networks were trained using 5-fold cross-validation, and the final predictions were aggregated using averaging.

3 Results and Discussion

The performance of our final model was evaluated on the CARE-MyoPS validation set. The results for scar, edema, and scar + edema segmentation are presented in Table 2. In Fig. 3, we present the performance of the final model on four representative cases from our holdout validation set. Examples a) and b) correspond to cases where the final model achieved the highest Dice scores for scar + edema, both scoring 0.90. In contrast, examples c) and d) illustrate cases with the lowest scores, 0.33 and 0.19, respectively. Challenging anatomical variability, motion artifacts, breath-hold position differences, and subtle intensity differences between pathological and healthy tissues contribute to diminished segmentation performance. In contrast, the high-performing cases typically exhibit well-defined scar and edema boundaries, minimal image artifacts, and consistent contrast across imaging modalities.

Table 2. Challenge validation results.

Metric	Scar	Edema	Scar + Edema
Dice score	0.6097	0.6419	0.6258
Sensitivity	0.5390	0.6306	0.5848
Precision	0.7501	0.6907	0.7204
Hausdorff distance	19.0409	21.0432	20.0421

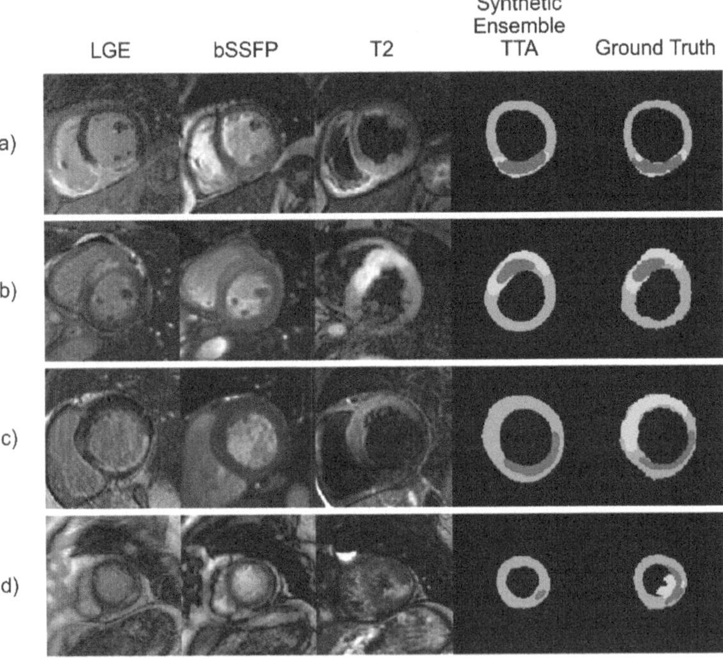

Fig. 3. Representative cases from the holdout validation set. **a** and **b** show examples with the highest Dice scores for combined scar and edema segmentation. **c** and **d** show examples with the lowest Dice scores. Healthy myocardium is shown in green, scar in red, and edema in pink.

To further assess the contribution of each component in the second stage of our pipeline, we conducted an ablation study on the holdout validation set. We considered the following model configurations:

- Baseline: A 2D nnU-Net was trained on LGE, bSSFP, T2, and binary myocardium masks to segment healthy myocardium, scar, and edema, using data exclusively from centers B and C (n = 381).
- Ensemble: Two 2D nnU-Nets were used. The primary model was trained only on the in vivo data from all modalities and binary myocardium (n = 381) to segment healthy myocardium, scar, and edema. The auxiliary model was trained on LGE and binary myocardium masks (n = 1954) to segment healthy myocardium and scar tissue. The final prediction was obtained by substituting the scar prediction from the primary model with the output from the auxiliary model.
- Synthetic: The primary model was trained on the extended dataset (n = 1954), where synthetic bSSFP and T2 sequences were generated for cases lacking in vivo acquisitions.
- Synthetic + Ensemble: Two 2D nnU-Nets were used with the primary network trained on the full dataset, including synthetic bSSFP and T2 (n = 1954).
- Synthetic + Ensemble + TTA: The full pipeline with test-time augmentation, incorporating spatial transformations (flips and rotations), Gaussian noise, and Gaussian blur during inference.

The Dice scores from the ablation study for both the challenge validation set (A) and the holdout validation set (B) are documented in Table 3. Figure 4 illustrates the distributions of the Dice scores from the ablation study conducted on our holdout validation set.

Table 3. Mean Dice scores of the ablation study on the challenge validation set (A) and the holdout validation set (B).

Model	Scar		Edema		Scar + Edema	
	A	B	A	B	A	B
Baseline	0.5794	0.6450	0.6335	0.4994	0.6065	0.6828
Ensemble	0.6097	0.7003	0.6358	0.5056	0.6228	0.6917
Synthetic	0.5802	0.6500	0.6358	0.5558	0.6080	0.7312
Synthetic + Ensemble	0.6097	0.7003	0.6377	0.5477	0.6237	0.7274
Synthetic + Ensemble + TTA	0.6097	0.7003	0.6419	0.5756	0.6258	0.7416

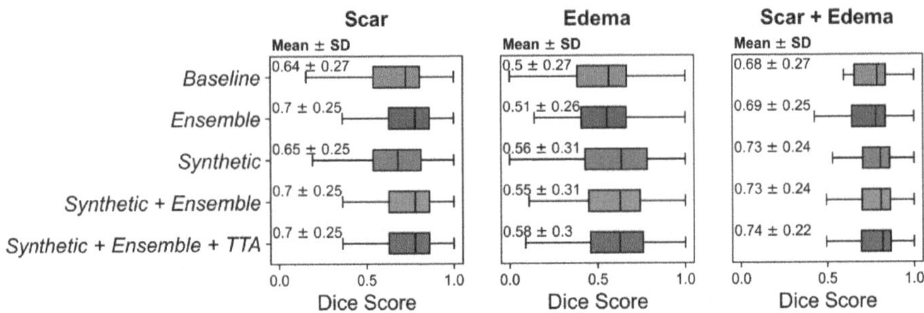

Fig. 4. Comparison of the Dice score distributions on the holdout validation set.

Furthermore, Fig. 5 presents qualitative segmentation outputs for each configuration considered in the ablation study, enabling a direct visual comparison of the contributions of individual components to overall performance. Quantitatively, the final model outperformed the baseline across all cases, achieving Dice score improvements of 0.03 for scar, 0.01 for edema, and 0.02 for scar + edema. A key factor contributing to this improvement was the inclusion of synthetic bSSFP and T2 sequences, which enabled training on an expanded dataset of 1954 samples, approximately five times larger than the 381 available in vivo multi-modal cases. This expansion effectively addressed the challenge of data heterogeneity and the limited availability of multi-sequence data across various clinical centers.

Moreover, the introduction of a dedicated auxiliary model for scar segmentation significantly improved the accuracy of scar boundary delineation. This model was trained exclusively on LGE images and binary myocardium masks, avoiding potential confounding features from bSSFP and T2 images, which are less informative for scar characterization. Additionally, this choice eliminates issues related to misalignment between modalities. By isolating the scar segmentation task, the model can fully leverage the strong contrast provided by LGE, leading to sharper and more precise predictions of scar tissue. These enhanced predictions were then used to replace the scar output of the primary model, which was trained on all available modalities. This design deliberately avoids segmenting the scar and edema as a single composite label within the primary model. In our experiments, when the two labels were spatially disconnected, the network trained to predict a merged label exhibited lower performance. By treating the labels separately, our approach likely improved the delineation of true edema boundaries, as the network was not required to infer edema from the residual region. This approach effectively combined the strengths of both specialized and multi-modal networks.

Finally, the application of test-time augmentation significantly enhanced the robustness and consistency of final predictions. This approach improved generalization by allowing the network to adapt to subtle variations in orientation and appearance that frequently occur in real-world clinical data. Overall, incorporating synthetic data generation, auxiliary modeling, and test-time augmentation collectively results in a more accurate and generalizable segmentation framework.

While our framework has shown promising results, several limitations still exist that require further investigation. First, although the use of synthetic bSSFP and T2 sequences substantially increased the size of the training dataset, it remains uncertain whether similar effective results could be achieved using simpler augmentation techniques directly applied to LGE images. Techniques such as intensity mapping, histogram equalization, or contrast transfer could reduce the computational overhead associated with generative models such as SPADE-GANs.

Moreover, our image augmentation approach can only be used during training, as it requires true labels for conditioning information. The limitation means it cannot be applied during inference, unlike the previously mentioned image augmentation methods that do not depend on label availability. Future work will explore whether such lightweight alternatives can serve as effective substitutes while reducing training complexity and resource demands.

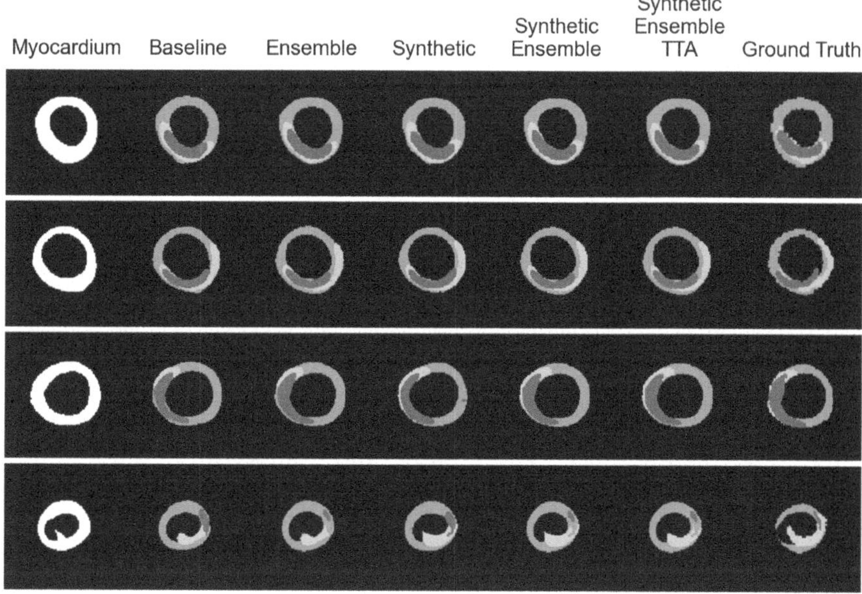

Fig. 5. Four examples from the holdout validation set for each individual method in the ablation study. The myocardium predictions from the first stage are shown in the first column. Healthy myocardium is shown in green, scar in red, and edema in pink.

Second, the current ensembling strategy aggregates predictions by combining outputs from separate models trained for scar and edema segmentation. While this method has improved performance, adopting more sophisticated ensembling techniques could yield even greater improvements in results.

Lastly, the test-time augmentation procedure used in our pipeline focused on basic spatial transformations and minor intensity perturbations. However, spatial augmentations often produce highly similar outputs in architectures such as nnU-Net, which limits their ability to improve robustness significantly. Future work could evaluate alternative TTA strategies to better capture uncertainty and variation in clinical scenarios.

4 Conclusion

In this work, we proposed a two-stage deep learning framework for joint scar and edema segmentation in multi-sequence cardiac MRI, incorporating sequence completion using synthetic bSSFP and T2, auxiliary networks, and test-time augmentation to improve performance. The results show that each component contributes to improved accuracy. The final model achieves Dice scores comparable to those of state-of-the-art methods reported in the literature, demonstrating the effectiveness of our approach for multi-sequence cardiac image segmentation.

Disclosure of Interests. The authors have no competing interests to declare that are relevant to the content of this article.

References

1. Brown, J., Gerhardt, T., Kwon, E.: Risk Factors for Coronary Artery Disease. StatPearls Publishing (2023). https://www.ncbi.nlm.nih.gov/books/NBK554410/
2. Toupin, S., Pezel, T., Bustin, A., Cochet, H.: Whole-heart high-resolution late gadolinium enhancement: techniques and clinical applications. J. Magn. Reson. Imaging **55**(4), 967–987 (2022)
3. West, A., Kramer, C.: Cardiovascular magnetic resonance imaging of myocardial infarction, viability, and cardiomyopathies. Curr. Probl. Cardiol. **35**(4), 176–220 (2010)
4. Kellman, P., Arai, A.: Cardiac imaging techniques for physicians: Late enhancement. J. Magn. Reson. Imaging **36**(3), 529–542 (2012)
5. Li, L., et al.: MyoPS: A benchmark of myocardial pathology segmentation combining three-sequence cardiac magnetic resonance images. Med. Image Anal. **87**, 102–808 (2023)
6. Qiu, J., et al.: MyoPS-Net: Myocardial pathology segmentation with flexible combination of multi-sequence CMR images. Med. Image Anal. **84**, 102694 (2023)
7. Ding, W., et al.: Aligning multi-sequence CMR towards fully automated myocardial pathology segmentation. IEEE Trans. Med. Imaging **42**(12), 3474–3486 (2023)
8. Zhuang, X.: Multivariate mixture model for myocardial segmentation combining multi-source images. IEEE Trans. Pattern Anal. Mach. Intell. **41**(12), 2933–2946 (2019)
9. Flett, A., Hasleton, J., Cook, C., Hausenloy, D., Quarta, G., Ariti, C., Muthurangu, V., Moon, J.: Evaluation of techniques for the quantification of myocardial scar of differing etiology using cardiac magnetic resonance. JACC: Cardiovasc. Imaging **4**(2), 150–156 (2011)
10. Wu, Y., Tang, Z., Li, B., Firmin, D., Yang, G.: Recent advances in fibrosis and scar segmentation from cardiac MRI: a state-of-the-art review and future perspectives. Front. Physiol. **12**, 46 (2021)
11. Lustermans, D., Amirrajab, S., Veta, M., Breeuwer, M., Scannell, C.: Optimized automated cardiac MR scar quantification with GAN-based data augmentation. Comput. Methods Programs Biomed. **226**, 107–116 (2022)
12. Wang, K., Yang, X., Miao, J., Li, L., Yao, J., Zhou, P., Xue, W., Zhou, G., Zhuang, X., Ni, D.: AWSnet: An auto-weighted supervision attention network for myocardial scar and edema segmentation in multi-sequence cardiac magnetic resonance images. Med. Image Anal. **77** (2022)
13. Liu, Y., Zhang, M., Zhan, Q., Gu, D., Liu, G.: Two-stage method for segmentation of the myocardial scars and edema on multi-sequence cardiac magnetic resonance. In: Zhuang, X., Li, L. (eds.) Myocardial Pathology Segmentation Combining Multi-Sequence Cardiac Magnetic Resonance Images. MyoPS 2020. LNCS, vol. 12554, pp. 26–36. Springer, Cham (2020)

14. Schwab, M., Pamminger, M., Kremser, C., Haltmeier, M., Mayr, A.: Deep learning pipeline for fully automated myocardial infarct segmentation from clinical cardiac MR scans. Radiol. Adv. (2025)
15. Ronneberger, O., Fischer, P., Brox, T.: U-Net: Convolutional networks for biomedical image segmentation. In: Navab, N., Hornegger, J., Wells, W., Frangi, A. (eds.) Medical Image Computing and Computer-Assisted Intervention—MICCAI 2015. MICCAI 2015. LNCS, vol. 9351, pp. 234–241. Springer, Cham (2015)
16. Isensee, F., Jaeger, P., Kohl, S., Petersen, J., Maier-Hein, K.: NnU-net: a self-configuring method for deep learning-based biomedical image segmentation. Nat. Methods **18**(2), 203–211 (2021)
17. Gao, J., Cai, Y., Zhao, Z., Lan, X., Huang, Q., Lan, L., et al.: RGU-Mamba: an U-mamba network with region-based training optimized for domain generalization applied to myocardial scar and edema segmentation. In: Zhuang, X., Ding, W., Wu, F., Gao, S., Li, L., Wang, S. (eds.) Comprehensive Analysis and Computing of Real-World Medical Images. LNCS, vol. 15548, pp. 77–86. Springer, Cham (2025)
18. Luo, Z., Wang, G.: Multi-model ensemble and region specific normalization for myocardial pathology segmentation with partial modalities. In: Zhuang, X., Ding, W., Wu, F., Gao, S., Li, L., Wang, S. (eds.) Comprehensive Analysis and Computing of Real-World Medical Images. LNCS, vol. 15548, pp. 106–115. Springer, Cham (2025)
19. Lin, H., Tavakoli, N., Schiffers, F., Lopez-Tapia, S., Kim, D., Katsaggelos, A.: GenSegNet: leveraging synthetic sequences and pseudo labels for multi-sequence myocardial pathology segmentation. In: Zhuang, X., Ding, W., Wu, F., Gao, S., Li, L., Wang, S. (eds.) Comprehensive Analysis and Computing of Real-World Medical Images. LNCS, vol. 15548, pp. 227–239. Springer, Cham (2025)
20. Nyul, L., Udupa, J., Zhang, X.: New variants of a method of MRI scale standardization. IEEE Trans. Med. Imaging **19**(2), 143–150 (2000)
21. Park, T., Liu, M.-Y., Wang, T.-C., Zhu, J.-Y.: Semantic image synthesis with spatially-adaptive normalization. In: Proceedings of the IEEE/CVF Conference on Computer Vision and Pattern Recognition (CVPR), pp. 2337–2346. IEEE (2019)
22. Isola, P., Zhu, J.-Y., Zhou, T., Efros, A.A.: Image-to-image translation with conditional adversarial networks. In: Proceedings of the IEEE Conference on Computer Vision and Pattern Recognition (CVPR), pp. 1125–1134. IEEE (2017)
23. Arjovsky, M., Chintala, S., Bottou, L.: Wasserstein GAN. In: Proceedings of the 34th International Conference on Machine Learning (ICML), pp. 214–223 (2017)
24. Johnson, J., Alahi, A., Fei-Fei, L.: Perceptual losses for real-time style transfer and super-resolution. In: European Conference on Computer Vision (ECCV), pp. 694–711. Springer (2016)

Semi-supervised Liver Segmentation and Patch-Based Fibrosis Staging with Registration-Aided Multi-parametric MRI

Boya Wang[1(✉)], Ruizhe Li[1,2,3], Chao Chen[1,2], and Xin Chen[1]

[1] Intelligent Modelling & Analysis Group (IMA), School of Computer Science, University of Nottingham, Nottingham, UK
boya.wang@nottingham.ac.uk
[2] Lab for Uncertainty in Data and Decision Making (LUCID), School of Computer Science, University of Nottingham, Nottingham, UK
[3] Nottingham Biomedical Research Centre (BRC), School of Medicine, University of Nottingham, Nottingham, UK

Abstract. Liver fibrosis poses a substantial challenge in clinical practice, emphasizing the necessity for precise liver segmentation and accurate disease staging. Based on the CARE Liver 2025 Track 4 Challenge, this study introduces a multi-task deep learning framework developed for liver segmentation (LiSeg) and liver fibrosis staging (LiFS) using multiparametric MRI. The LiSeg phase addresses the challenge of limited annotated images and the complexities of multi-parametric MRI data by employing a semi-supervised learning model that integrates image segmentation and registration. By leveraging both labeled and unlabeled data, the model overcomes the difficulties introduced by domain shifts and variations across modalities. In the LiFS phase, we employed a patch-based method which allows the visualization of liver fibrosis stages based on the classification outputs. Our approach effectively handles multimodality imaging data, limited labels, and domain shifts. The proposed method has been tested by the challenge organizer on an independent test set that includes in-distribution (ID) and out-of-distribution (OOD) cases using three-channel MRIs (T1, T2, DWI) and seven-channel MRIs (T1, T2, DWI, GED1-GED4). The code is freely available. Github link: https://github.com/mileywang3061/Care-Liver.

Keywords: Liver fibrosis · Multi-parametric MRI · Patch-based classification

1 Introduction

Liver fibrosis can progress to cirrhosis or hepatocellular carcinoma if not detected early. The CARE Liver 2025 challenge (Track 4) [3,8,14] aims to develop AI-based methods for liver segmentation and fibrosis staging, using multi-center,

X. Zhuang et al. (Eds.): CARE 2025, LNCS 16257, pp. 124–134, 2026.
https://doi.org/10.1007/978-3-032-16271-7_12

multi-vendor MRI data from 610 patients with liver fibrosis. The dataset includes T1-weighted (T1), T2-weighted (T2), diffusion-weighted (DWI), and Gd-EOB-DTPA-enhanced dynamic phases (GED1–GED4), covering arterial, portal venous, delayed, and hepatobiliary phases. All data include GED4, which is always available, while other phases may be missing and are not spatially aligned.

This study addresses both segmentation and classification tasks, which are interconnected but require different modeling strategies. For the segmentation task, we focus on a semi-supervised setting, where only a small subset of GED4 images have annotated liver masks, while all other phases remain unlabeled. The multi-vendor and multi-phase nature of the dataset poses challenges such as domain shifts and misalignment between modalities. Previously developed supervised methods perform well on fully labeled, single-modality datasets but struggle with limited annotations and large modality variations. Semi-supervised approaches (e.g., Mean Teacher [9], pseudo-labeling [2,6]) leverage unlabeled data, but often fail to ensure spatial and structural consistency across modalities. In contrast, joint registration–segmentation frameworks [5,7,15] have shown promise by maintaining geometric structure and label consistency through spatial alignment.

Recent advancements in liver fibrosis classification have increasingly leveraged deep learning and radiomics to improve diagnostic accuracy and clinical interpretability. Convolutional neural networks (CNNs) applied to gadoxetic acid-enhanced MR images have demonstrated promising performance [16]. More recently, transformer-based architectures, such as the Vision Transformer (ViT), have exploited self-attention mechanisms to enhance feature representation [1,10]. Complementary to deep learning, radiomics extracts high-dimensional quantitative features from medical images, including texture, shape, and intensity [11,13]. Current trends emphasize the integration of multi-view learning and uncertainty modeling to simultaneously improve accuracy and interpretability. For example, Gao et al. [3] proposed a framework combining local and global features to achieve reliable and interpretable results, while MERIT [8] further incorporates feature-specific evidential fusion and class-distribution-aware calibration, outperforming traditional CNN and radiomics based approaches.

In this study, we propose a framework for liver segmentation and fibrosis staging from multi-phase and multi-vendor liver MRI data. For segmentation, the BRBS framework [5] is adopted and improved to jointly learn registration and segmentation in a semi-supervised manner, enabling label propagation across modalities and improving performance with limited annotations. For classification, a patch-based strategy is introduced to capture fine-grained intensity and texture features, where Stage 1 and Stage 4 image patches serve as the surrogates for healthy and unhealthy tissues, and subject-level stages are inferred from the proportion of Stage 4 patches. By integrating both tasks, the framework ensures that segmentation outputs support classification, enhancing reliability and clinical applicability.

2 Methods

As illustrated in Fig. 1, the overall framework consists of two main stages: semi-supervised multi-parametric MRI segmentation and patch-based fibrosis classification. The multi-parametric MRI with the labeled GED4 masks are first input into the Better Registration Better Segmentation (BRBS) framework [5] to generate the masks for unlabeled GED4 images. The multi-parametric MRI is also input to the ANTs algorithm [12] to be spatially aligned. Subsequently, the aligned MRIs and their corresponding GED4 masks are used in the patch-based classification model based on the ResNet18 architecture to achieve fibrosis classification.

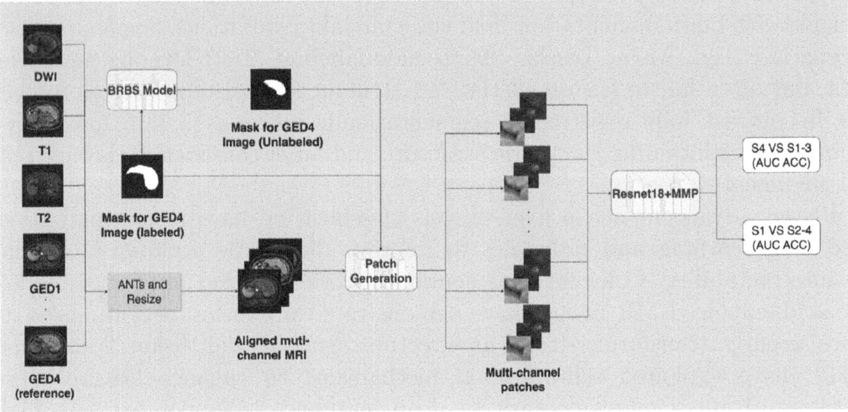

Fig. 1. Overview of the proposed framework. Multi-parametric MRI (DWI, T1, T2, GED1–GED4 with GED4 as reference) are aligned using ANTs [12], and the liver masks of unlabeled GED4 are generated by the BRBS model. Multi-channel patches are extracted by ResNet18 and probability mapping for cirrhosis (S4 vs. S1–3) and substantial (S1 vs. S2–4) fibrosis classification

2.1 Semi-supervised Liver Segmentation and MRI Alignment

The liver segmentation of GED4 images is performed using the BRBS framework [5], which jointly learns registration and segmentation in a semi-supervised setting. In the CARE Liver 2025 dataset, only the hepatobiliary phase (GED4) provides manual annotations, while other phases remain unlabeled. BRBS addresses this by registering each unlabeled modality to GED4 and warping the manual mask to generate pseudo-labels, thereby enabling the segmentation network to be supervised across all phases.

To improve pseudo-label reliability, BRBS introduces two mechanisms. The **Weighted Consistency Constraint (WCC)** requires the warped atlas mask to match the segmentation prediction, while the estimated deformation fields are constrained to be smooth and cycle-consistent. The **Space–Style Sampling Program (S3P)** augments supervision by interpolating spatial deformations and style displacements between atlas and another unlabeled image. The resulting synthetic pairs capture intermediate anatomical shapes and contrast variations. Together, WCC and S3P enhance the authenticity, diversity, and robustness of pseudo-labels, enabling reliable semi-supervised liver segmentation across all MRIs.

In the original BRBS design, the registration sub-network is trained using Normalized Cross-Correlation (NCC) as the similarity loss. However, due to the multi-modal nature of the CARE Liver dataset, we replace NCC with a local, patch-based Mutual Information (MI) loss [4], which is more robust to modality-dependent intensity variations.

For each patch p, we compute the mutual information between the fixed image X and the moving image Y as:

$$\mathrm{MI}^{(p)}(X,Y) = \sum_{i,j} P_{XY}^{(p)}(i,j) \log\left(\frac{P_{XY}^{(p)}(i,j)+\varepsilon}{P_X^{(p)}(i)P_Y^{(p)}(j)+\varepsilon}\right) \tag{1}$$

where $P_{XY}^{(p)}(i,j)$ is the joint histogram over intensity bins i and j in patch p, and $P_X^{(p)}(i)$ and $P_Y^{(p)}(j)$ are the marginal histograms. The constant $\varepsilon = 10^{-6}$ ensures numerical stability.

The final local mutual information loss is defined as the negative mean MI across all N_{patch} patches, which is fully differentiable and compatible with deep learning frameworks.

$$\mathcal{L}\mathrm{MI} = 1 - \frac{1}{N_{\text{patch}}} \sum_{p=1}^{N_{\text{patch}}} \mathrm{MI}^{(p)}(X,Y) \tag{2}$$

The segmentation network is supervised using Dice loss on the labeled images, while pseudo-labels generated for the unlabeled images extend supervision across all modalities. We used the BRBS method mainly to achieve semi-supervised liver segmentation. The multi-modality MRI alignment results are generated by applying ANTs [12] rigid registration, which are found to be better than the BRBS deformable registration results for this task.

The aligned multi-parametric MRIs and their corresponding liver masks are then used in the classification model for patch extraction from the liver region.

2.2 Patch-Based Liver Fibrosis Staging

A patch-based classification strategy was employed, leveraging the pathological manifestations of liver fibrosis across different stages. Based on the aligned multi-parametric MRIs, overlapping and multi-channel patches are extracted from the liver region. Several patch sizes (8×8, 16×16, and 32×32) were evaluated, with 16×16 achieving the best performance given the input image size. The multi-channel patches for non-contrast data are three channels (i.e. T1, T2, DWI), and for contrast-enhanced data are seven channels (i.e. T1, T2, DWI, GED1-GED4). To handle missing modalities, zero-filled channels were used.

We hypothesize that liver fibrosis occurs in a local region rather than necessarily affecting the whole liver region, especially for the intermediate stages 2 and 3. Hence, for model training, we only sample patches from Stage 1 and Stage 4 subjects to form the "good" and "bad" patches, respectively, for a binary classification. The Stage 2 and Stage 3 subjects are excluded from the training and used only for validation purposes. A simplified ResNet-18 backbone was employed for patch-level feature extraction, followed by an MLP classifier.

During model inference, overlapping patches are extracted from the whole liver region of an unseen subject, and the patch-level classification is performed. The subject-level fibrosis stage is estimated by the percentage of Stage 4 patches over all patches. Thresholds τ_1 and τ_2 are determined based on a validation set and applied to the percentage value for classifying Stage 1 vs. Stage 2–4 and Stage 4 vs. Stage 1–3, respectively. This percentage value is then converted to a likelihood value between 0 to 1 using piecewise mapping functions based on the thresholds of τ_1 and τ_2. The resulting probabilities are denoted as $\hat{y}_1$ for substantial fibrosis detection (Stage 1 vs. Stage 2–4) and $\hat{y}_4$ for cirrhosis detection (Stage 4 vs. Stage 1–3). Here is the pipeline of the classification process:

Given a subject with modalities $\{M_i\}_{i=1}^{K}$ and segmentation mask Ω:

1. **Patch extraction:**

$$\mathcal{P} = \left\{ p_j(M_i \odot \Omega) \;\middle|\; i = 1, \ldots, K,\ j = 1, \ldots, N \right\}$$

$\mathcal{P}$ contains N overlapping 16×16 patches from all K modalities, with zero-filling to handle missing channels.

2. **Patch-level classification:**

$$z_j = f_{\text{ResNet18+MLP}}(p_j), \quad z_j \in \{0, 1\}$$

where $z_j = 1$ denotes a Stage 4-like patch.

3. **Subject-level scoring:**

$$s = \frac{1}{N} \sum_{j=1}^{N} z_j$$

s is the proportion of Stage 4-like patches.

4. **Fibrosis probability mapping:**

$$\hat{y}_1 = \begin{cases} 1 - \frac{0.5}{\tau_1} s, & 0 \leq s \leq \tau_1 \\ 0.5 - \frac{0.5}{1-\tau_1} (s - \tau_1), & \tau_1 < s \leq 1 \end{cases}$$

$$\hat{y}_4 = \begin{cases} \frac{0.5s}{\tau_2}, & 0 \leq s \leq \tau_2 \\ \frac{0.5(s-\tau_2)}{(1-\tau_2)} + 0.5, & \tau_2 < s \leq 1 \end{cases}$$

with threshold τ_1 and τ_2 optimized on the validation set.

3 Experiments and Results

3.1 Dataset

The experiments were conducted on the **CARE Liver 2025 Track 4** dataset [8], which contains multi-parametric MRI scans from 610 patients diagnosed with liver fibrosis. Each subject may include part or all of the modalities: T1-weighted (T1), T2-weighted (T2), diffusion-weighted imaging (DWI), and Gd-EOB-DTPA-enhanced dynamic phases (GED1–GED4). Some modalities are missing for certain subjects; however, GED4 is consistently available for all subjects. As summarized in Table 1, the dataset is collected from multiple centers and vendors, forming three in-distribution (ID) groups: A, B1, and B2.

Table 1. Summary of dataset splits in CARE Liver 2025 Track 4. Values are shown as total cases (labeled liver mask cases)

Dataset	**A**	**B1**	**B2**	**OOD (C)**	**Total**
Training	130 (10)	170 (10)	60 (10)	–	360 (30)
Validation	20 (20)	20 (20)	20 (20)	–	60 (60)
Test	60 (60)	60 (60)	60 (60)	70 (70)	250 (250)

The training set contains 360 cases, with each group contributing 10 cases with manually annotated liver masks and the remaining cases left unlabeled. The validation set comprises 60 cases (20 per group). The test set includes 190 cases, with 60 from each ID group and 70 out-of-distribution (OOD) cases from vendor C, center C, which are used to assess model generalization.

For the segmentation experiments, we used 62 images (31 from T1 and 31 from T2) as a validation set, while all remaining images (566) were included in the training set.

For training the classification model, only 87 Stage 1 and 150 Stage 4 subjects were used. To address the substantial class imbalance, geometric transformations, such as flipping and rotation, were applied to both liver masks and all corresponding modality channels. This augmentation strategy balanced the number of patches between classes and mitigated the potential bias in model training. The validation phase included subjects from all four stages, comprising 10 Stage 1, 32 Stage 2, 64 Stage 3, and 17 Stage 4 subjects.

3.2 Parameter Setting

All segmentation experiments were conducted using a learning rate of 1×10^{-4}, with training performed for 500 epochs, each epoch consisting of 200 iterations. The network was trained from scratch using all available data (both labeled and unlabeled), as described in Sect. 3.1.

In the classification model, a learning rate of 1×10^{-4} was employed. Given the large number of patches and their high similarity, training was limited to 10 epochs. All models were trained from scratch using the cross-entropy loss.

Dynamic learning rate scheduling was applied at the iteration level, with the learning rate adjusted every 5000 iterations. We employed 4-fold cross-validation to determine the thresholds τ_1 and τ_2, which were set to 0.37 and 0.66 for non-contrast MRIs and 0.35 and 0.70 for contrast MRIs.

3.3 Liver Segmentation Results

In the challenge of liver segmentation subtasks (LiSeg), our method was evaluated on all MRI modalities of both ID and OOD tasks.

Table 2. Segmentation results on the CARE Liver 2025 validation set

Method	**GED4**		**T1**		**T2**		**DWI**	
	Dice↑	HD↓	Dice↑	HD↓	Dice↑	HD↓	Dice↑	HD↓
BRBS-NCC	0.9047	42.12	0.8935	73.90	0.7423	52.30	0.6521	45.67
BRBS-MI	0.9518	36.81	0.9345	66.75	0.8323	35.95	0.8323	35.95

Table 3. Comparison of leaderboard results on the test set for Non-Contrast subtasks. The In-Distribution data (vendors A, B1, and B2) and Out-of-Distribution data (vendor C) are evaluated separately. Only the top five teams are shown

Team	Dice(%)	HD(mm)
BIGS2	94.34	38.06
Sigma(Ours)	**93.18**	**58.99**
CitySJTU	92.62	27.80
BioDreamer	91.96	31.83
MIHL	86.42	163.91

(a) T1 (In-Distribution)

Team	Dice(%)	HD(mm)
BIGS2	95.48	22.11
Sigma(Ours)	**95.03**	**29.04**
CitySJTU	94.44	25.54
BioDreamer	94.18	28.24
MIHL	73.51	102.79

(b) T1 (Out-Of-Distribution)

Team	Dice(%)	HD(mm)
CitySJTU	88.90	34.60
BIGS2	87.22	35.24
BioDreamer	82.01	37.16
Sigma(Ours)	**75.68**	**75.44**
MIHL	20.24	121.48

(c) T2 (In-Distribution)

Team	Dice(%)	HD(mm)
BIGS2	90.15	35.17
CitySJTU	88.94	24.52
BioDreamer	84.57	25.84
Sigma(Ours)	**62.08**	**72.29**
MIHL	7.14	118.06

(d) T2 (Out-Of-Distribution)

Team	Dice(%)	HD(mm)
CitySJTU	83.74	26.96
Sigma(Ours)	**82.34**	**34.19**
BIGS2	80.29	31.04
BioDreamer	72.10	31.33
MIHL	26.12	99.25

(e) DWI (In-Distribution)

Team	Dice(%)	HD(mm)
Sigma(Ours)	**90.41**	**19.72**
CitySJTU	88.57	11.21
BIGS2	84.81	11.21
BioDreamer	78.12	15.96
MIHL	45.67	51.76

(f) DWI (Out-Of-Distribution)

We first evaluated our method on the validation set for refining our model. We compared two configurations of the BRBS framework: (1) **BRBS-NCC**, the original BRBS using NCC loss, trained with 30 annotated GED4 images and all unlabeled in the CARE Liver 2025 dataset; (2) **BRBS-MI**, where NCC is replaced by the MI loss, using the same training data as BRBS-NCC.

As shown in Table 2, replacing NCC by MI led to consistent improvement across all MRI sequences. The MI-based model (BRBS-MI) achieved higher Dice scores (Dice) and lower Hausdorff Distances (HD), especially on T2 and DWI, where modality differences were more pronounced. This demonstrates that MI better handles cross-modality variations during registration and improves label propagation.

Our method was further evaluated and compared to other teams using the test set, as shown in Table 3. Our method produced Dice values of 93.18% and 95.03% for T1 ID and T1 OOD respectively, and ranked the second place. The DWI results were particularly noteworthy: our model achieved the second best ID segmentation performance (Dice = 82.34%), and the best OOD segmentation performance (Dice = 90.41%), confirming its robustness to domain shifts and signal variations. However, segmentation on the T2 modality remained a relative lower performance compared to other methods, with Dice scores of 75.68% (ID) and 62.08% (OOD), which ranked us the fourth place. This decreased performance on T2 MRI, could be caused by the higher intensity heterogeneity and its limited representation in the training data.

3.4 Liver Fibrosis Classification Results

Based on the segmentation results, we further evaluated the classification performance of liver fibrosis staging task, and compared to other teams. Task 1 refers to the classification of Stage 4 vs. Stage 1–3, and Task 2 refers to the classification of Stage 1 vs. Stage 2–4. The area under the ROC (AUC) and classification accuracy (ACC) were calculated based on the results obtained by running our docker file on the challenge organizer's server. Table 4 presents the top five teams' performance across all fibrosis staging subtasks on the test set.

For the contrast-enhanced modality results (Table 4 (a) (d)), our method achieved the best performance in ID cases (ACC = 75.83%) for Task 1, and ranked the third for Task 2 with an ACC of 77.50%. For the OOD cases, our method achieved the second best (ACC=58.57%) and the best performance (ACC=92.86%) on Task 1 and Task 2 respectively. The results show that the model achieved high accuracies in both ID and OOD cases, demonstrating its ability to correctly stage liver fibrosis in both tasks.

For the non-contrast modality results (Table 4 (e)-(h)), our method achieved relatively lower performance than other methods for the ID cases (ranked the 5th). However, it achieved the best performance for OOD cases on both Task 1 (ACC=71.43%) and Task 2 (ACC=92.86%). This indicates that our model generalized well on test cases of unseen centers.

One advantage of using our patch-based method is that the percentage of Stage-4 patches can be visualized for certain interpretability. Figure 2 shows the

Table 4. Comparison of leaderboard results on the test set for liver fibrosis staging tasks. The In-Distribution data (vendors A, B1, and B2) and Out-of-Distribution data (vendor C) are evaluated separately. Only the top five teams are shown

Team	ACC(%)	AUC(%)
Sigma(Ours)	**75.83**	**83.92**
WSQ	72.50	78.31
Team space	71.67	79.39
CitySJTU	70.83	75.10
BioDreamer	68.33	77.19

(a) Contrast-Enhanced in S4 vs. S1-S3 (In-Distribution)

Team	ACC(%)	AUC(%)
WSQ	80.83	84.50
Team space	79.17	80.24
Sigma(Ours)	**77.50**	**83.42**
CitySJTU	75.00	78.45
BioDreamer	74.58	78.11

(b) Contrast-Enhanced in S1 vs. S2-S4 (In-Distribution)

Team	ACC(%)	AUC(%)
BioDreamer	63.71	67.40
Sigma(Ours)	**58.57**	**54.12**
Team space	52.86	60.22
CitySJTU	41.43	46.81
WSQ	41.43	66.95

(c) Contrast-Enhanced in S4 vs. S1-S3 (Out-Of-Distribution)

Team	ACC(%)	AUC(%)
Sigma(Ours)	**92.86**	**75.38**
NW-Radio	92.86	52.62
BioDreamer	92.86	47.68
WSQ	82.86	37.23
Team space	64.29	64.62

(d) Contrast-Enhancedin S1 vs. S2-S4 (Out-Of-Distribution)

Team	ACC(%)	AUC(%)
Team space	74.17	81.33
potato	72.50	77.22
CitySJTU	71.67	78.61
BioDreamer	70.83	77.89
Sigma(Ours)	**70.00**	**77.22**

(e) Non-Contrast in S4 vs. S1-S3 (In-Distribution)

Team	ACC(%)	AUC(%)
Team space	76.67	83.93
TeamZhang	74.17	68.48
potatp	71.67	78.51
BioDreamer	70.00	77.11
CitySJTU	70.00	73.71

f) Non-Contrast in S1 vs. S2-S4 (In-Distribution)

Team	ACC(%)	AUC(%)
Sigma(Ours)	**71.43**	**69.47**
potato	70.00	71.51
TeamZhang	64.29	68.83
Team space	64.29	52.73
CitySJTU	42.86	49.31

(g) Non-Contrast in S4 vs. S1-S3 (Out-Of-Distribution)

Team	ACC(%)	AUC(%)
Sigma(Ours)	**92.86**	**86.31**
NW-Radio	92.86	40.31
TeamZhang	91.43	71.38
Team space	88.57	61.23
BioDreamer	88.29	59.40

(h) Non-Contrast in S1 vs. S2-S4 (Out-Of-Distribution)

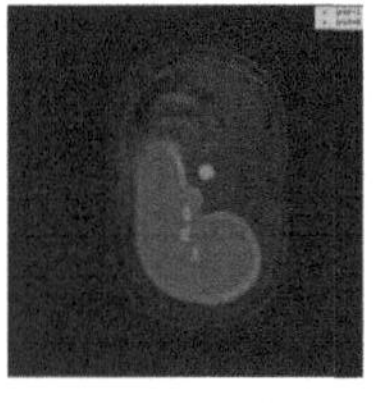

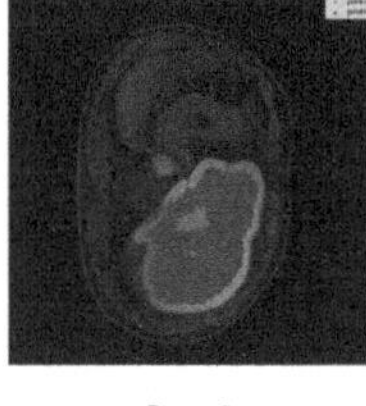

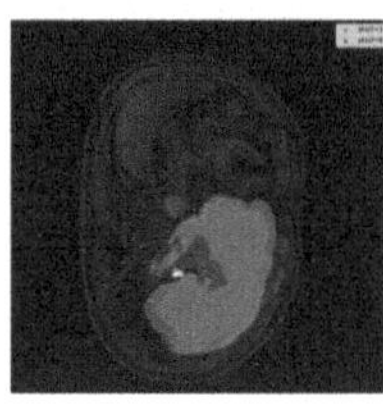

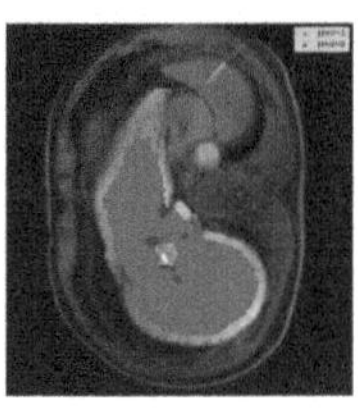

Fig. 2. Visualization of patch-level predictions at different fibrosis stages (Stage 1–4). Blue represents stage 1 patches (pred = 0), while red represents stage 4 patches (pred = 1). The percentage of blue and red patches varies with disease stage, reflecting the progression from early stages to advanced stages

visualization of the patch-level prediction for one example subject in each stage. Red presents the stage 4 patch, and blue refers to the stage 1 patch. It can be seen that as the fibrosis severity increases, the percentage of stage-4 patches increases as well.

Overall, the liver fibrosis staging results reveal that our method achieves top-tier performance in both contrast-enhanced and non-contrast modalities, with strong OOD generalization. The classification accuracy could be dependent on the liver segmentation performance (e.g. particularly lower for T2 MRI), as inaccurate liver region of interest could affect the precision of patch sampling.

4 Conclusions

We proposed a fully automated framework for liver fibrosis staging that integrates semi-supervised segmentation, multi-modality registration and a patch-based classifier. The method achieves robust segmentation across GED4, T1, T2, and DWI MRIs, and demonstrates strong performance in liver fibrosis staging, particularly using three-channel non-contrast MRIs. Importantly, the patch-based design enables visualization of localized pathological regions, offering clinically meaningful insights for objective liver fibrosis assessment. Future work will focus on streamlining the framework to improve the efficiency and accuracy.

References

1. Dai, Y., Gao, Y., Liu, F.: Transmed: transformers advance multi-modal medical image classification. Diagnostics **11**(8), 1384 (2021)
2. Deng, G., Sun, H., Xie, W.: Correlation-based switching mean teacher for semi-supervised medical image segmentation. Neurocomputing **633**, 129818 (2025)
3. Gao, Z., Liu, Y., Wu, F., Shi, N., Shi, Y., Zhuang, X.: A reliable and interpretable framework of multi-view learning for liver fibrosis staging. In: International Conference on Medical Image Computing and Computer-Assisted Intervention, pp. 178–188 (2023)
4. Guo, C.K.: Multi-modal image registration with unsupervised deep learning. Ph.D. thesis, Massachusetts Institute of Technology (2019)
5. He, Y., Ge, R., Qi, X., Chen, Y., Wu, J., Coatrieux, J.L., Yang, G., Li, S.: Learning better registration to learn better few-shot medical image segmentation: authenticity, diversity, and robustness. IEEE Trans. Neural Netw. Learn. Syst. **35**(2), 2588–2601 (2022)
6. Jia, D.: Semi-supervised multi-organ segmentation with cross supervision using siamese network. In: MICCAI Challenge on Fast and Low-Resource Semi-supervised Abdominal Organ Segmentation, pp. 293–306. Springer (2022)
7. Li, R., Figueredo, G., Auer, D., Dineen, R., Morgan, P., Chen, X.: A unified framework for semi-supervised image segmentation and registration. In: 2025 IEEE 22nd International Symposium on Biomedical Imaging (ISBI), pp. 1–5. IEEE (2025)
8. Liu, Y., Gao, Z., Shi, N., Wu, F., Shi, Y., Chen, Q., Zhuang, X.: Merit: multi-view evidential learning for reliable and interpretable liver fibrosis staging. Med. Image Anal. **102**, 103507 (2025)
9. Lou, Q., Lin, T., Qian, Y., Lu, F.: Semi-supervised liver segmentation based on local regions self-supervision. Med. Phys. **51**(5), 3455–3463 (2024)
10. Manzari, O.N., Ahmadabadi, H., Kashiani, H., Shokouhi, S.B., Ayatollahi, A.: Medvit: a robust vision transformer for generalized medical image classification. Comput. Biol. Med. **157**, 106791 (2023)
11. Park, H.J., Lee, S.S., Park, B., Yun, J., Sung, Y.S., Shim, W.H., Shin, Y.M., Kim, S.Y., Lee, S.J., Lee, M.G.: Radiomics analysis of gadoxetic acid-enhanced mri for staging liver fibrosis. Radiology **290**(2), 380–387 (2019)

12. Tustison, N.J., Cook, P.A., Holbrook, A.J., Johnson, H.J., Muschelli, J., Devenyi, G.A., Duda, J.T., Das, S.R., Cullen, N.C., Gillen, D.L., et al.: The antsx ecosystem for quantitative biological and medical imaging. Sci. Rep. **11**(1), 9068 (2021)
13. Wang, K., Lu, X., Zhou, H., Gao, Y., Zheng, J., Tong, M., Wu, C., Liu, C., Huang, L., Jiang, T., et al.: Deep learning radiomics of shear wave elastography significantly improved diagnostic performance for assessing liver fibrosis in chronic hepatitis b: a prospective multicentre study. Gut **68**(4), 729–741 (2019)
14. Wu, F., Zhuang, X.: Minimizing estimated risks on unlabeled data: a new formulation for semi-supervised medical image segmentation. IEEE Trans. Pattern Anal. Mach. Intell. **45**(5), 6021–6036 (2023)
15. Xu, Z., Niethammer, M.: Deepatlas: joint semi-supervised learning of image registration and segmentation. In: International Conference on Medical Image Computing and Computer-Assisted Intervention, pp. 420–429. Springer (2019)
16. Yasaka, K., Akai, H., Abe, O., Kiryu, S.: Deep learning with convolutional neural network for differentiation of liver masses at dynamic contrast-enhanced ct: a preliminary study. Radiology **286**(3), 887–896 (2018)

A Two-Stage Myocardial Pathology Segmentation Method Based on Multi-sequence CMR Images

Yonghui Wang, Chanyue Zhao, Patrice Monkam, and Shouliang Qi(✉)

College of Medicine and Biological Information Engineering, Northeastern University, Shenyang, China
2410579@stu.neu.edu.cn

Abstract. Myocardial pathology segmentation is crucial for quantifying myocardial danger zones in the diagnosis of acute myocardial infarction. However, effective segmentation remains challenging due to incomplete image sequences, the need to view different pathologies on different CMR sequences, difficulties in aligning pathology regions, the limited resolution of some clinical CMR sequences and the small size of myocardial lesions. To address these issues, we propose a two-stage method for segmenting myocardial lesions in CMR images. This method considers the inherent incompleteness of CMR sequences and the distinct characteristics of edema and scar tissue, enabling the segmentation of normal myocardium and two pathological regions: edema and scar tissue. We validated our method using CARE 2025 Challenge CMR images, and the results on the validation set demonstrate its effectiveness in segmenting complex myocardial pathologies. Validation showed Dice scores of 0.5302 and 0.5308 for edema and scar, respectively. These findings highlight the effectiveness and broad applicability of our segmentation approach in clinical settings.

Keywords: Multi-center learning · Late gadolinium enhancement · Two-stage segmentation · Myocardial infarction

1 Introduction

Acute myocardial infarction (AMI) is one of the leading causes of morbidity and mortality worldwide. It is primarily triggered by the rupture or detachment of an atherosclerotic plaque in the coronary arteries, resulting in acute vascular occlusion and subsequent myocardial ischemia. If blood flow is not promptly restored, the ischemic myocardium first develops interstitial edema, and sustained ischemia eventually leads to irreversible necrosis, forming a myocardial infarction (MI) [1]. Cardiac magnetic resonance (CMR) imaging is the gold standard for non-invasive characterization of myocardial tissue pathology [2]. Among its various sequences, late gadolinium enhancement (LGE) and T2-weighted imaging (T2WI) are particularly useful for detecting scar and edema, respectively. In LGE images, infarcted myocardium appears as high signal regions due to delayed washout of gadolinium contrast in fibrotic tissue [3]. In T2-weighted sequences,

X. Zhuang et al. (Eds.): CARE 2025, LNCS 16257, pp. 135–144, 2026.
https://doi.org/10.1007/978-3-032-16271-7_13

myocardial edema also presents as high signal intensity due to increased water content in the tissue [4]. Both LGE and T2 sequences offer excellent tissue contrast and spatial resolution, allowing clear delineation of the myocardium and associated pathologies. Notably, both scar and edema are localized within the myocardial region, and in many cases, edema surrounds the scar core, reflecting the "area at risk" during the acute phase of AMI. These imaging features are not only valuable for diagnosis and risk stratification, but also provide critical prior knowledge for automated segmentation models in CMR-based myocardial pathology analysis.

With the rapid advancement of deep learning techniques, an increasing number of models have been applied to the segmentation of myocardial pathologies. Among these, convolutional neural network (CNN)-based architectures remain the most prevalent, with U-Net [5] serving as the dominant framework. Nevertheless, myocardial scars and edema present considerable segmentation challenges due to their small volumes, irregular morphologies, and heterogeneous distribution within the myocardium. Leveraging prior anatomical knowledge can partially alleviate these difficulties: as both scars and edema are confined to the myocardial region, a coarse-to-fine segmentation strategy can be employed, first delineating the myocardium, followed by the localization of pathological regions. In this study, myocardial pathology segmentation is formulated as a two-stage process: (1) segmentation of the myocardium and (2) segmentation of myocardial scars and edema. The latter are typically visualized using distinct cardiac magnetic resonance (CMR) sequences, late gadolinium enhancement (LGE) for scars and T2-weighted imaging for edema. Owing to cardiac motion during CMR acquisition, these sequences often require post-processing registration to achieve spatial correspondence [6]. However, registration is hindered by the small size and irregular shapes of the target lesions. To address this, we develop independent segmentation models for the automatic detection of myocardial scars and edema.

2 Methods

2.1 Dataset

The CARE Challenge dataset comprises data from seven centers, with considerable variation in sequence types across sites. Centers A and H contain only LGE sequences, with 81 and 35 participants, respectively; notably, Centre H provides annotations solely for the scar region. Centers B and C offer more comprehensive data, including CINE, LGE, and T2 sequences, with 50 and 45 participants, respectively. Centre D, designated for testing, includes 20 participants. Centers E, F, and G contain only CINE and LGE sequences, with 7, 9, and 8 participants, respectively. Among these centers, only B and C provide T2 sequences for training. For participants with LGE sequences from centers other than H, annotations include the left and right ventricles, myocardium, and scar; for those with T2 sequences, annotations include edema. Furthermore, substantial intercenter variation exists in the distribution of CMR sequences, as illustrated in Fig. 1. Differences are evident in both image intensity distribution and short-axis resolution: Centers C and D achieve a resolution of approximately 0.7 mm in the short-axis plane, whereas the other centers have a resolution of around 1.3 mm.

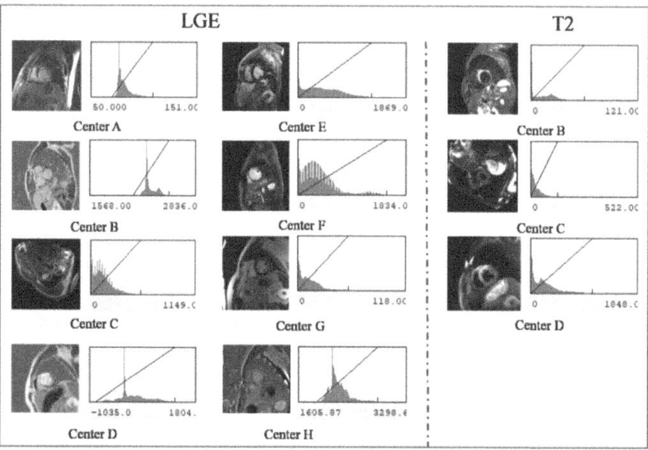

Fig. 1. The CARE2025 Myops dataset includes multi-center LGE and T2 sequences and intensity distributions. The LGE sequences include data from eight centers, and the T2 sequences include data from three centers. Centre D is used for testing, and the other centers are used for training.

There is a certain degree of misalignment between different sequences, and the myocardium in the T2 sequence does not perfectly correspond to that in the LGE sequence. As shown in Fig. 2, there is a marked difference in myocardial thickness between the two sequences. In the right T2 sequence, the region labelled as myocardial scar actually corresponds to the left ventricle, which is entirely due to misalignment between the sequences. Because edema and scar occupy relatively small areas, registration errors are visually amplified. Consequently, different sequences are employed to segment different pathological regions of the myocardium: LGE sequences are used for myocardial scar, whereas T2 sequences are used for edema.

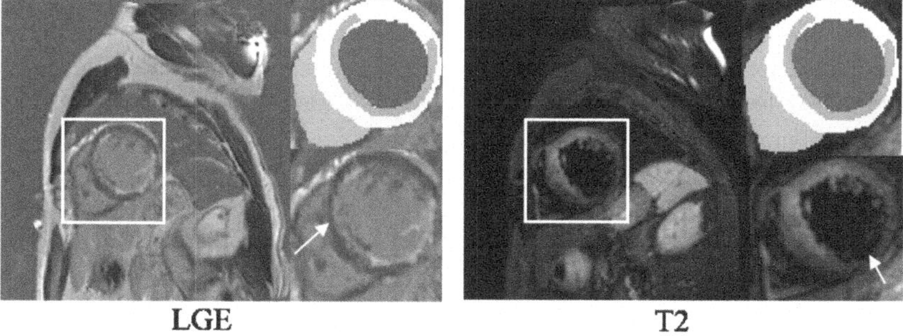

Fig. 2. This is a schematic diagram showing the registration failures of the LGE and T2 sequences in the CARE2025Myops dataset. The white arrows indicate areas with significant registration inaccuracies, which result in incorrect labeling. The labelled locations include the left and right ventricles, the left ventricular myocardium, edema and scars.

2.2 Overview

This section presents an overview of the proposed segmentation framework, as illustrated in Fig. 3. It details the overall pipeline, the segmentation architecture, and the loss functions employed during training. The algorithm consists of two stages: Stage-myo and Stage-mi.

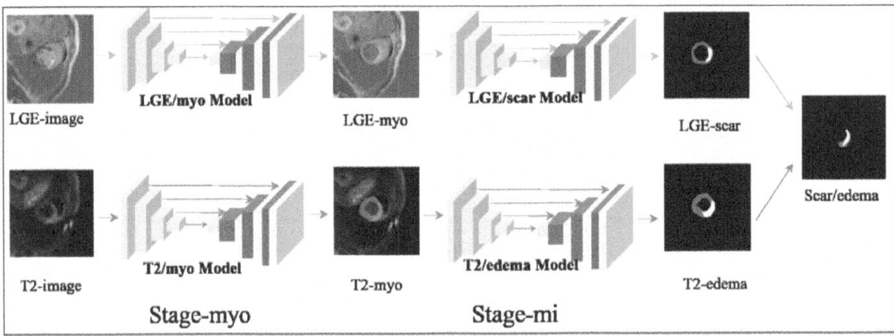

Fig. 3. The proposed two-stage framework segments myocardial pathology using LGE and T2 sequences independently for scars and edema, respectively. It comprises two stages: Stage-myo and Stage-mi.

We adopt a two-stage approach to segment the myocardium and associated pathologies. In the first stage, the myocardium is segmented. In the second stage, pathological regions within the myocardium are segmented. Because different pathologies are best visualized in different sequences, for instance, scar is more apparent in LGE sequences, while edema is more apparent in T2 sequences. We employ independent sequence-specific models for each pathology. An LGE myocardial segmentation model was trained using short-axis LGE images from multiple centers, with each center's data normalized independently. Likewise, a T2 myocardial segmentation model was trained using short-axis T2 images from multiple centers, also normalized independently. The resulting myocardial masks from the LGE and T2 models were then used to train dedicated segmentation models for scar and edema, respectively. All models were implemented using the U-Net architecture.

2.3 Model Structure

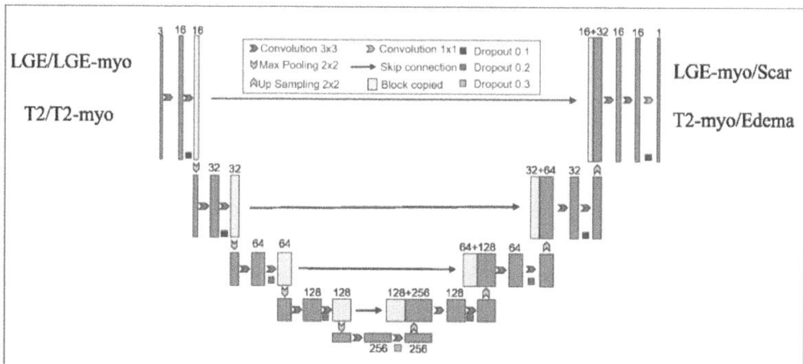

Fig. 4. The U-shaped network is a commonly used segmentation model in two-stage myocardial pathology segmentation.

We segment scars and edema through two independent branches, each comprising two stages, resulting in a total of four models. All models share the same architecture, illustrated in Fig. 4, which is a validated and widely adopted design for segmentation tasks. Each stage is built on a backbone network consisting of an encoder, a decoder, and skip connections. The encoder–decoder structure follows the U-Net design, incorporating five down-sampling and five up-sampling layers. A 3D convolutional neural network (CNN) is employed to preserve myocardial continuity along the heart's longitudinal axis. This approach effectively addresses both the anatomical continuity of the myocardium and the irregular spatial distribution of myocardial scar.

2.4 Loss Function

We employed a combination of cross-entropy loss [7] and Dice loss [8] for all four segmentation models. While cross-entropy loss is widely used for pixel-level classification, it is less sensitive to spatial continuity within the same semantic region. To mitigate this limitation, we incorporated Dice loss, which enhances spatial consistency and improves the delineation between different anatomical structures. The overall loss function is defined as:

$$L_c = -\frac{1}{N}\sum_{i=0}^{C-1} w_i y_i \log(p_i) \tag{1}$$

$$L_d = \frac{1}{N}\sum_{i=0}^{C-1} 1 - Dice_i \tag{2}$$

$$L = \lambda_c \cdot L_c + \lambda_d \cdot L_d \tag{3}$$

where p_i and y_i represent the predicted probability and label, respectively, w_i represents the weight of each class and $Dice_i$ represents the Dice value for the ith class. λ_c and λ_d represent the cross-entropy and Dice loss weights, respectively.

3 Experiments

In this section, we validate the effectiveness of our method. The experimental setup mainly consists of data preprocessing, training details, and evaluation metrics.

3.1 Data Preprocessing

Data preprocessing primarily involved normalizing sequences from different centers and standardizing image sizes. Although the same normalization approach was applied across centers, the specific normalization parameters varied. Data preprocessing primarily involved normalizing sequences from different centers and adjusting image sizes. Although the same normalization strategy was applied across centers, the specific parameters varied. For the LGE sequence at Centre A, voxel values were clipped to [0,100] and divided by 100 to scale to [0, 1]. At Centre B, values were reduced by 1500, clipped to [0, 1500], and then divided by 1500. At Centre C, values were clipped to [0,800] and divided by 800, while at Centre D, values were increased by 1000, clipped to [0, 3000], and divided by 3000. For Centre E, values were clipped to [0, 2000] and divided by 2000, and for Centers F and G, values were clipped to [0,200] and divided by 200. For the T2 sequence at Centers B and C, voxel values were standardized by subtracting the mean and dividing by the standard deviation.

During the myocardial segmentation stage, substantial variations in image size and short-axis resolution were observed across different centers. Initially, the original images were padded along the z-axis to 12 slices and then cropped into $12 \times 128 \times 128$ patches for model training. In the subsequent pathological segmentation stage, the myocardial center images obtained from the previous stage were similarly cropped to $12 \times 128 \times 128$ and input into the pathological segmentation model. Consistent data augmentation strategies were applied to both datasets during the Stage-myo and Stage-mi training phases, primarily involving a set of geometric transformations, including translation, flipping, rotation, and scaling. Rotation and scaling were restricted to the short-axis plane, with rotation angles ranging from -180° to 180°. These augmentation procedures are designed to improve the model's robustness against inter-individual variability and imaging inconsistencies.

3.2 Train Detail

We used the same optimizer and hyperparameter settings to train the four segmentation models. The models were trained using the Adam optimizer [9] for 500 epochs with an initial learning rate of 0.001. The learning rate was then reduced by a factor of 0.1 at iterations 50, 100 and 150. The momentum parameters β_1 and β_2 were set to 0.9 and 0.999, respectively, with a batch size of 4, and the code was implemented using the PyTorch framework. The runtime environment configuration is as follows: The Central Processing Unit (CPU) is an Intel(R) Core(TM) i7–7700 processor running at 3.60 GHz; the Graphics Processing Unit (GPU) is an NVIDIA GeForce RTX 3090; and the memory is 24 GB.

3.3 Evaluation Metrics

We used the main evaluation metrics of the CARE Challenge, which combine clinical and geometric metrics, including the Dice coefficient and Hausdorff distance (HD) [10]. The Dice coefficient is used to measure the degree of overlap between two sets and is defined as follows:

$$\text{Dice} = \frac{2|P \cap G|}{|P| + |G|} \tag{4}$$

where P is the final predicted result, and G is the label. The Dice lies between 0 (no overlap) and 1 (perfect overlap). HD is another commonly used metric for evaluating the degree of mismatch between two sets and is defined as follows:

$$\text{HD} = \max\{\max_{p \in P} d(p, G), \max_{g \in G} d(g, P)\} \tag{5}$$

where d(a, b) $= min_{b \in B}\|a - b\|$ denotes the minimum Euclidean distance from point a $\in$ A to set B.

4 Results

This section presents the segmentation results achieved by the two-stage myocardial pathology segmentation method on CARE2025 datasets.

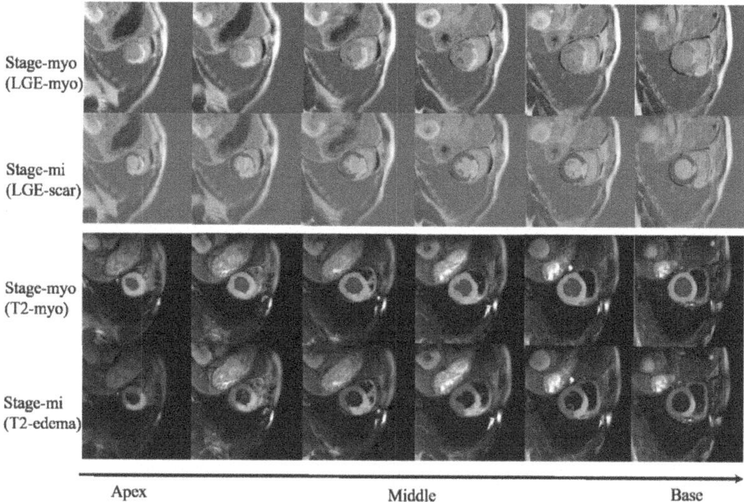

Fig. 5. Segmentation results for Case 1 from center D of the CARE2025 validation set, including LGE and T2 sequences. The LGE sequence depicts segmentation of myocardial tissue and scars, while the T2 sequence depicts segmentation of myocardial tissue and edema.

As shown in Fig. 5, we visualized the segmentation results for Case 1 in the validation set, including myocardial tissue and scar in the LGE sequence, as well as myocardial tissue and edema in the T2 sequence. Examination of myocardial tissue segmentation in the validation set indicated satisfactory performance, with nearly all tissue correctly encompassing the scarred areas. The T2 sequence, being a black-blood sequence, provides clear myocardial structure, which facilitates accurate segmentation. Across subjects, the myocardium consistently appears as a ring-shaped structure in CMR sequences, contributing to the robustness of the segmentation. In the validation set, the Dice score for scar segmentation was 0.5308 with a HD of 21.96, while for edema, the Dice score was 0.5302 with an HD of 29.45 (Fig. 6).

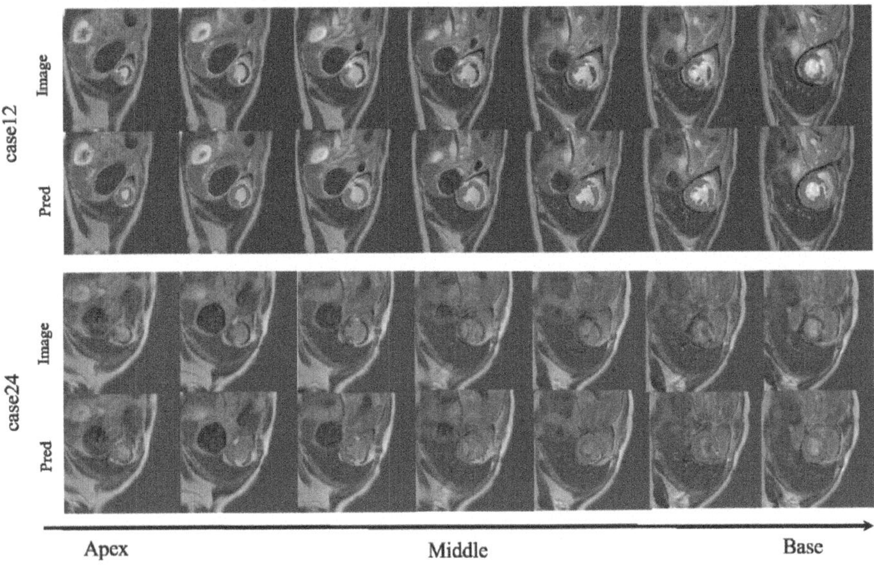

Fig. 6. Visualization of segmentation results for Cases 12 and 24 from center D of the CARE2025 validation set. In the LGE sequence, red indicates normal myocardial tissue and green indicates scar tissue. Both cases exhibit a large MVO region.

The segmentation of certain scar regions remains suboptimal, as these regions would typically fully encircle the MVO. When the MVO is large, it may be misclassified as myocardial tissue rather than scar tissue, whereas small MVO regions are not affected. As illustrated in cases 12 and 24 of the validation set, the MVO nearly spans from the endocardium to the epicardium, resulting in failed scar segmentation by the model. For edema segmentation, the model can accurately delineate high-contrast regions within the myocardium once the T2 myocardial region is extracted. Nevertheless, artefacts in some myocardial areas are the main source of inaccurate edema segmentation.

5 Discussion and Conclusion

In this study, we developed a two-stage model for segmenting myocardial scar and edema in multi-sequence CMR images, enabling the identification of both myocardial scars and edema. Due to registration errors between LGE and T2 sequences, these sequences were processed separately for scar and edema segmentation, respectively. Since both pathologies are confined to the myocardial region, we first segmented the myocardium and subsequently segmented the scar and edema within it. All models employed 3D U-Net for segmentation. Given that the CARE2025 dataset comprises sequences from multiple centers, we applied sequence-specific normalization parameters during training and validation. On the CARE2025 validation set, the Dice scores for scar and edema segmentation were 0.5308 and 0.5302, respectively.

The two-stage myocardial pathology segmentation model demonstrates accurate delineation of myocardial scarring and edema, primarily because initial myocardial segmentation effectively reduces false-positive pathology regions. Furthermore, in cross-center segmentation, careful pre-processing of multi-center CMR sequences is crucial. We selected widely used medical image segmentation models to achieve robust segmentation of myocardial scarring and edema. While the proposed workflow is simple and logically structured, there remains considerable room for improvement in segmentation accuracy, particularly in multi-center data integration, which will be the main focus of future work.

Declaration of Competing Interest. The authors declare that they have no known competing financial interests or personal relationships that could have appeared to influence the work reported in this paper.

References

1. Thygesen, K., Alpert, J.S., White, H.D., et al.: Universal definition of myocardial infarction[J]. J. Am. Coll. Cardiol. **50**(22), 2173–2195 (2007)
2. Muraki, R., Teramoto, A., Sugimoto, K., et al.: Automated detection scheme for acute myocardial infarction using convolutional neural network and long short-term memory[J]. PLoS ONE **17**(2), e0264002 (2022)
3. Li, W., Wang, L., Qin, S.: CMS-UNet: cardiac multi-task segmentation in MRI with a u-shaped network [M]. In: Myocardial Pathology Segmentation Combining Multi-Sequence CMR Challenge. Cham: Springer International Publishing, 92–101 (2020)
4. Ferreira, V.M., Piechnik, S.K., Dall'Armellina, E., Karamitsos, T.D., Francis, J.M., Ntusi, N., Holloway, C., Choudhury, R.P., Kardos, A., Robson, M.D., et al.: T1 mapping for the diagnosis of acute myocarditis using CMR: comparison to T2-weighted and late gadolinium enhanced imaging. JACC: Cardiovasc. Imaging **6**, 1048–1058 (2013)
5. Ronneberger, O, Fischer. P, Brox, T.U-net: Convolutional networks for biomedical image segmentation[C]. In: Medical image computing and computer-assisted intervention–MICCAI 2015: 18th international conference, Munich, Germany, October 5–9, 2015, proceedings, part III 18. Springer international publishing, 234–241 (2015)
6. Zhuang, X.: Multivariate mixture model for myocardial segmentation combining multi-source images. IEEE Trans. Pattern Anal. Mach. Intell. **41**(12), 2933–2946 (2018)

7. Mao, A., Mohri, M., Zhong, Y.: Cross-entropy loss functions: theoretical analysis and applications[C]. In: International conference on Machine learning. PMLR, 23803–23828 (2023)
8. Li, X., Sun, X., Meng, Y., et al. : Dice loss for data-imbalanced NLP tasks[J] (2019). arXiv: 1911.02855
9. Kingma, D.P., Ba, J.A.: A method for stochastic optimization[J] (2014) arXiv:1412.6980
10. Vesal, S., Ravikumar, N., Maier, A.: Automated multi-sequence cardiac MRI segmentation using supervised domain adaptation[C]. In; International workshop on statistical atlases and computational models of the heart. Cham: Springer International Publishing, 300–308 (2019)

Decoupled Teacher-Student Framework for Few-Shot Liver Segmentation with Boundary-Aware Learning

Yu Xie, Zhenyu Chen, Yuxin Lin, Yan Huang, and Mingjing Yang(✉)

College of Physics and Information Engineering, Fuzhou University, Fuzhou 350108, China
yangmj5@fzu.edu.cn

Abstract. Accurate segmentation of the liver from Hepatobiliary Phase (HBP) Magnetic Resonance Imaging (MRI) is of significant clinical importance for non-invasive liver fibrosis assessment. Deep learning-based approaches, however, are often constrained by the limited availability of annotated data, leading to suboptimal model performance in few-shot learning scenarios. To address this challenge, we propose a decoupled teacher-student learning framework featuring a two-stage training strategy. Initially, a teacher model is trained on a small set of labeled images to generate pseudo-labels for a larger, unlabeled dataset. Subsequently, we train a structurally enhanced student model on the combined set of original labels and generated pseudo-labels. A key innovation of our framework is the decoupling of the pseudo-label generation and student learning stages, which effectively mitigates error reinforcement. To further enhance segmentation quality, we introduce a comprehensive enhancement scheme for the student model. This scheme incorporates three key components: a Signed Distance Function (SDF)-based loss as the cornerstone of our boundary-aware learning approach, which compels the model to leverage rich geometric information at organ contours; an Atrous Spatial Pyramid Pooling (ASPP) module to capture multi-scale structures; and a progressive training paradigm tailored for datasets of heterogeneous quality. Our proposed method was evaluated on the CARE2025 challenge dataset, and the experimental results demonstrated the effectiveness of our framework for robust segmentation in data-limited medical imaging contexts.

Keywords: Few-shot Liver Segmentation · Decoupled Teacher-Student Learning · Boundary-Aware Learning

1 Introduction

The non-invasive quantitative assessment of liver fibrosis holds significant importance for clinical diagnosis and treatment [6,15], for which automated analysis based on Hepatobiliary Phase (HBP) Magnetic Resonance Imaging (MRI) offers

X. Zhuang et al. (Eds.): CARE 2025, LNCS 16257, pp. 145–155, 2026.
https://doi.org/10.1007/978-3-032-16271-7_14

a promising technological path. A critical prerequisite is the precise segmentation of the liver region. Manual delineation, the current gold standard, is a time-consuming and labor-intensive process that suffers from considerable inter- and intra-observer variability. To address these limitations, automated segmentation methods based on deep learning, particularly Convolutional Neural Networks (CNNs) like U-Net [18], have achieved remarkable success [4,9]. However, their reliance on large-scale annotated data remains a key limitation, especially in few-shot scenarios where performance often declines substantially.

To tackle data scarcity, Semi-Supervised Learning (SSL) [3,24,27] has emerged as a dominant paradigm. SSL strategies largely fall into two categories: pseudo-labeling [14,25] and consistency regularization [11,13,16,22]. The latter category includes co-training and mutual-learning frameworks [21,29], such as the Mutual Correction Framework (MCF) [23], which leverage consistency checks between diverse network branches or augmented views to learn from unlabeled data. Despite their effectiveness, both paradigms are vulnerable to a critical failure mode under extreme data scarcity: a detrimental self-reinforcing error loop. In this loop, a model trained on insufficient labeled data generates inherently noisy pseudo-labels. This leads to confirmation bias, where the model continuously reinforces its own initial mistakes, causing the propagation of blurred or inaccurate contours and severely compromising clinical utility [20,25,26].

To break this performance bottleneck, we propose a decoupled teacher-student learning framework. By completely separating the generation of pseudo-labels (by the teacher) from the training of the final model (the student), our approach severs the confirmation bias cycle. However, this decoupling introduces a new challenge: the student model must learn effectively from the teacher's imperfect pseudo-labels, which often suffer from ambiguous boundaries. Therefore, we further enhance the student model to contend with this challenge. Our principal enhancement is a dedicated boundary-aware learning mechanism, inspired by prior work on boundary-focused losses [10,12]. This is complemented by an optimized network architecture and a specialized training strategy to bolster the student's ability to learn robustly from the imperfect teacher.

The main contributions of our work are:

- We propose a decoupled teacher-student learning framework that effectively utilizes unlabeled data through a generate-then-train strategy, mitigating the confirmation bias problem common in traditional semi-supervised methods.
- We design a comprehensive enhancement scheme for the student model, headlined by a boundary-aware learning module with an SDF loss to sharpen contours. This is supported by an ASPP module to enrich feature perception and a progressive training strategy to stabilize learning.
- We provide extensive experimental validation on the CARE2025 challenge dataset, where results demonstrate the effectiveness and superiority of our proposed method in the context of few-shot medical image segmentation.

2 Methods

The proposed method is a decoupled two-stage teacher-student framework designed to break the confirmation bias loop found in conventional self-training methods. The overall architecture is illustrated in Fig. 1. The core principle is the complete separation of pseudo-label generation from the optimization of the final student model, preventing a weak model from corrupting its own training process with low-quality pseudo-labels.

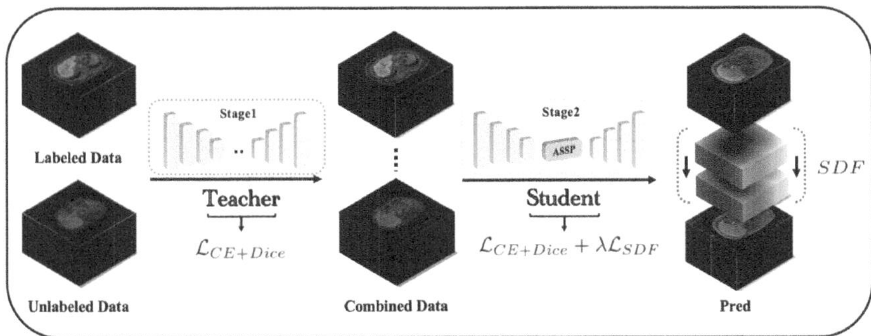

Fig. 1. The proposed two-stage decoupled teacher-student framework. In Stage 1, a teacher model is trained on limited labeled data to generate pseudo-labels for unlabeled data. In Stage 2, a student model, enhanced with an ASPP module, is trained using both the original ground-truth labels and the generated pseudo-labels to produce the final segmentation. This decoupling is key to preventing the error reinforcement seen in traditional self-training methods.

2.1 Stage 1: Teacher Training and Pseudo-Label Generation

The objective of the first stage is to extract foundational knowledge from the limited high-quality annotated data. To this end, an initial teacher model is trained using the full set of manually labeled data. The teacher model is built upon the nnU-Net framework [8], a robust, self-configuring architecture renowned for its state-of-the-art performance across numerous biomedical segmentation tasks. After training, this model performs inference on the large set of unlabeled images, and the resulting segmentation predictions are saved as pseudo-labels. This stage effectively transfers knowledge from a few expert-annotated samples to a much broader dataset, providing rich supervisory signals for the student model.

2.2 Stage 2: Enhanced Student Learning

To overcome the challenge of learning from imperfect pseudo-labels—specifically their noisy boundaries—we introduce a comprehensive enhancement scheme for the student model. First, a data-driven filtering strategy (detailed in Sect. 3.1) is employed to select a high-confidence subset of pseudo-labels, ensuring the student learns from reliable signals. Then, the student model is trained on this combined dataset of ground-truth and high-confidence pseudo-labels using a multifaceted enhancement strategy focused on boundary-aware learning, architectural optimization, and a robust training paradigm.

Loss Function Optimization for Boundary-Awareness. To explicitly address the boundary ambiguity inherent in pseudo-labels, we augment the standard segmentation loss with a term that enforces geometric consistency at object contours. Our baseline loss function, inherited from nnU-Net, is a combination of Cross-Entropy (CE) and Dice loss, denoted as $\mathcal{L}_{CE+Dice}$.

$$\mathcal{L}_{CE} = -\frac{1}{N}\sum_{i=1}^{N}\sum_{c=1}^{C} G_{ic}\log(P_{ic}) \tag{1}$$

$$\mathcal{L}_{Dice} = 1 - \frac{2\sum_{i=1}^{N} G_i P_i + \epsilon}{\sum_{i=1}^{N} G_i + \sum_{i=1}^{N} P_i + \epsilon} \tag{2}$$

To this baseline, we add a loss based on the Signed Distance Function (SDF), a technique adapted from shape representation learning [17] that is highly effective for refining boundaries in medical segmentation [28]. The total loss function $\mathcal{L}_{total}$ is a weighted sum:

$$\mathcal{L}_{total} = \mathcal{L}_{CE+Dice} + \lambda\mathcal{L}_{SDF} \tag{3}$$

where λ balances the region-based and boundary-based losses. Following prior work that utilizes SDF-based losses for medical segmentation, we set the balancing weight λ to 0.01. This value has been shown to provide an effective trade-off between region-based and boundary-based objectives [17,28] (Fig. 2).

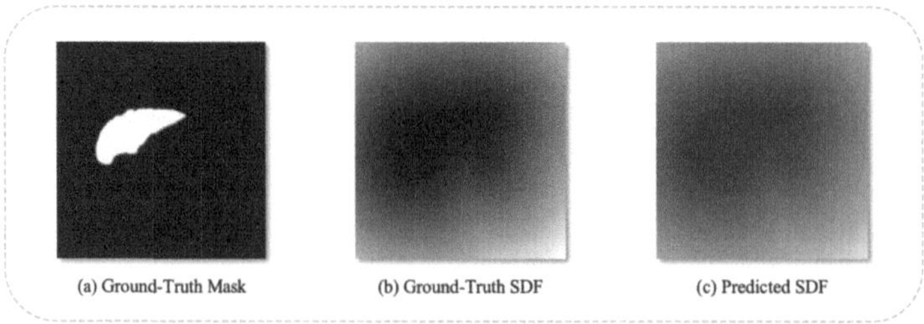

Fig. 2. Illustration of the Signed Distance Function (SDF) and the boundary loss calculation. (a) A binary ground-truth mask. (b) The corresponding SDF representation, where grayscale intensity indicates the signed distance to the boundary (darker inside, lighter outside). (c) The SDF loss is computed as the difference between the ground-truth SDF (b) and the model's predicted SDF.

The $\mathcal{L}_{SDF}$ term is the Mean Absolute Error between the model's predicted SDF map (S_{pred}) and the ground-truth SDF map (S_{gt}) over the image domain Ω:

$$\mathcal{L}_{SDF} = \frac{1}{|\Omega|} \sum_{p \in \Omega} |S_{\text{pred}}(p) - S_{\text{gt}}(p)| \tag{4}$$

Architecture Optimization for Multi-Scale Perception. To improve the student model's ability to handle significant variations in liver shape and scale, we integrate an Atrous Spatial Pyramid Pooling (ASPP) module [2] into the network's bottleneck, as shown in Fig. 3. The ASPP module employs multiple parallel atrous convolutions with different dilation rates (e.g., r=1, 6, 12, 18), allowing it to probe features at multiple receptive fields simultaneously. The resulting multi-scale feature maps are concatenated and fused, enabling the model to be sensitive to both fine details and large-scale structures, thereby enhancing segmentation accuracy.

Progressive Training Strategy. To manage the heterogeneous quality of the combined dataset, we introduce a progressive training paradigm. This involves a balanced sampling strategy, where the initial epochs alternate between samples from the ground-truth pool (L_t) and the pseudo-labeled pool (L_p). This ensures stable initial learning from high-fidelity data before heavy exposure to noisier labels. Furthermore, an asymmetric data augmentation scheme [19] is applied, where significantly more aggressive spatial and intensity transformations (e.g., elastic deformations, random rotations) are applied exclusively to the pseudo-labeled data. This acts as a form of regularization, compelling the model to learn core, invariant anatomical features and reducing its susceptibility to overfitting on the noise inherent in the teacher's predictions.

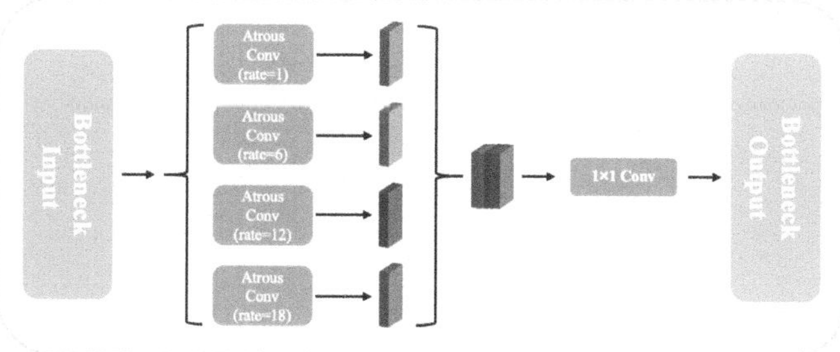

Fig. 3. The structure of the Atrous Spatial Pyramid Pooling (ASPP) module. It consists of four parallel atrous convolution branches with varying rates, which are concatenated and then fused by a 1x1 convolution.

3 Experiments and Results

3.1 Dataset and Experimental Settings

The data is from the CARE2025 liver segmentation challenge, which provides 30 cases with manual annotations (labeled set) and 330 cases without (unlabeled set). After the teacher model generated initial pseudo-labels for all 330 cases, we employed a data-driven filtering strategy to select a reliable subset for student training. We performed a cluster analysis on the unlabeled data based on their grayscale histograms using PCA (Fig. 4), revealing three distinct groups corresponding to variations in image brightness. To select the most reliable pseudo-labels, we assumed that the teacher model would perform best on images distributionally similar to its training data. We computed a prototype histogram from the 30 labeled cases and then calculated the Bhattacharyya distance D_B between this prototype and each unlabeled case's histogram:

$$D_B(H_{proto}, H_u) = -\ln\left(\sum_{k=0}^{K-1} \sqrt{H_{proto}(k) \cdot H_u(k)}\right) \tag{5}$$

We selected the top 72 cases with the smallest distance, forming a high-confidence pseudo-labeled set. This was crucial for stabilizing student training.

The final dataset for Stage 2 thus consisted of 102 cases (30 labeled, 72 pseudo-labeled), on which we performed 5-fold cross-validation (81 training, 21 validation per fold). All experiments were implemented in PyTorch on an NVIDIA GeForce RTX 3080 (12GB). The student model, based on nnU-Net v2, was trained for 800 epochs with a batch size of 1 using the AdamW optimizer. Evaluation metrics were the Dice Similarity Coefficient (DSC) and the 95% Hausdorff Distance (HD95).

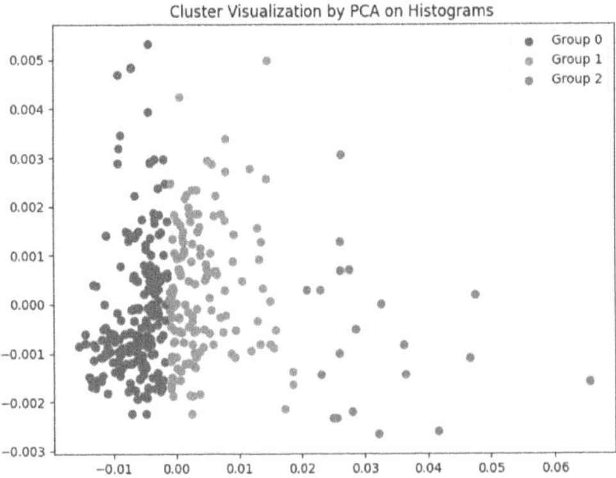

Fig. 4. Cluster visualization of the unlabeled dataset based on PCA of grayscale histograms. The data is grouped into three distinct clusters, primarily corresponding to variations in image brightness, which guided our pseudo-label selection strategy.

3.2 Results

Comparative Experiments and Analysis. We compared our framework against several powerful fully-supervised (Swin-UNet [1], Res-UNet [5]) and semi-supervised (MCF [23], GVSL [7]) methods. The results in Table 1 and Fig. 5 confirm the superiority of our method. While advanced supervised models are constrained by limited data, semi-supervised methods like MCF and GVSL leverage unlabeled data to achieve better performance. However, they often exhibit boundary errors (yellow regions in Fig. 5). This may be because their consistency-based learning mechanisms can struggle to correct systematic boundary noise from the initial teacher and may even reinforce it if different branches of the model develop a shared bias. In contrast, our framework's explicit, SDF-driven boundary-aware learning directly rectifies these contour imperfections. This explains why our method yields a result that is both quantitatively superior and visually cleaner, with minimal boundary errors.

Ablation Study. To validate the contribution of each component, we conducted an ablation study. Starting from a baseline model, we sequentially added the Progressive Training strategy, the ASPP module, and the SDF loss. As summarized in Table 2, the full model achieved substantial improvements, increasing the DSC from 0.9512 to 0.9655 and reducing the HD95 by 53.6% (from 41.25mm to 19.16mm). The drastic reduction in HD95 highlights the critical role of boundary-aware learning in enhancing contour precision. The final model outperformed all intermediate variants, demonstrating a strong synergy among the proposed enhancements.

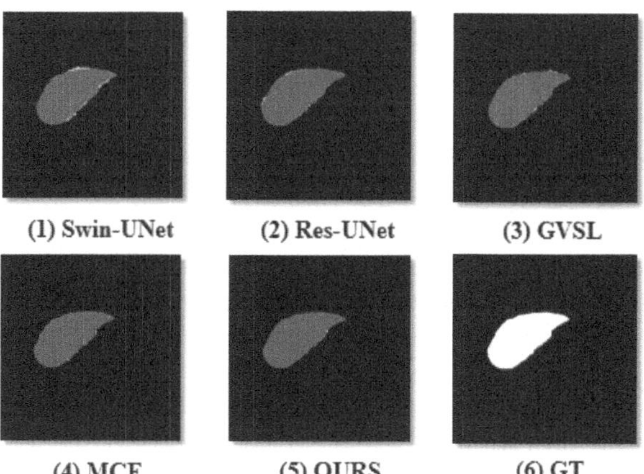

Fig. 5. Visual comparison of segmentation results. Gray indicates the correctly segmented region (true positive), while yellow highlights error regions (over- and under-segmentation).

Table 1. Comparison of segmentation performance with different methods. The best results are highlighted in bold.

Method	Dice (↑)	HD95 (mm) (↓)
Swin-UNet	0.9472	23.46
Res-UNet	0.9485	27.51
GVSL	0.9555	21.80
MCF	0.9592	24.71
Ours	**0.9655**	**19.16**

Table 2. Ablation study of our proposed modules on the CARE2025 validation set. We report mean values and show the cumulative effect of each enhancement. The best results are highlighted in bold.

Method	DSC (↑)	HD95 (mm) (↓)
Baseline	0.9512	41.25
+ Progressive Training	0.9539	36.70
+ Progressive Training + ASPP	0.9590	32.38
+ All Enhancements	**0.9655**	**19.16**

Official Challenge Results. Our method (team name: SuperIdols) was evaluated on the two official CARE 2025 test sets: an In-Distribution (ID) set and an Out-of-Distribution (OOD) set from an unseen center to assess model generalization.

On the ID test set, our approach achieved a Dice score of 0.9610 and an HD95 of 23.30 mm. Notably, it demonstrated strong robustness and generalization on the OOD test set, achieving a Dice score of 0.9770 and an HD95 of 14.65 mm. These results further validate the effectiveness of our decoupled framework and boundary-aware learning strategy in achieving reliable and generalizable segmentation performance.

4 Conclusion

In this paper, we proposed a decoupled teacher-student framework that effectively addresses the challenge of few-shot liver segmentation by breaking the error reinforcement cycle common in semi-supervised learning. Our work demonstrates that by explicitly enhancing a student model, it can surpass its teacher and correct the noise inherent in pseudo-labels. Specifically, our framework empowers the student by incorporating a multi-scale ASPP module for robust feature extraction, a progressive training strategy for stable learning, and crucially, a boundary-aware SDF loss that instills a strong geometric prior of the object's contours. Our experimental results underscore the critical importance of this boundary-aware approach, confirming that our framework significantly outperforms representative supervised and semi-supervised methods.

However, we acknowledge several limitations that open avenues for future research. Firstly, the quality of pseudo-labels still fundamentally depends on the initial teacher model, meaning the student may inherit some of the teacher's inherent biases. Secondly, our pseudo-label filtering strategy, while effective, is a heuristic based on global grayscale histograms. This approach may preferentially select typical cases and might not be robust to domain shifts involving more complex features like texture. While we prioritized pseudo-label quality over quantity to ensure training stability, this led to a lower utilization rate of the available unlabeled data. Future work should explore more advanced filtering techniques, such as incorporating uncertainty estimation (e.g., via Monte Carlo Dropout), to create a larger, more diverse, yet still reliable pseudo-labeled dataset. Finally, a detailed sensitivity analysis on key hyperparameters, such as the SDF loss weight λ and the number of selected pseudo-labels, would be valuable for assessing the method's generalizability. This work presents a robust paradigm for semi-supervised segmentation, and addressing these limitations will be a key focus of our future investigations.

References

1. Cao, H., Wang, Y., Chen, J., Jiang, D., Zhang, X., Tian, Q., Wang, M.: Swin-unet: Unet-like pure transformer for medical image segmentation. In: European Conference on Computer Vision, pp. 205–218. Springer (2022)
2. Chen, L.C., Zhu, Y., Papandreou, G., Schroff, F., Adam, H.: Encoder-decoder with atrous separable convolution for semantic image segmentation. In: Proceedings of the European Conference on Computer Vision (ECCV), pp. 801–818 (2018)
3. Cheplygina, V., De Bruijne, M., Pluim, J.P.: Not-so-supervised: a survey of semi-supervised, multi-instance, and transfer learning in medical image analysis. Med. Image Anal. **54**, 280–296 (2019)
4. Christ, P.F., Elshaer, M.E.A., Ettlinger, F., Tatavarty, S., Bickel, M., Bilic, P., Rempfler, M., Armbruster, M., Hofmann, F., D'Anastasi, M., et al.: Automatic liver and lesion segmentation in ct using cascaded fully convolutional neural networks and 3d conditional random fields. In: International Conference on Medical Image Computing and Computer-Assisted Intervention, pp. 415–423. Springer (2016)
5. Diakogiannis, F.I., Waldner, F., Caccetta, P., Wu, C.: Resunet-a: a deep learning framework for semantic segmentation of remotely sensed data. ISPRS J. Photogramm. Remote. Sens. **162**, 94–114 (2020)
6. Gao, Z., Liu, Y., Wu, F., Shi, N., Shi, Y., Zhuang, X.: A reliable and interpretable framework of multi-view learning for liver fibrosis staging. In: International Conference on Medical Image Computing and Computer-Assisted Intervention, pp. 178–188. Springer (2023)
7. He, Y., Yang, G., Ge, R., Chen, Y., Coatrieux, J.L., Wang, B., Li, S.: Geometric visual similarity learning in 3d medical image self-supervised pre-training. In: Proceedings of the IEEE/CVF Conference on Computer Vision and Pattern Recognition, pp. 9538–9547 (2023)
8. Isensee, F., Jaeger, P.F., Kohl, S.A., Petersen, J., Maier-Hein, K.H.: nnu-net: a self-configuring method for deep learning-based biomedical image segmentation. Nat. Methods **18**(2), 203–211 (2021)

9. Jansen, M.J., Kuijf, H.J., Niekel, M., Veldhuis, W.B., Wessels, F.J., Viergever, M.A., Pluim, J.P.: Liver segmentation and metastases detection in mr images using convolutional neural networks. J. Med. Imaging **6**(4), 044003–044003 (2019)
10. Karimi, D., Salcudean, S.E.: Reducing the hausdorff distance in medical image segmentation with convolutional neural networks. IEEE Trans. Med. Imaging **39**(2), 499–513 (2019)
11. Ke, Z., Qiu, D., Li, K., Yan, Q., Lau, R.W.: Guided collaborative training for pixel-wise semi-supervised learning. In: European Conference on Computer Vision, pp. 429–445. Springer (2020)
12. Kervadec, H., Bouchtiba, J., Desrosiers, C., Granger, E., Dolz, J., Ayed, I.B.: Boundary loss for highly unbalanced segmentation. In: International Conference on Medical Imaging with Deep Learning, pp. 285–296. PMLR (2019)
13. Laine, S., Aila, T.: Temporal ensembling for semi-supervised learning. arXiv preprint arXiv:1610.02242 (2016)
14. Lee, D.H., et al.: Pseudo-label: the simple and efficient semi-supervised learning method for deep neural networks. In: Workshop on Challenges in Representation Learning, ICML,. vol. 3, p. 896. Atlanta (2013)
15. Liu, Y., Gao, Z., Shi, N., Wu, F., Shi, Y., Chen, Q., Zhuang, X.: Merit: multi-view evidential learning for reliable and interpretable liver fibrosis staging. Med. Image Anal. **102**, 103507 (2025)
16. Ouali, Y., Hudelot, C., Tami, M.: Semi-supervised semantic segmentation with cross-consistency training. In: Proceedings of the IEEE/CVF Conference on Computer Vision and Pattern Recognition, pp. 12674–12684 (2020)
17. Park, J.J., Florence, P., Straub, J., Newcombe, R., Lovegrove, S.: Deepsdf: learning continuous signed distance functions for shape representation. In: Proceedings of the IEEE/CVF Conference on Computer Vision and Pattern Recognition, pp. 165–174 (2019)
18. Ronneberger, O., Fischer, P., Brox, T.: U-net: convolutional networks for biomedical image segmentation. In: International Conference on Medical Image Computing and Computer-Assisted Intervention, pp. 234–241. Springer (2015)
19. Shorten, C., Khoshgoftaar, T.M.: A survey on image data augmentation for deep learning. J. Big Data **6**(1), 1–48 (2019)
20. Sohn, K., Berthelot, D., Carlini, N., Zhang, Z., Zhang, H., Raffel, C.A., Cubuk, E.D., Kurakin, A., Li, C.L.: Fixmatch: simplifying semi-supervised learning with consistency and confidence. Adv. Neural. Inf. Process. Syst. **33**, 596–608 (2020)
21. Su, J., Luo, Z., Lian, S., Lin, D., Li, S.: Mutual learning with reliable pseudo label for semi-supervised medical image segmentation. Med. Image Anal. **94**, 103111 (2024)
22. Tarvainen, A., Valpola, H.: Mean teachers are better role models: weight-averaged consistency targets improve semi-supervised deep learning results. Adv. Neural Inf. Process. Syst. **30** (2017)
23. Wang, Y., Xiao, B., Bi, X., Li, W., Gao, X.: Mcf: mutual correction framework for semi-supervised medical image segmentation. In: Proceedings of the IEEE/CVF Conference on Computer Vision and Pattern Recognition, pp. 15651–15660 (2023)
24. Wu, F., Zhuang, X.: Minimizing estimated risks on unlabeled data: a new formulation for semi-supervised medical image segmentation. IEEE Trans. Pattern Anal. Mach. Intell. **45**(5), 6021–6036 (2022)
25. Xie, Q., Luong, M.T., Hovy, E., Le, Q.V.: Self-training with noisy student improves imagenet classification. In: Proceedings of the IEEE/CVF Conference on Computer Vision and Pattern Recognition, pp. 10687–10698 (2020)

26. Yu, L., Wang, S., Li, X., Fu, C.W., Heng, P.A.: Uncertainty-aware self-ensembling model for semi-supervised 3d left atrium segmentation. In: International Conference on Medical Image Computing and Computer-Assisted Intervention, pp. 605–613. Springer (2019)
27. Zhai, X., Oliver, A., Kolesnikov, A., Beyer, L.: S4l: self-supervised semi-supervised learning. In: Proceedings of the IEEE/CVF International Conference on Computer Vision, pp. 1476–1485 (2019)
28. Zhang, Y., Jiao, R., Liao, Q., Li, D., Zhang, J.: Uncertainty-guided mutual consistency learning for semi-supervised medical image segmentation. Artif. Intell. Med. **138**, 102476 (2023)
29. Zhou, Z.H., Li, M.: Tri-training: exploiting unlabeled data using three classifiers. IEEE Trans. Knowl. Data Eng. **17**(11), 1529–1541 (2005)

Label-Efficient Cross-Modality Generalization for Liver Segmentation in Multi-phase MRI

Quang-Khai Bui-Tran[1], Minh-Toan Dinh[2], Thanh-Huy Nguyen[3], Ba-Thinh Lam[1], Mai-Anh Vu[4], and Ulas Bagci[5](✉)

[1] Ho Chi Minh University of Science, Ho Chi Minh City, Vietnam
[2] National Central University, Taoyuan City, Taiwan
[3] Carnegie Mellon University, Pittsburgh, PA, USA
[4] University of Houston, Houston, TX, USA
[5] Northwestern University, Evanston, IL, USA
ulas.bagci@northwestern.edu

Abstract. Accurate liver segmentation in multi-phase MRI is vital for liver fibrosis assessment, yet labeled data is often scarce and unevenly distributed across imaging modalities and vendor systems. We propose a *label-efficient* segmentation approach that promotes *cross-modality generalization* under real-world conditions, where GED4 hepatobiliary-phase annotations are limited, non-contrast sequences (T1WI, T2WI, DWI) are unlabeled, and spatial misalignment and missing phases are common. Our method integrates a foundation-scale 3D segmentation backbone adapted via fine-tuning, co-training with cross pseudo supervision to leverage unlabeled volumes, and a standardized preprocessing pipeline. Without requiring spatial registration, the model learns to generalize across MRI phases and vendors, demonstrating robust segmentation performance in both labeled and unlabeled domains. Our results exhibit the effectiveness of our proposed label-efficient baseline for liver segmentation in multi-phase, multi-vendor MRI and highlight the potential of combining foundation model adaptation with co-training for real-world clinical imaging tasks.

Keywords: Cross-modality · Multi-phase MRI · Liver segmentation · Co-training

1 Introduction

Medical image segmentation has existed and been an important task for a long time, primarily due to its inherent interpretable nature, which is helpful to doctors in early diagnosis and treatment [1,13,15]. To date, there have been numerous medical image segmentation studies that were conducted on various organs

Q.-K. Bui-Tran, M.-T. Dinh and T.-H. Nguyen—Equal contribution.

X. Zhuang et al. (Eds.): CARE 2025, LNCS 16257, pp. 156–167, 2026.
https://doi.org/10.1007/978-3-032-16271-7_15

of the human body, and one of them is the liver [6,9,13,22]. Especially, under the label-scarce scenario, many noticeable works [16–18] have tackled the partially annotated medical datasets and shown promising results on various settings.

The liver is one of the most important internal organs responsible for critical physiological functions. Additionally, the liver has complex anatomical structures [10]. This complexity is further exacerbated by coupling with various pathological changes and high heterogeneity in medical images. One of the common liver diseases with such pathological changes today is liver fibrosis, a progressive condition resulting from chronic liver injury. Therefore, to diagnose effectively, it is crucial to segment the liver and accurately assess the fibrosis stage.

In response to these clinical needs, the CARE (Comprehensive Analysis & computing of REal-world medical images) 2025 challenge [5,12,21], in conjunction with MICCAI 2025, aims to advance real-world medical image analysis. In the CARE 2025 challenge, there are a total of five tracks that focus on distinct organs and their specific problems. In these tracks, CARE-Liver aims to advance the progress of Liver Fibrosis quantification and analysis methods. This track includes a crucial task, LiSeg - the automatic liver segmentation for liver MRI scans from multi-sequence and multi-center with limited ground truth.

The overall objective of the LiSeg task is to utilize the multi-modality MRI scans with the limitation of ground truth to segment the liver accurately. The challenges in this task are the limited liver mask annotations, along with the distribution shift due to the collection of data from multiple centers. Furthermore, the LiSeg task is divided into two sub-tasks corresponding to the segmentation of two different types of data: contrast and non-contrast data. However, only the ground truth for contrast data is provided. Therefore, the LiSeg task not only requires effective segmentation with limited ground truth data for a single data type, but also requires effective segmentation with unannotated non-contrast data. In view of the aforementioned considerations, we provide a comprehensive and standardized assessment of semi-supervised learning methods in this challenging task of liver segmentation.

In this paper, we propose a label-efficient liver segmentation framework tailored for multi-phase, multi-vendor MRI under limited annotation and cross-modality domain shift. To address the scarcity of annotated hepatobiliary-phase (GED4) data and the distributional gap across imaging centers, we leverage a suite of semi-supervised learning techniques, including Cross Pseudo Supervision (CPS) [3], Bidirectional Copy-Paste (BCP) [2], and MiDSS[14], to exploit unlabeled GED4 and non-contrast sequences effectively. As our backbone, we adopt STU-Net [7], a scalable and transferable segmentation model pretrained on large-scale multi-organ datasets, and further fine-tune it on the ATLAS liver segmentation dataset to improve adaptation to the target domain. This fine-tuning step provides a strong initialization prior to applying semi-supervised strategies. We validate our approach on the CARE-Liver challenge LiSeg task and conduct extensive ablation studies to analyze the contribution of each component in our pipeline, demonstrating strong generalization across MRI modalities and scanner vendors with minimal supervision.

2 Methodology

2.1 Problem Definition

The LiSeg Task of CARE-Liver 2025 challenge requires segmenting the liver in multi-phase fibrosis across multiple modalities, which specifically are categorized into two types: contrast (Gadolinium ethoxybenzyl diethylenetriamine pentaacetic acid enhanced fourth phase - GED4), and non-contrast data (T1-weighted imaging - T1WI, T2-weighted imaging - T2WI). The dataset of this challenge comprises several centers (Vendor A, B, and C), a total of 610 patients. All patients were diagnosed with liver fibrosis and underwent multi-phase MRI scans. However, only GED4 images of ten patients from each center are annotated, while other modalities and patients' counterparts are labeled.

Let $\mathsf{V}_n^{(p)} \in \mathbb{R}^{D\times W\times H}$ denote the volume for patient n at phase $p \in \mathcal{P}$ and $\mathcal{P} = \{\text{GED4}, \text{T1WI}, \text{T2WI}\}$. Formally, we define the training labeled set as $\mathcal{D}^l = \{(\mathsf{V}_n^{(\text{GED4})}, \mathsf{G}_n)\}_{n=1}^N$ where $\mathsf{G}_n \in \{0,1\}^{D\times W\times H}$ represents the binary liver segmentation mask and $N = 30$ (10 annotations per center). The training unlabeled set comprises $\mathcal{D}^u = \{\mathsf{V}_m^{(p)}\}_{m=1,p\in\mathcal{P}}^M$ where M represents the vast majority of patients whose unlabeled volumes across all phases and $M = 330$.

The primary objective is to learn two distinct segmentation functions corresponding two types of data, contrast and non-contrast: $f_\theta^{(\text{contrast})} : \mathbb{R}^{D\times W\times H} \rightarrow [0,1]^{D\times W\times H}$ for GED4 volumes and $f_\phi^{(\text{non-contrast})} : \mathbb{R}^{D\times W\times H} \rightarrow [0,1]^{D\times W\times H}$ for T1WI, and T2WI phases. While the challenge in GED4 images training is excessively limited labels, other modalities' counterparts do not have any direct supervision, requiring knowledge transfer from the limited GED4 annotations.

2.2 Scalable and Transferable Medical Image Segmentation Models

Although nnU-Net [8] has demonstrated strong performance across various tasks by automatically adapting to dataset-specific properties (e.g., input patch size, spacing), its reliance on dynamic hyperparameter selection limits the transferability of pretrained models. Core architectural parameters such as the number of resolution stages, kernel sizes, and downsampling/upsampling ratios are derived from dataset heuristics, making nnU-Net models less generalizable across tasks without retraining.

To address this, STU-Net [7] introduces a scalable and transferable framework by categorizing hyperparameters into two types: (i) *weight-related* (e.g., resolution stages), and (ii) *weight-unrelated* (e.g., input patch size). The former are fixed (e.g., six resolution stages and $(3\times3\times3)$ convolution kernels), ensuring consistent model weights across tasks, while the latter follow nnU-Net's robust defaults.

STU-Net further incorporates several architectural improvements: **(1) Residual blocks** replace basic Conv-IN-LeakyReLU blocks in the encoder and decoder, using two $3\times3\times3$ convolutions with a skip connection to stabilize deep training and preserve gradient flow. **(2) Downsampling blocks** employ a dual-branch design: a main branch with two convolutions (stride 1 then 2) and a skip branch with a $1\times1\times1$ convolution (stride 2), and their outputs are summed to retain spatial features. **(3) Upsampling blocks** use nearest-neighbor interpolation followed by a $1\times1\times1$ convolution, avoiding learnable parameters and improving transferability across resolutions. **(4) Compound scaling**, inspired by EfficientNet [20], jointly increases network depth and width at each resolution stage, enhancing both receptive field and representational capacity.

Together, these design choices make pretrained STU-Net a more generalizable and weight-compatible backbone for transfer across diverse medical tasks (Table 1).

Table 1. STU-Net configurations at different scales.

Model	Depth	Width	Parameters (M)	FLOPs (T)
STU-Net-S	(1,1,1,1,1,1)	(16,32,64,128,256,256)	14.60	0.13
STU-Net-B	(1,1,1,1,1,1)	(32,64,128,256,512,512)	58.26	0.51
STU-Net-L	(2,2,2,2,2,2)	(64,128,256,512,1024,1024)	440.30	3.81

Large-Scale Supervised Pretraining: STU-Net is pretrained on the *TotalSegmentator* dataset, which includes 104 anatomical classes. The pretraining is conducted for 4000 epochs, which is four times longer than standard nnU-Net training and incorporates mirror data augmentation to enhance generalization for downstream tasks.

2.3 Cross Pseudo Supervision for 3D Segmentation

We utilize a dual-network training strategy based on the *STU-Net* architecture, which is a strong foundation model and suitable for various tasks and data. The framework consists of two identical 3D segmentation networks with independent parameters:

$$\mathsf{P}_1 = \text{STU-Net}(\mathsf{V}; \boldsymbol{\theta}_1), \tag{1}$$

$$\mathsf{P}_2 = \text{STU-Net}(\mathsf{V}; \boldsymbol{\theta}_2), \tag{2}$$

where $\mathsf{P}_1, \mathsf{P}_2 \in \mathbb{R}^{C\times D\times W\times H}$ are voxel-wise confidence maps after softmax normalization over C classes.

The same augmented input volume V is provided to both networks to encourage consistent learning while enabling complementary supervision. To simplify notation, the forward path can be expressed as:

$$\begin{aligned} \mathsf{V} \rightarrow \text{STU-Net}(\boldsymbol{\theta}_1) \rightarrow \mathsf{P}_1 \rightarrow \mathsf{Y}_1, \\ \searrow \text{STU-Net}(\boldsymbol{\theta}_2) \rightarrow \mathsf{P}_2 \rightarrow \mathsf{Y}_2, \end{aligned} \tag{3}$$

where Y_1 and Y_2 are pseudo segmentation maps obtained by applying the argmax operation to P_1 and P_2, respectively. Each pseudo label $\mathbf{y}_{1i}$ ($\mathbf{y}_{2i}$) is a one-hot vector corresponding to the predicted class at voxel i (Fig. 1).

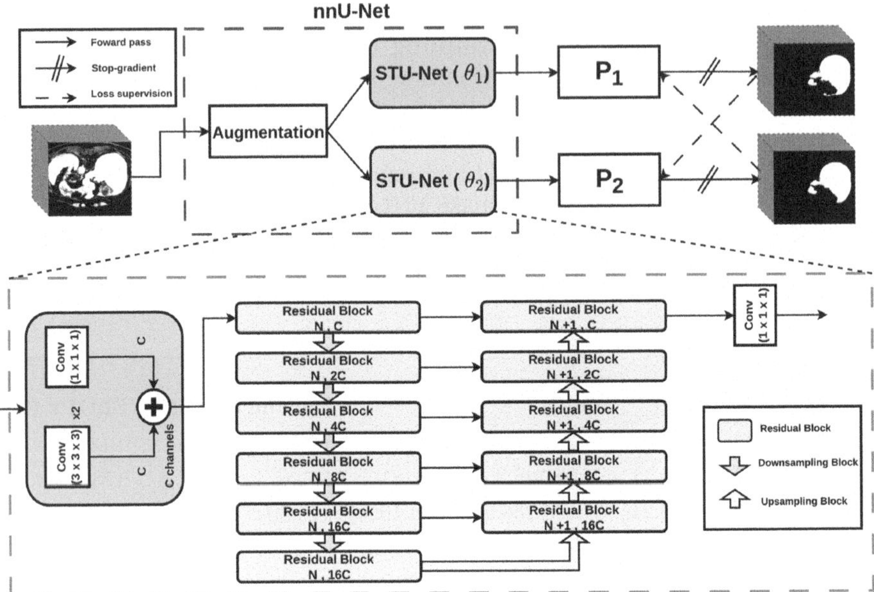

Fig. 1. Overview of the semi-supervised segmentation cross pseudo supervision framework. The framework utilizes the auto configurations of nnU-Net for loading data and augmentation, while the backbone uses the STU-Net model with a strong pretrained weight. Then deploy cross pseudo supervised between the two models.

The total training loss consists of two components: (i) a **supervised loss** $\mathcal{L}_s$ applied to labeled data, and (ii) a **cross pseudo supervision loss** $\mathcal{L}_{cps}$ applied to both labeled and unlabeled data.

Supervised Loss: For labeled volumes, we employ the standard voxel-wise cross-entropy loss for each network:

$$\mathcal{L}_s = \frac{1}{|\mathcal{D}^l|} \sum_{V \in \mathcal{D}^l} \frac{1}{W \times H \times D} \sum_{i=0}^{W \times H \times D} \Big(\ell_{ce}(\mathbf{p}_{1i}, \mathbf{y}^*_{1i}) + \ell_{ce}(\mathbf{p}_{2i}, \mathbf{y}^*_{2i}) \Big), \tag{4}$$

where ℓ_{ce} denotes the cross-entropy function, $\mathbf{p}_{1i}$ and $\mathbf{p}_{2i}$ are the softmax probability vectors for voxel i, and $\mathbf{y}^*_{1i}$, $\mathbf{y}^*_{2i}$ are the corresponding ground truth one-hot vectors.

Cross Pseudo Supervision Loss: In the unlabeled case, pseudo labels are generated from one network and used to supervise the other. This bidirectional supervision is defined as:

$$\mathcal{L}_{cps}^{u} = \frac{1}{|\mathcal{D}^u|} \sum_{\mathsf{V} \in \mathcal{D}^u} \frac{1}{W \times H \times D} \sum_{i=0}^{W \times H \times D} \Big(\ell_{ce}(\mathbf{p}_{1i}, \mathbf{y}_{2i}) + \ell_{ce}(\mathbf{p}_{2i}, \mathbf{y}_{1i}) \Big), \tag{5}$$

where $\mathbf{y}_{1i}$ and $\mathbf{y}_{2i}$ are pseudo labels produced by the other network.

Similarly, we define $\mathcal{L}_{cps}^{l}$ for labeled volumes using the same formulation. The total cross pseudo supervision loss is a combination of the losses on both the labeled and unlabeled data, which is:

$$\mathcal{L}_{cps} = \mathcal{L}_{cps}^{l} + \mathcal{L}_{cps}^{u}. \tag{6}$$

Final Objective The complete loss function is:

$$\mathcal{L} = \mathcal{L}_{s} + \lambda \mathcal{L}_{cps}, \tag{7}$$

where λ is a balancing hyperparameter controlling the contribution of cross pseudo supervision, which allows the networks to improve their predictions mutually, leveraging information from both labeled and unlabeled 3D volumes.

3 Experiments

3.1 Dataset

LiQA Dataset The dataset comprises a multi-center cohort of 610 patients diagnosed with liver fibrosis, including 170 new cases beyond the CARE2024 challenge [5,12,21]. Patients were scanned across four clinical centers using three MRI vendors *Philips Ingenia 3.0T*, *Siemens Skyra 3.0T*, and *Siemens Aera 1.5T*, resulting in realistic multi-vendor variability. Each patient underwent multi-phase MRI, including T2-weighted (T2WI), diffusion-weighted (DWI), T1-weighted (T1WI), and Gd-EOB-DTPA-enhanced dynamic imaging at four phases: arterial (GED1, 25s post-injection), portal venous (GED2, 1min), delayed (GED3, 4min), and hepatobiliary (GED4, 20min). The training set includes 360 cases (vendor A: 130, B1: 170, B2: 60), but only 30 GED4 scans (8.3%) have segmentation labels, posing a strong annotation scarcity challenge. Consequently, *subtask 1* (T1WI, T2WI, DWI) operates fully unsupervised, while *subtask 2* (GED4) requires label-efficient or semi-supervised strategies. The validation set contains 60 fully annotated cases (20 per vendor A, B1, B2). The test set includes 190 cases from all vendors (A: 40, B1: 40, B2: 40, C: 70), with vendor C held out to assess generalization. Key challenges include missing sequences (except GED4), inter-vendor protocol differences, and the lack of spatial pre-alignment, reflecting the heterogeneity of clinical liver MRI data.

ATLAS Dataset The ATLAS dataset from the MICCAI 2023 ATLAS challenge [19], includes 60 public and 30 private patient cases. Each case contains multiple NIFTI-format MRI scans and corresponding labels. Images were acquired using various MRI machines and sequences, with one of three post-contrast phases (arterial, portal, or delayed) selected. Liver and tumour masks were merged into a single foreground for the accurate liver segmentation task.

Table 2. Sub-Task 1 – GED4 segmentation results on the private validation set from the organizers with STU-Net-S backbone. ↑: higher is better, ↓: lower is better. Bold indicates the best result, underline indicates the second best.

Method	DSC ↑	HD ↓
CPS	**0.9685**	**25.56**
BCP	<u>0.9553</u>	<u>86.69</u>
MiDSS	0.9142	126.17

3.2 Experimental Setup

Due to computational constraints, only 3D STU-Net-S is adopted as the backbone network initialized with pretrained weights and fine-tuned on the ATLAS dataset to adapt the foundation model to the task-specific setting. MRI data are preprocessed and augmented using the nnU-Net pipeline, including z-score normalization, random spatial transformations, and other standard augmentations. Adam optimizer is employed for all training. Fine-tuning on ATLAS is performed for 100 epochs with a learning rate of 1×10^{-2} and a batch size of 2. Semi-supervised model training is carried out with a learning rate of 1×10^{-3} for a maximum of 36 epochs and a batch size of 4. All experiments are implemented in PyTorch and executed on a single NVIDIA GeForce RTX 3090 Ti GPU.

Evaluation Metrics: For the LiSeg task, liver segmentation performance of our methods is assessed by using the Dice Similarity Coefficient (DSC) and Hausdorff Distance (HD), in accordance with the evaluation criteria of the challenge.

3.3 Results

Sub-Task 1: Contrast-Enhanced Liver Segmentation (GED4) The Table 2 shows the results on contrast-enhanced hepatobiliary phase (GED4) using the private validation set. Three methods compared include the state-of-the-art semi-supervised model CPS [3], BCP [2], and MiDSS [14]. Specifically, CPS achieves superior performance with a DSC of 0.9685 and an HD of 25.56. Both BCP and MiDSS, which adopt teacher-student architectures, achieved competitive results but still underperform compared to CPS.

Sub-Task 2: Non-Contrast Liver Segmentation Table 3 reports segmentation results on non-contrast modalities without annotations. For T1WI, CPS with STU-Net-S fine-tuned on ATLAS achieves the best performance (DSC: 0.9465, HD: 62.84), outperforming the non-fine-tuned counterpart (DSC: 0.9392,

HD: 89.90). Results on T2WI are notably lower (DSC: 0.7673, HD: 81.76), highlighting the additional difficulty of segmenting this modality in the absence of annotations. This can be explained by two different groups of reasons, including the difference in characteristics between the modality and our training scenario.

Regarding the different features, physically, T2WI exhibits completely reversed signal characteristics compared to GED4 and T1WI. Specifically, while the liver appears hyperintense (bright) on GED4 due to hepatocytes' uptake of Gd-EOB-DTPA intermediate-to-high signal on T1WI, the liver appears hypointense (dark) on T2WI [4]. This contrast pattern reversal creates a fundamental challenge for CNN feature transfer [11]. CNN, which learns from 30 annotated GED4 images, tends to detect bright-to-dark transitions such as liver-to-background. In contrast, when it is applied to T2WI with dark liver regions, its features fail catastrophically with significant performance drops for the cross-modality medical image segmentation task.

In terms of training scenarios, despite our efforts to address label scarcity for cross-modality medical images, it still cannot completely address the domain gap problem. The external dataset used for pretraining was ATLAS, which included only T1 CE-MRI and no T2, resulting in a significant bias toward T1/contrast-enhanced patterns. A pseudo-labeling strategy with 220 cases was generated only for unlabeled GED4, with no direct supervision signal for the T2WI domain. As a result, our models have no chance to self-correct on the T2 distribution.

Table 3. Sub-Task 2 – Segmentation results on non-contrast modalities (T1WI, T2WI) from the private validation set provided by the organizers.

Modality	Method	DSC ↑	HD ↓
T1WI	CPS with STU-Net-S (fine-tuned on ATLAS)	**0.9465**	**62.84**
	CPS with STU-Net-S	0.9392	89.90
	MiDSS with STU-Net-S + nnU-Net preprocessing	0.8948	128.93
T2WI	CPS with STU-Net-S (fine-tuned on ATLAS)	0.7673	81.76

Ablation Study. Table 4 highlights the impact of foundation model pre-training and task-specific fine-tuning. The baseline CPS with a 3D U-Net backbone performs poorly (DSC: 0.7752, HD: 141.07), highlighting the limitations of training from scratch, particularly in semi-supervised settings with a large amount of unlabeled data. Replacing the backbone with STU-Net-S substantially improves performance (DSC: 0.9685, HD: 25.56). Further initializing the model with ATLAS fine-tuning weights yields the best results.

Different processing pipelines are also employed to investigate their contributions to the overall performance. Following the MiDSS pipeline, full augmentation substantially degrades performance (DSC: 0.9142, HD: 126.17), while weak augmentation by disabling Elastic Transform, Random Crop & Rotate, and Random Crop Zoom leads to an even larger drop (DSC: 0.8665, HD: 130.04). In contrast, adopting nnU-Net preprocessing with its automatically configured data

Table 4. Ablation study on Sub-Task 1. Comparison of different backbones, ATLAS fine-tuning, and augmentation strategies on the private validation set.

Method	**DSC ↑**	**HD ↓**
CPS with 3D U-Net	0.7752	141.07
CPS with STU-Net-S	0.9685	25.56
CPS with STU-Net-S (fine-tuned on ATLAS)	**0.9705**	**19.55**
MiDSS with STU-Net-S + nnU-Net preprocessing	0.9578	37.85
MiDSS with STU-Net-S + full augmentation	0.9142	126.17
MiDSS with STU-Net-S + weak augmentation	0.8665	130.04

loader achieves competitive results (DSC: 0.9578, HD: 37.85), highlighting the robustness of the nnU-Net pipeline compared to manual augmentation design.

Table 5. LiSeg evaluation results across different MRI modalities for liver segmentation. Results are reported for In-Domain (ID) and Out-of-Domain (OOD) test sets using Dice Similarity Coefficient (DSC) and Hausdorff Distance (HD) metrics.

Modality	**ID Test**		**OOD Test**	
	DSC ↑	**HD ↓**	**DSC ↑**	**HD ↓**
GED4	94.56	56.59	97.26	21.52
T1	86.42	163.91	73.51	102.79

3.4 Discussion

To clarify the performance gap between the methods, the limited annotated GED4 data is split into 5 cases for validation and the remaining cases for training. The qualitative results shown in Figs. 3 demonstrate that the CPS method closely follows the liver boundaries in the ground truth. Additionally, Fig. 2 further illustrates the benefits of fine-tuning the foundation model on ATLAS and leveraging nnU-Net preprocessing.

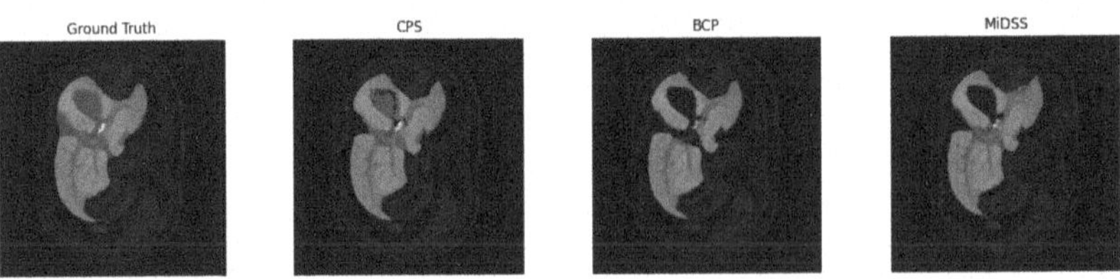

Fig. 2. Qualitative results on GED4 under different pretraining weights and preprocessing pipelines.

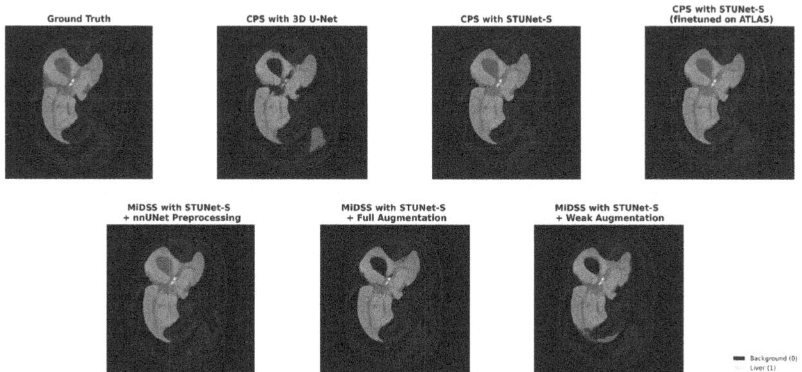

Fig. 3. Qualitative results on GED4 using different semi-supervised methods.

Our models are designed to address multiple subtasks concurrently. As reported in Tables 3, 2, and 5, performance on non-contrast modalities lags behind that of GED4, likely due to the scarcity of annotated data for these modalities. In future work, strategies that enhance cross-modality generalization will be investigated, with a particular focus on improving performance for non-contrast data.

Our models are also evaluated on a private dataset from the CARE-Liver challenge to validate the robustness, and their results are shown in Table 5. These results suggest that the models generalize well to out-of-distribution data, supporting their potential for use in clinical practice.

4 Conclusion

In this work, we present a comprehensive study on liver MRI segmentation under the extreme annotation scarcity and multi-vendor heterogeneity of the LiQA dataset. By combining nnU-Net preprocessing, the STU-Net backbone with foundation model fine-tuning from ATLAS, and carefully designed semi-supervised strategies, we demonstrate substantial improvements in both contrast-enhanced and non-contrast settings. Our results on the LiQA dataset demonstrate the strength of the baseline, which integrates foundation model fine-tuning with semi-supervised learning for robust liver segmentation in real-world clinical settings.

Acknowledgement. This research is partially supported by the following NIH grants: R01-HL171376 and U01-CA268808. We thank AI VIETNAM for supporting GPUs for training experiments.

References

1. Azad, R., Aghdam, E.K., Rauland, A., Jia, Y., Avval, A.H., Bozorgpour, A., Karimijafarbigloo, S., Cohen, J.P., Adeli, E., Merhof, D.: Medical image segmentation review: the success of u-net. IEEE Trans. Pattern Anal. Mach. Intell. (2024)
2. Bai, Y., Chen, D., Li, Q., Shen, W., Wang, Y.: Bidirectional copy-paste for semi-supervised medical image segmentation. In: Proceedings of the IEEE/CVF Conference on Computer Vision and Pattern Recognition, pp. 11514–11524 (2023)
3. Chen, X., Yuan, Y., Zeng, G., Wang, J.: Semi-supervised semantic segmentation with cross pseudo supervision. In: Proceedings of the IEEE/CVF Conference on Computer Vision and Pattern Recognition, pp. 2613–2622 (2021)
4. Curvo-Semedo, L., Brito, J.B., Seco, M.F., Costa, J.F., Marques, C.B., Caseiro-Alves, F.: The hypointense liver lesion on t2-weighted mr images and what it means. Radiographics **30**(1), e38 (2010)
5. Gao, Z., Liu, Y., Wu, F., Shi, N., Shi, Y., Zhuang, X.: A reliable and interpretable framework of multi-view learning for liver fibrosis staging. In: International Conference on Medical Image Computing and Computer-Assisted Intervention, pp. 178–188 (2023)
6. Heller, N., Isensee, F., Trofimova, D., Tejpaul, R., Zhao, Z., Chen, H., Wang, L., Golts, A., Khapun, D., Shats, D., et al.: The kits21 challenge: automatic segmentation of kidneys, renal tumors, and renal cysts in corticomedullary-phase ct. arXiv preprint arXiv:2307.01984 (2023)
7. Huang, Z., Wang, H., Deng, Z., Ye, J., Su, Y., Sun, H., He, J., Gu, Y., Gu, L., Zhang, S., et al.: Stu-net: scalable and transferable medical image segmentation models empowered by large-scale supervised pre-training. arXiv preprint arXiv:2304.06716 (2023)
8. Isensee, F., Jaeger, P.F., Kohl, S.A., Petersen, J., Maier-Hein, K.H.: nnu-net: a self-configuring method for deep learning-based biomedical image segmentation. Nat. Methods **18**(2), 203–211 (2021)
9. Isensee, F., Wald, T., Ulrich, C., Baumgartner, M., Roy, S., Maier-Hein, K., Jaeger, P.F.: nnu-net revisited: a call for rigorous validation in 3d medical image segmentation. In: International Conference on Medical Image Computing and Computer-Assisted Intervention, pp. 488–498. Springer (2024)
10. Juza, R.M., Pauli, E.M.: Clinical and surgical anatomy of the liver: a review for clinicians. Clin. Anat. **27**(5), 764–769 (2014)
11. Kang, B., Nam, H., Kang, M., Heo, K.S., Lim, M., Oh, J.H., Kam, T.E.: Target-aware cross-modality unsupervised domain adaptation for vestibular schwannoma and cochlea segmentation. Sci. Rep. **14**(1), 27883 (2024)
12. Liu, Y., Gao, Z., Shi, N., Wu, F., Shi, Y., Chen, Q., Zhuang, X.: Merit: multi-view evidential learning for reliable and interpretable liver fibrosis staging. Med. Image Anal. **102**, 103507 (2025)
13. Ma, J., He, Y., Li, F., Han, L., You, C., Wang, B.: Segment anything in medical images. Nat. Commun. **15**(1), 654 (2024)
14. Ma, Q., Zhang, J., Qi, L., Yu, Q., Shi, Y., Gao, Y.: Constructing and exploring intermediate domains in mixed domain semi-supervised medical image segmentation. In: Proceedings of the IEEE/CVF Conference on Computer Vision and Pattern Recognition, pp. 11642–11651 (2024)
15. Nguyen, T.H., Kha, Q.H., Truong, T.N.T., Lam, B.T., Ngo, B.H., Dinh, Q.V., Le, N.Q.K.: Towards robust natural-looking mammography lesion synthesis on ipsilateral dual-views breast cancer analysis. In: Proceedings of the IEEE/CVF International Conference on Computer Vision, pp. 2564–2573 (2023)

16. Nguyen, T.H., Nguyen, T., Nguyen, X.B., Vu, N.L.V., Dinh, V.Q., Meriaudeau, F.: Semi-supervised skin lesion segmentation under dual mask ensemble with feature discrepancy co-training. In: Medical Imaging with Deep Learning
17. Nguyen, T.H., Vu, N.L.V., Nguyen, H.T., Dinh, Q.V., Li, X., Xu, M.: Semi-supervised histopathology image segmentation with feature diversified collaborative learning. In: AAAI Bridge Program on AI for Medicine and Healthcare, pp. 165–172. PMLR (2025)
18. Pham, H.H., Nguyen, H.T., Vu, N.L.V., Dinh, Q.V., Nguyen, T.H., Li, X., Xu, M., et al.: Fetal-bcp: addressing empirical distribution gap in semi-supervised fetal ultrasound segmentation. In: 2025 IEEE 22nd International Symposium on Biomedical Imaging (ISBI), pp. 1–4. IEEE (2025)
19. Quinton, F., Popoff, R., Presles, B., Leclerc, S., Meriaudeau, F., Nodari, G., Lopez, O., Pellegrinelli, J., Chevallier, O., Ginhac, D., et al.: A tumour and liver automatic segmentation (atlas) dataset on contrast-enhanced magnetic resonance imaging for hepatocellular carcinoma. Data **8**(5), 79 (2023)
20. Tan, M., Le, Q.E., et al.: Rethinking model scaling for convolutional neural networks. In: Proceedings of the International Conference on Machine Learning, Long Beach, CA, USA, vol. 15 (2019)
21. Wu, F., Zhuang, X.: Minimizing estimated risks on unlabeled data: a new formulation for semi-supervised medical image segmentation. IEEE Trans. Pattern Anal. Mach. Intell. **45**(5), 6021–6036 (2023)
22. Zhu, J., Hamdi, A., Qi, Y., Jin, Y., Wu, J.: Medical sam 2: segment medical images as video via segment anything model 2. arXiv preprint arXiv:2408.00874 (2024)

UniCarSeg: A Unified Framework for Multi-task Cardiac Image Segmentation

Wenzhen Zhang[1], Xifeng Hu[1], Wenmiao Wang[2], Xiaoxiao Cui[3], Bangjun Li[1(✉)], and Yujun Li[1]

[1] School of Information Science and Engineering, Shandong University, Qingdao 266237, China
libangjun@mail.sdu.edu.cn

[2] Department of Thoracic Surgery, The Second Hospital, Cheeloo College of Medicine, Shandong University, Jinan 250033, China

[3] School of Software & Joint SDU-NTU Centre for Artificial Intelligence Research (C-FAIR), Shandong University, Jinan 250101, China

Abstract. Medical image analysis has demonstrated significant value in the diagnosis and treatment of cardiovascular diseases, highlighting the urgent need for accurate and robust cardiac image segmentation. However, a fundamental challenge in clinical practice lies in the simultaneous execution of multiple segmentation tasks required for comprehensive evaluation, such as delineating individual cardiac structures, the whole heart structure, or both anatomical structures and pathological regions (e.g., scars). Existing methods are typically tailored to a specific imaging modality or task, limiting their generalizability, while the simple combination of separate models often results in fragmented workflows. To address this issue, we propose UniCarSeg, a unified framework for multi-task cardiac image segmentation. Specifically, UniCarSeg leverages a pre-trained medical image segmentation foundation model to effectively extract universal, shared feature representations and incorporates a Kolmogorov-Arnold Network (KAN)-based mask decoder (KMD) for task-specific segmentation. This design enables an effective feature transformation from generic visual embeddings to precise cardiac segmentation output. Extensive experiments on the multi-center, multi-modality cardiac structure and pathology segmentation dataset (CARE-Cardiac) from the CARE2025 Challenge, along with additional public cardiac datasets, demonstrate that UniCarSeg consistently achieves superior performance. By enabling the segmentation of diverse cardiac regions within a single unified framework, our method demonstrates substantial potential to advance both cardiac diagnostics and treatment planning.

Keywords: Cardiac segmentation · Medical image analysis · Multi-tasks · Unified Model

X. Zhuang et al. (Eds.): CARE 2025, LNCS 16257, pp. 168–179, 2026.
https://doi.org/10.1007/978-3-032-16271-7_16

1 Introduction

Cardiovascular diseases remain one of the leading causes of morbidity and mortality worldwide, highlighting the urgent need for accurate and efficient cardiac image analysis [11,28]. Cardiac imaging techniques, such as computed tomography (CT) and magnetic resonance imaging (MRI), provide comprehensive information on both structure and function, allowing early diagnosis, treatment planning, and prognosis assessment [12]. Moreover, medical image segmentation plays a pivotal role in medical image analysis, which involves identifying and delineating the boundaries of organs, lesions, and other anatomical regions, facilitating precise clinical diagnosis and analysis. However, the inherent complexity of cardiac anatomy, together with variations introduced by respiratory motion, cardiac contraction, and multi-center acquisition protocols, makes automated segmentation highly challenging [4,10,16].

Deep learning-based approaches have demonstrated remarkable success in medical image segmentation, with U-Net and its numerous variants becoming the de facto standard. Variants such as attention-based architectures [19] and multi-scale feature fusion networks [23] have significantly improved performance. Previous studies on left atrium segmentation have shown its clinical value for the analysis of atrial fibrillation [15]. Similarly, automatic delineation of myocardial structures and scar regions plays a crucial role in evaluating myocardial diseases and supporting clinical decision-making [26,27]. Meanwhile, incorporating multi-modality and multi-center data improves the potential for real-world applicability but also introduces substantial domain shifts that reduce model robustness [8]. This poses a greater challenge, requiring models that not only achieve accurate segmentation performance but also generalize effectively across different domains and modalities. To this end, several recent studies have explored various strategies to enhance robustness and generalization. Probabilistic perturbation modules have been proposed to increase tolerance to domain shifts [16]. Strong data augmentation combined with calibration techniques has been shown to mitigate data heterogeneity and improve predictive confidence [24]. Synthetic data generation and pseudo-labeling approaches have also been introduced to alleviate the shortage of annotated datasets [17]. Although these contributions push the field forward, they remain largely focused on isolated structures [22] or pathologies [21], without offering a holistic solution for real-world clinical analysis. This is because cardiac diagnosis typically involves multiple interrelated tasks, such as delineating anatomical structures (e.g., atria, ventricles, vessels) and identifying pathological regions (e.g., scars) in various imaging modalities and acquisition protocols. Relying on separate models for each task leads to fragmented workflows, limited knowledge transfer, and poor adaptability to missing or heterogeneous data.

In this paper, we propose a unified cardiac segmentation method, UniCarSeg, which provides an all-in-one solution by employing a single model to address multiple segmentation tasks. Specifically, we employ a pretrained image encoder from the foundation segmentation model as the backbone to extract shared feature representations and introduce a Kolmogorov-Arnold Network (KAN)-based

Mask Decoder (KMD) to segment different anatomical structures. This design effectively bridges general-purpose visual features with task-specific cardiac segmentation, enabling precise delineation of diverse cardiac anatomical regions across tasks. Experiments on large and comprehensive cardiac datasets demonstrate the promising performance of the proposed model.

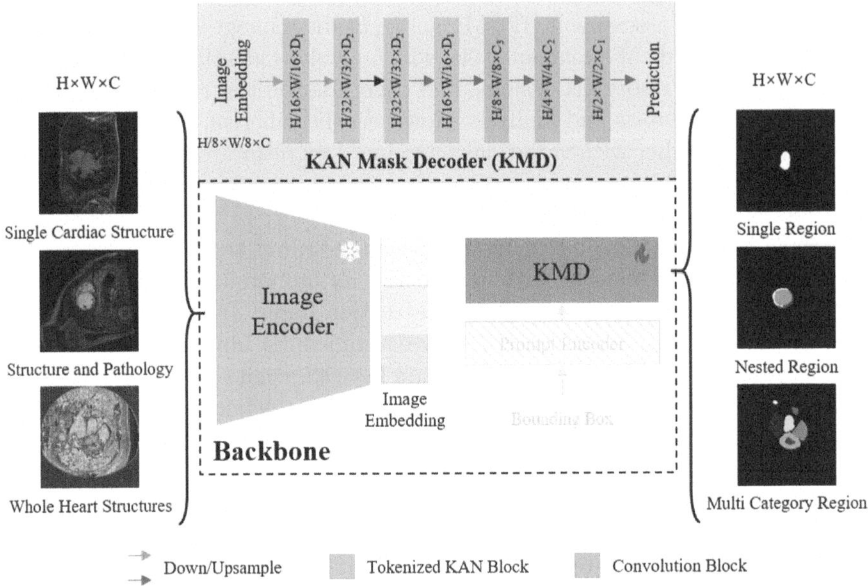

Fig. 1. Overview of the proposed UniCarSeg, a united solution for different cardiac structure segmentation tasks. The model is based on a shared pretrained image encoder and possesses different mask decoders (KMD) for different tasks.

2 Method

This paper proposes UniCarSeg, a unified cardiac segmentation method for comprehensive analysis of cardiac structures and pathologies. As illustrated in Fig. 1, UniCarSeg provides an all-in-one solution to address multiple segmentation tasks. It adopts a pre-trained universal image encoder as the backbone to extract shared feature representations, while multiple task-specific decoders are employed to predict different anatomical regions. By integrating the image encoder from the foundation segmentation model, our framework leverages the powerful representation learning of large-scale pretraining while maintaining the domain adaptability required for medical applications, thereby achieving a balance between generalization and precision. To further enhance model generalization across modalities and centers, we introduce intensity normalization and resolution harmonization during preprocessing, ensuring that the backbone receives standardized input. Notably, existing interactive foundation models typically rely on bounding box prompts to segment individual targets in medical images. Such reliance limits their applicability to scenarios involving mixed single-region segmentation, nested region segmentation, and multi-category region segmentation. Therefore, we disabled the prompt encoder. In addition, the shared features extracted by the image encoder are passed to separate mask decoders for different segmentation tasks. Finally, UniCarSeg provides a unified model that allows for the segmentation of individual cardiac structures, the whole cardiac structure, or both anatomical structures and pathological regions simultaneously.

2.1 Universal Image Encoder

Recent vision foundation models have demonstrated promising performance across various medical image analysis tasks, providing generalist and versatile solutions through models trained on large-scale datasets [20,25]. A representative work is SAM [9], which can segment arbitrary objects in images in an interactive manner. To bridge the gap between natural and medical images, MedSAM [20] was further developed by fine-tuning the pretrained SAM on medical images. Correspondingly, our framework adopts the same image encoder as MedSAM for universal feature extraction. Specifically, this backbone encoder consists of 12 Transformer layers and operates on resampled medical images (CT/MRI), extracting hierarchical feature representations that are robust to modality differences and imaging artifacts. Compared with conventional CNN-based backbones, the Transformer-based encoder provides stronger modeling of long-range dependencies, which is critical for capturing the complex anatomical context of cardiac structures. Finally, the pre-trained encoder delivers shared feature representations for subsequent multi-task predictions.

2.2 KAN Mask Decoder

The Kolmogorov-Arnold Network (KAN) has proven effective in approximating high-dimensional complex functions, demonstrating robust performance across diverse applications [13]. After feature extraction by the universal image encoder, we employ a KAN-based mask decoder (KMD) to generate task-specific segmentation outputs. As illustrated in Fig. 1, the decoder integrates a stack of tokenized KAN blocks with down-sampling, up-sampling, and convolutional blocks to enable progressive segmentation. The structure of the tokenized KAN block is shown in Fig. 2. First, tokenization is performed by reshaping the encoder's output features into a flattened sequence of 2D patches. These vectorized patches are then mapped into a latent multidimensional embedding space via a trainable linear projection, implemented as a convolutional layer with a kernel size of 3. The resulting tokens are subsequently fed into a series of KAN layers (N=3). Following each KAN layer, the features are processed by a depth-wise convolutional layer (DwConv), batch normalization, and a ReLU activation. Residual connections are incorporated by adding the original tokens, after which layer normalization is applied and the output features are passed to the next block. In addition, each convolutional block consists of three components: a convolutional layer, batch normalization, and a ReLU activation.

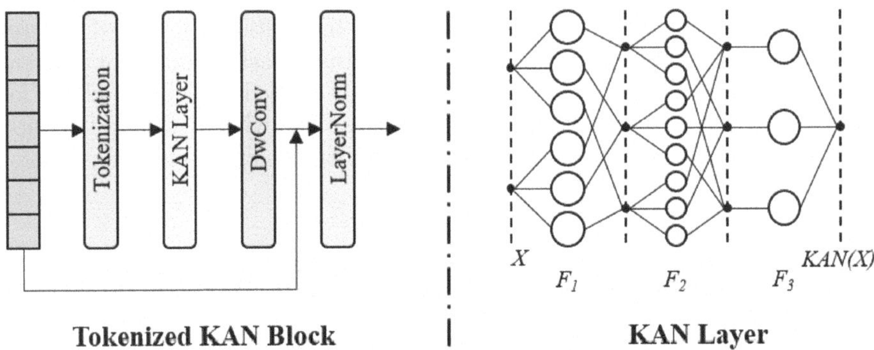

Fig. 2. Structure of tokenized KAN block and KAN layer.

2.3 Model Training

Training Strategy In order to leverage the powerful feature representation capability of MedSAM while avoiding overfitting, the image encoder is frozen throughout the training, and only the KMD parameters are updated. This training strategy ensures that the KMD learns to transform the frozen MedSAM features into accurate anatomical and pathological delineations while maintaining robustness across heterogeneous multi-center and multi-modality datasets.

Loss Function Training is carried out in a fully supervised manner. Given an input cardiac image I with the corresponding ground truth label Y, the frozen image encoder generates high-level visual embeddings F, which are subsequently decoded by the KMD into segmentation predictions $\hat{Y}$. To optimize the network, we employ a hybrid loss function $\mathcal{L}$ that combines the cross-entropy loss $\mathcal{L}_{\mathrm{CE}}$ and the Dice loss $\mathcal{L}_{\mathrm{Dice}}$ as follows:

$$\mathcal{L} = \mathcal{L}_{\mathrm{CE}}(\hat{Y}, Y) + \mathcal{L}_{\mathrm{Dice}}(\hat{Y}, Y) \tag{1}$$

3 Experiments

3.1 Dataset and Preprocessing

Dataset We conducted experiments on the multi-center, multi-modality cardiac structure and pathology segmentation dataset (CARE-Cardiac) from the CARE2025 Challenge [6,14,28,29]. This dataset was specifically curated to encompass three interrelated sub-tasks: (1) Single Cardiac Structure (left atrium) Segmentation, (2) Whole Heart Structure Segmentation, and (3) Structure and Pathology (left ventricle, myocardium, and scar) Segmentation. The CARE-Cardiac dataset captures the heterogeneity of real-world clinical practice by including CT and MRI acquisitions collected from multiple institutions and scanner vendors, thereby presenting substantial challenges in domain generalization and robustness. The detailed experimental settings for each sub-task are as follows:

- **Single Cardiac Structure Segmentation:** A total of 130 late gadolinium enhancement (LGE) MRI cases from Center A are provided for training. For validation, 20 cases from Centers A and C are available, and 44 cases from Centers A, B, and C constitute the test set.
- **Whole Heart Structure Segmentation:** Training data consists of 20 CT cases from Center A, 20 CT cases from Center B, and 20 MRI cases from Centers C&D, along with 26 MRI cases from Center E. Validation data include 50 cases (20 CT cases from Center A, 10 CT cases from Center B, and 20 MRI cases from Centers C&D). The test set expands to 90 cases that span five centers (A, B, C&D, F, and G) and includes both CT and MRI acquisitions.
- **Structure and Pathology Segmentation:** Training data include 200 LGE MRI cases collected from seven centers (A-G), covering various acquisition protocols. The validation consists of 25 cases from Center D, and the test set provides 41 cases from Centers D and B.

In addition, the Automatic Cardiac Diagnosis Challenge (ACDC) dataset [1] is added to the model segmentation task to test its generalization ability. The tasks for ACDC include manual expert segmentation of the right ventricular (RV) and left ventricular (LV), as well as the myocardium (Myo). Training data include 70 MRI cases. The validation consists of 10 cases, and the test set provides 20 cases.

Preprocessing To further enhance model generalization across modalities and centers, we introduce intensity normalization and resolution harmonization during preprocessing, ensuring that the backbone receives standardized input. For segmentation of the whole heart, all anatomical structures are unified into seven target classes: left ventricle, right ventricle, left atrium, right atrium, myocardium, ascending aorta, and pulmonary artery. For pathology segmentation, scar regions are delineated as additional labels.

3.2 Implementation Details

Our method is implemented using PyTorch, using MedSAM as the backbone model. The model is trained on an NVIDIA RTX 3090 24GB GPU for up to 1000 epochs of training with a batch size of 24. Both the image encoder and the mask decoder in the baseline model are included in gradient updates. The model accepts images of size 512×512. We used the AdamW [18] optimizer with a weight decay of 0.01 and a learning rate of 0.0001.

3.3 Evaluation Metrics

To comprehensively assess the performance of the proposed unified segmentation model, we employ multiple quantitative metrics commonly used in medical image segmentation:

- **Dice Similarity Coefficient (DSC):** Measures volumetric overlap between prediction and ground truth, serving as the primary metric for evaluation.
- **Hausdorff Distance (HD, 95%):** Evaluates the accuracy of boundaries by computing the 95th percentile of the distances between the predicted and reference contours.

Model performance is first validated on the dedicated validation set, followed by blind evaluation on the held-out test set, which includes unseen centers and modalities to assess domain generalization.

3.4 Results and Analysis

Table 1 presents the quantitative results of UniCarSeg in different tasks under two testing scenarios (ID and OOD). Here, in-distribution (ID), also referred to as seen centers, indicates that the training and test sets originate from the same data sources, while out-of-distribution (OOD), termed unseen centers, indicates that the test set comes from previously unseen data acquisition centers and exhibits a distribution shift compared to the training data. For the left atria segmentation task, an average DSC of 75.84% and an average HD of 55.7614 were achieved. In the whole heart structure segmentation task, the average DSC reached 75.66% and the average HD was 42.3493. For the structure and pathology segmentation task, the results were an average DSC of 60.67% and an average HD of 22.4493. In general, UniCarSeg demonstrates competitive performance in various cardiac segmentation tasks.

Table 1. Quantitative evaluation of UniCarSeg across different tasks, with DSC and HD reported under in-distribution (In-dist.) and out-of-distribution (Out-of-dist.) settings, respectively. Task 1:Single Cardiac Structure Segmentation; Task 2: Whole Heart Structure Segmentation; Task 3: Structure and Pathology Segmentation

	In-dist.		Out-of-dist.		Average	
Segmentation Task	DSC↑	HD(mm)↓	DSC↑	HD(mm)↓	DSC↑	HD(mm)↓
Task 1	0.8708	68.5828	0.7059	49.7781	0.7584	55.7614
Task 2	0.8486	28.3754	0.6187	63.3101	0.7566	42.3493
Task 3	0.5483	25.9150	0.6417	20.3698	0.6067	22.4493

Figure 3 illustrates the visual segmentation results of UniCarSeg on various images in different testing scenarios. Through comparative analysis of multiple dimensions, including segmentation boundaries, structural integrity, and cross-type consistency, the effectiveness and robustness of the method are validated. Specifically, on both MRI and CT images, the proposed method accurately segments different anatomical structures of the heart, with clear boundaries that closely align with the true morphology. This demonstrates UniCarSeg's capability to perceive features across various cardiac regions. Meanwhile, in different tasks, such as left atria segmentation, whole heart segmentation, structure, and pathology segmentation, the segmentation results exhibit strong structural consistency and semantic discriminability, confirming that the KMD mechanism employed effectively models both commonalities and differences among tasks. The proposed method maintains high generalization capability in cross-modality and multi-center cardiac imaging scenarios, reflecting its strong adaptability to multi-source data.

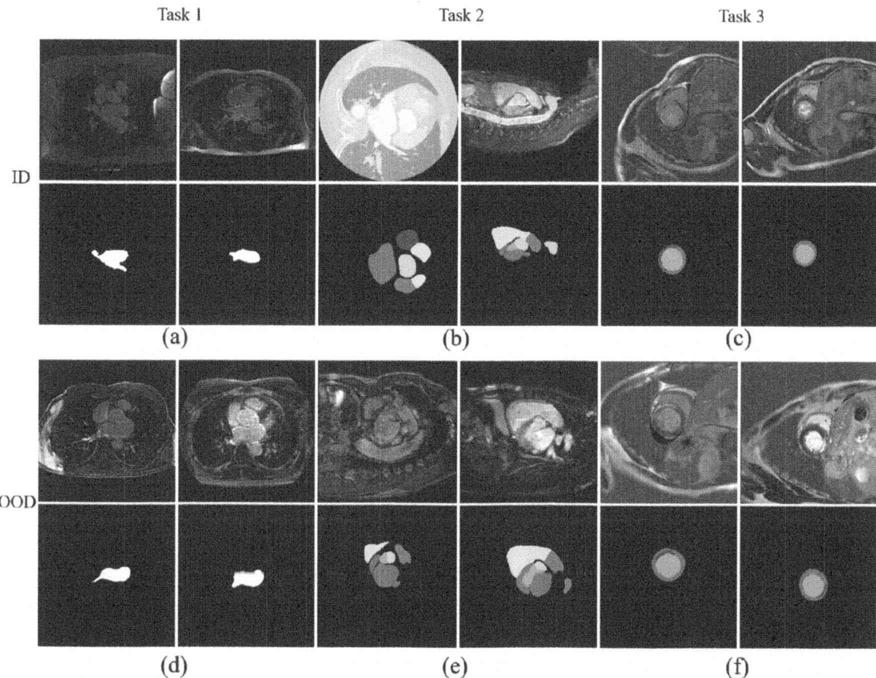

Fig. 3. Visualization of cardiac segmentation examples across different tasks and scenarios. Task 1: Single Cardiac Structure Segmentation (a, d); Task 2: Whole Heart Structure Segmentation (b, e); Task 3: Structure and Pathology Segmentation (c, f). The top two rows show segmentation results in the in-distribution (ID) setting, while the bottom two rows show results in the out-of-distribution (OOD) setting.

Table 2 presents the quantitative comparison results of different methods on the ACDC dataset. It can be seen that the average DSC of the proposed method reached 0.9027, achieving the best performance. Although the RV and LV of the segmentation results did not reach the optimal level, other models have specific advantages in segmenting certain parts, but UniCarSeg has a more balanced segmentation ability for various parts of cardiac MRI images.

Table 2. Quantitative comparison of different methods on the ACDC dataset in terms of the DSC metric.

Methods	Average	RV	Myo	LV
VIT-CUP [5]	0.8145	0.8146	0.7071	0.9218
R50-VIT-CUPP [5]	0.8757	0.8607	0.8188	0.9475
TransUNet [3]	0.8971	**0.8886**	0.8454	**0.9573**
SwinUNet [2]	0.9000	0.8855	0.8562	0.9583
UNETR [7]	0.8861	0.8529	0.8652	0.9402
Ours	**0.9027**	0.8844	**0.8872**	0.9365

Figure 4 shows the visualization segmentation results and ground truth of various types of cardiac MRI images using the proposed method on the ACDC dataset. UniCarSeg can achieve precise segmentation of various cardiac MRI images. No matter what shape the heart appears in MRI, the proposed method can accurately segment the region of interest.

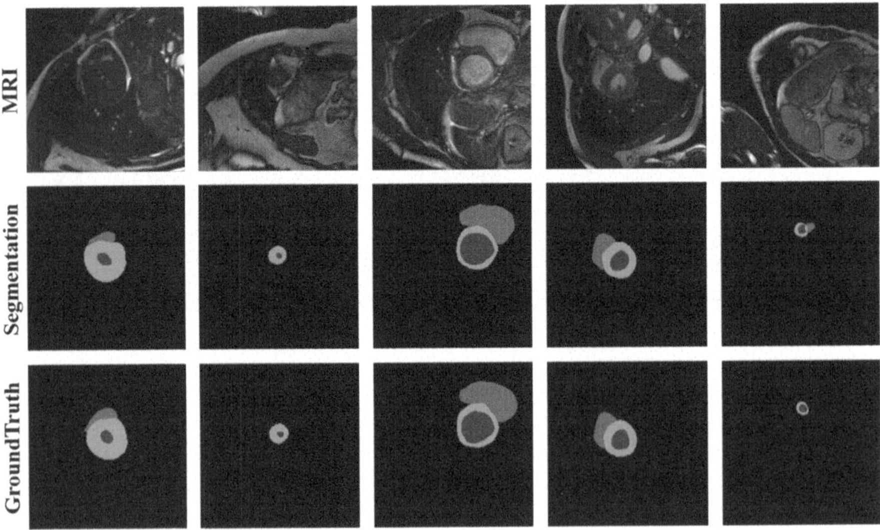

Fig. 4. Visualization of cardiac segmentation examples on the ACDC dataset. Note: Red represents the right ventricle, green represents the myocardium, and blue represents the left ventricle.

In summary, the proposed method not only achieves state-of-the-art segmentation accuracy but also demonstrates notable robustness and versatility in multi-task and multi-modality cardiac image analysis, showing broad potential for clinical application.

4 Conclusion

In this paper, we proposed UniCarSeg, a unified cardiac segmentation method capable of delineating diverse cardiac anatomical structures for clinical disease analysis. UniCarSeg integrates a pretrained image encoder from the foundation segmentation model with a newly designed KAN-based mask decoder (KMD), effectively transforming universal visual embeddings into precise, task-specific medical segmentations. Extensive experiments on the CARE-Cardiac challenge and extra cardiac datasets demonstrate that UniCarSeg achieves competitive and robust performance in simultaneously segmenting different cardiac structures and pathological regions, underscoring its potential for real-world clinical applications.

Future work will focus on enhancing the model's generalization across more imaging modalities and tasks. Meanwhile, exploring a more lightning-fast and flexible decoder to better adapt to diverse segmentation scenarios provides further insights into its practical utility and clinical relevance.

Disclosure of Interests. The authors have no competing interests to declare that are relevant to the content of this article.

References

1. Bernard, O., Lalande, A., Zotti, C., Cervenansky, F., Yang, X., Heng, P.A., Cetin, I., Lekadir, K., Camara, O., Ballester, M.A.G., et al.: Deep learning techniques for automatic mri cardiac multi-structures segmentation and diagnosis: is the problem solved? IEEE Trans. Med. Imaging **37**(11), 2514–2525 (2018)
2. Cao, H., Wang, Y., Chen, J., Jiang, D., Zhang, X., Tian, Q., Wang, M.: Swin-unet: Unet-like pure transformer for medical image segmentation. In: European Conference on Computer Vision, pp. 205–218. Springer (2022)
3. Chen, J., Lu, Y., Yu, Q., Luo, X., Adeli, E., Wang, Y., Lu, L., Yuille, A.L., Zhou, Y.: Transunet: transformers make strong encoders for medical image segmentation. arXiv preprint arXiv:2102.04306 (2021)
4. Cui, X., Cao, Y., Liu, Z., Sui, X., Mi, J., Zhang, Y., Cui, L., Li, S.: Trsa-net: task relation spatial co-attention for joint segmentation, quantification and uncertainty estimation on paired 2d echocardiography. IEEE J. Biomed. Health Inform. **26**(8), 4067–4078 (2022)
5. Dosovitskiy, A., Beyer, L., Kolesnikov, A., Weissenborn, D., Zhai, X., Unterthiner, T., Dehghani, M., Minderer, M., Heigold, G., Gelly, S., et al.: An image is worth 16x16 words: transformers for image recognition at scale. arXiv preprint arXiv:2010.11929 (2020)
6. Gao, S., Zhou, H., Gao, Y., Zhuang, X.: Bayeseg: Bayesian modeling for medical image segmentation with interpretable generalizability. Med. Image Anal. **89**, 102889 (2023)

7. Hatamizadeh, A., Tang, Y., Nath, V., Yang, D., Myronenko, A., Landman, B., Roth, H.R., Xu, D.: Unetr: transformers for 3d medical image segmentation. In: Proceedings of the IEEE/CVF Winter Conference on Applications of Computer Vision, pp. 574–584 (2022)
8. Huang, J., Sun, X., Wang, L.: Enhancing foundation model robustness for multi-center real-world medical image analysis. In: MICCAI Challenge on Comprehensive Analysis and Computing of Real-World Medical Images, pp. 13–23. Springer (2025)
9. Kirillov, A., Mintun, E., Ravi, N., Mao, H., Rolland, C., Gustafson, L., Xiao, T., Whitehead, S., Berg, A.C., Lo, W.Y., et al.: Segment anything. In: Proceedings of the IEEE/CVF International Conference on Computer Vision, pp. 4015–4026 (2023)
10. Li, B., Hu, W., Feng, C.M., Li, Y., Liu, Z., Xu, Y.: Multi-contrast complementary learning for accelerated mr imaging. IEEE J. Biomed. Health Inform. **28**(3), 1436–1447 (2024)
11. Li, B., Zhang, P., Cao, Y., Sun, L., Feng, J., Zhang, Y., Yang, Q., Li, Y., Liu, Z.: Aivus: Guidewire artifacts inpainting for intravascular ultrasound imaging with united spatiotemporal aggregation learning. IEEE Trans. Comput. Imaging **8**, 679–692 (2022)
12. Li, B., Zhang, W., Mukhopadhyay, S.C., Li, Y., Liu, Z.: Spatial frequency adaptive spatiotemporal learning for accelerating cmr reconstruction. IEEE Trans. Instrum. Meas. **74**, 1–13 (2025)
13. Li, C., Liu, X., Li, W., Wang, C., Liu, H., Liu, Y., Chen, Z., Yuan, Y.: U-kan makes strong backbone for medical image segmentation and generation. In: Proceedings of the AAAI Conference on Artificial Intelligence, vol. 39, pp. 4652–4660 (2025)
14. Li, L., Zimmer, V.A., Schnabel, J.A., Zhuang, X.: Atrialjsqnet: a new framework for joint segmentation and quantification of left atrium and scars incorporating spatial and shape information. Med. Image Anal. **76**, 102303 (2022)
15. Li, X., Gao, R., Zheng, Y., Zheng, S., Chen, W.: A left atrial automatic segmentation based on rescaunet. In: MICCAI Challenge on Comprehensive Analysis and Computing of Real-World Medical Images, pp. 139–148. Springer (2025)
16. Lin, B., Dong, J., Zheng, Y., Xiang, Y., Yang, M.: Enhancing domain generalization for cardiac image segmentation with probabilistic perturbation. In: MICCAI Challenge on Comprehensive Analysis and Computing of Real-World Medical Images, pp. 1–12. Springer (2024)
17. Lin, H., Tavakoli, N., Schiffers, F., López-Tapia, S., Kim, D., Katsaggelos, A.K.: Gensegnet: Leveraging synthetic sequences and pseudo labels for multi-sequence myocardial pathology segmentation. In: MICCAI Challenge on Comprehensive Analysis and Computing of Real-World Medical Images, pp. 227–239. Springer (2024)
18. Loshchilov, I., Hutter, F.: Decoupled weight decay regularization. ArXiv Preprint ArXiv:1711.05101 (2017)
19. Lyu, Y., Tian, X.: Mwg-unet: hybrid deep learning framework for lung fields and heart segmentation in chest x-ray images. Bioengineering **10**(9), 1091 (2023)
20. Ma, J., He, Y., Li, F., Han, L., You, C., Wang, B.: Segment anything in medical images. Nat. Commun. **15**(1), 654 (2024)
21. Margolis, I., Toso, L.D., Buoso, S., Kozerke, S.: Two-stage weighted ensemble method for myocardial edema and scar segmentation. In: MICCAI Challenge on Comprehensive Analysis and Computing of Real-World Medical Images, pp. 55–65. Springer (2025)

22. Salgado-Garcia, R.J., Vila-Blanco, N., Carreira, M.J., Nuñez-Garcia, M.: Efficient multi-modal whole heart segmentation via cascaded u-net: a practical solution for clinical settings. In: MICCAI Challenge on Comprehensive Analysis and Computing of Real-World Medical Images, pp. 158–167. Springer (2024)
23. Tang, M., Li, N., Pan, L.: Improved nn-unet: generalizable multi-scale attention-driven segmentation of multi-sequence myocardial pathology. In: MICCAI Challenge on Comprehensive Analysis and Computing of Real-World Medical Images, pp. 96–105. Springer (2024)
24. Tran, C., Li, A., Espinoza, A., Kamal, S., Samuel, A., Jiang, C., Zhuang, J., Shi, Y., Xu, X.: Enhance multi-modal and multi-center whole heart segmentation using data augmentation and model calibration. In: MICCAI Challenge on Comprehensive Analysis and Computing of Real-World Medical Images, pp. 126–138. Springer (2024)
25. Zhang, S., Zhang, Q., Zhang, S., Liu, X., Yue, J., Lu, M., Xu, H., Yao, J., Wei, X., Cao, J., et al.: A generalist foundation model and database for open-world medical image segmentation. Nat. Biomed. Eng. 1–16 (2025)
26. Zhang, Y., Cheng, H., Li, D., Pan, L.: Left atrial scar segmentation and quantification using residual cbam-eam attention unet for lge mri. In: MICCAI Challenge on Comprehensive Analysis and Computing of Real-World Medical Images, pp. 149–157. Springer (2025)
27. Zhu, Z., Lin, Y., Yang, M.: Me-unet: Enhancing mamba for myocardial pathology segmentation in multi-center multi-sequence cmr images. In: MICCAI Challenge on Comprehensive Analysis and Computing of Real-World Medical Images, pp. 66–76. Springer (2025)
28. Zhuang, X.: Multivariate mixture model for myocardial segmentation combining multi-source images. IEEE Trans. Pattern Anal. Mach. Intell. **41**(12), 2933–2946 (2019)
29. Zhuang, X., Shen, J.: Multi-scale patch and multi-modality atlases for whole heart segmentation of mri. Med. Image Anal. **31**, 77–87 (2016)

Improved mmFormer for Liver Fibrosis Staging via Missing-Modality Compensation

Zhejia Zhang(✉), Junjie Wang, and Le Zhang

School of Engineering, College of Engineering and Physical Sciences, University of Birmingham, Birmingham, UK

zhejiazhang2026@u.northwestern.edu

Abstract. In real-world clinical settings, magnetic resonance imaging (MRI) frequently suffers from missing modalities due to equipment variability or patient cooperation issues, which can significantly affect model performance. To address this issue, we propose a multimodal MRI classification model based on the mmFormer architecture with an adaptive module for handling arbitrary combinations of missing modalities. Specifically, this model retains the hybrid modality-specific encoders and the modality-correlated encoder from mmFormer to extract consistent lesion features across available modalities. In addition, we integrate a missing-modality compensation module which leverages zero-padding, modality availability masks, and a Delta Function with learnable statistical parameters to dynamically synthesize proxy features for recovering missing information. To further improve prediction performance, we adopt a cross-validation ensemble strategy by training multiple models on different folds and applying soft voting during inference. This method is evaluated on the test set of Comprehensive Analysis & Computing of REal-world medical images (CARE) 2025 challenge, targeting the Liver Fibrosis Staging (LiFS) task based on non-contrast dynamic MRI scans including T1-weighted imaging (T1WI), T2-weighted imaging (T2WI), and diffusion-weighted imaging (DWI). For Cirrhosis Detection and Substantial Fibrosis Detection on in-distribution vendors, our model obtains accuracies of 66.67% and 74.17%, and corresponding area under the curve (AUC) scores of 71.73% and 68.48%, respectively.

Keywords: 3D medical image analysis · Liver fibrosis staging · Multimodal deep learning

1 Introduction

Liver fibrosis results from the sustained overproduction and accumulation of extracellular matrix (ECM) proteins and is common across chronic liver diseases, such as viral hepatitis, alcohol-related liver disease, and metabolic steatohepatitis [1]. This sustained overaccumulation of ECM causes fibrotic scarring and distortion of the normal liver architecture, while the development of regenerative nodules marks the transition to cirrhosis [1]. Timely and accurate diagnostic and therapeutic strategies are crucial for slowing the progression of liver cirrhosis [2].

X. Zhuang et al. (Eds.): CARE 2025, LNCS 16257, pp. 180–189, 2026.
https://doi.org/10.1007/978-3-032-16271-7_17

Although liver biopsy has been regarded as the "gold standard" for diagnosing liver fibrosis, its limitations—including sampling variability, interpretative subjectivity, risk of complications, and high cost—have driven the development and widespread adoption of non-invasive alternatives such as imaging test and elastography to reduce the reliance on biopsy [3, 4]. Notably, multimodal MRI scans have become one of the most effective methods for liver fibrosis assessment, as they can capture complementary diagnostic information [5].

With the development of technology, increasingly advanced methods have been developed and integrated with existing non-invasive diagnostic tools for liver fibrosis assessment. Among these, artificial intelligence (AI) and deep learning have demonstrated significant potential in medical image analysis. Compared to traditional diagnostic approaches, AI-based methods provide not only improved efficiency and accuracy, but also enhanced robustness to external variability, enabling more consistent and reliable decision-making across diverse clinical settings [6].

However, the practical application of AI models has proven to be less straightforward than initially expected. In clinical practice, one or more MRI modalities may be missing due to hardware failures, patient non-cooperation, or inconsistent procedures, which result in the loss of specific information and prevents the model from fully capturing target features, thereby significantly compromising its accuracy and generalizability [5]. To address the challenge of missing MRI modalities, researchers have proposed various strategies, including modality imputation, modality synthesis and feature distillation to improve the performance of models [7–9].

In this study, we improve upon the original mmFormer architecture by replacing the segmentation head with a classification head and incorporating a missing-modality compensation module which generates proxy features to recover missing modality information [7]. To increase robustness while improving generalization performance, we adopt a cross-validation strategy during training and apply soft voting ensemble inference at validation, achieve more stable and reliable classification performance in real-world clinical scenarios.

2 Method

2.1 Dataset

The non-contrast subtasks of the LiFS challenge are based solely on three non-enhanced MRI modalities: T1WI, T2WI, and DWI, selected from the LiQA dataset of CARE 2025 challenge for the development and evaluation of liver fibrosis staging models [10–12]. This dataset includes MRI scans from 610 patients diagnosed with liver fibrosis, acquired using three different scanner vendors: Philips Ingenia 3.0T, Siemens Skyra 3.0T, and Siemens Aera 1.5T. The dataset is partitioned into 360 cases for training, 60 for validation, and 190 for testing. To assess out-of-vendor generalization, the test set includes 70 cases acquired on a fourth scanner from a manufacturer not represented in the training data. All data are provided in NIfTI format without preprocessing, and some cases contain randomly missing modalities. Our objective is to classify patients into four pathological stages (S1–S4), along with two binary subtasks:

1. Cirrhosis Detection (S1–S3 vs. S4)
2. Substantial Fibrosis Detection (S1 vs. S2–S4)

The training dataset comprising 360 patients was initially split into an internal training set and an internal validation set with a ratio of 0.75:0.25. To ensure robust evaluation, we further applied a 4-fold cross-validation strategy and stratified sampling was employed to guarantee that samples from each fibrosis stage were proportionally represented in each fold, preserving the stage distribution across all subsets [13].

2.2 Model Architecture

We adopt modality-specific and modality-correlated encoders from mmFormer, keeping their architectures largely consistent with the original design [7]. Our modifications center on a modality-compensation mechanism and a classification-oriented redesign (Fig. 1).

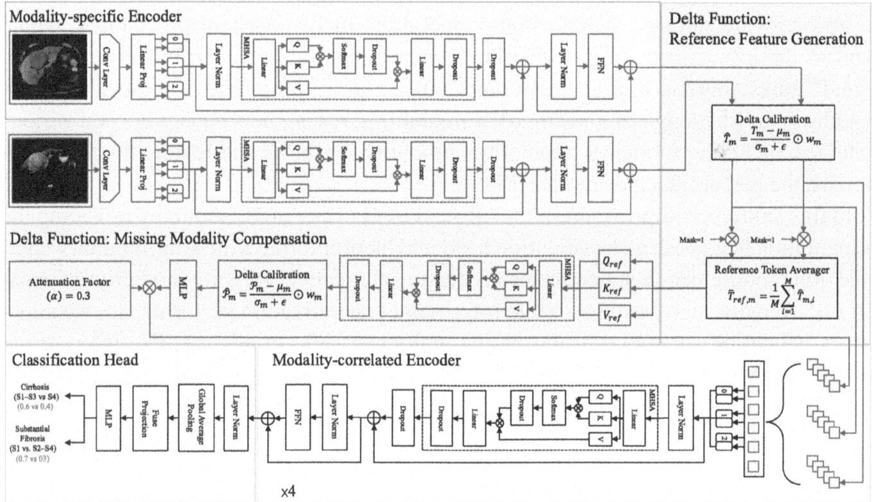

Fig. 1. The overall architecture of the model includes mmFormer's original modality-specific encoder, modality-correlated encoder, Delta Function for generating proxy features, and classification head [7].

2.3 Modality-Specific Encoder

Modality-specific encoder integrates a convolutional encoder with an intra-modality Transformer: local patterns are captured by the convolutional encoder; the produced feature maps are then processed by an intra-modality Transformer to learn long-range dependencies. For each available modality$m \in \{T1WI, T2WI, DWI\}$, it is processed by an identical modality-specific encoder with independent parameters from input volume $X_m \in \mathbb{R}^{1\times D\times H\times W}$.

Convolutional Encoder. The convolutional encoder $\mathcal{F}_m^{conv}$ stacks five residual 3D convolutional stages. Each stage begins with an entry 3D convolution. Stage 1 keeps unit stride, whereas stages 2 to 5 begin with an entry normalized convolution of stride 2 with reflect padding. At stage s, the cumulative down-sampling factor is 2^{s-1}; thus, at the top stage $s = 5$, it is 16. Thus, the top-stage spatial dimension is $\frac{D}{16} \times \frac{H}{16} \times \frac{W}{16}$. Within each stage, we apply two normalized convolutional units. Each unit consists of instance normalization, LeakyReLU, and dropout. The unit output is added to the stage input via an identity skip connection. Denoting the base width by $C_{base} = 8$, the channel schedule across stages follows

$$C_s = 2^{s-1} C_{base}, s \in \{1,2,3,4,5\} \tag{1}$$

The resulting local-context feature maps are given by

$$F_m^{local} = \mathcal{F}_m^{conv}\left(X_m; \theta_m^{conv}\right), F_m^{local} \in \mathbb{R}^{C_5 \times \frac{D}{16} \times \frac{H}{16} \times \frac{W}{16}} \tag{2}$$

The top-stage feature is then projected to a fixed embedding dimension and flattened into tokens for the intra-modality Transformer [7].

Intra-modality Transformer. To capture long-range dependencies within each modality, we use an intra-modality Transformer to explicitly model global context. For modality m, the branch tokenizes features and applies pre-norm residual blocks of multi-head self-attention (MSA) and a position-wise feed-forward network (FFN). We apply a $1 \times 1 \times 1$ convolution acting as a linear projection to obtain $C_t = 256$ channels and flatten voxels into a token sequence:

$$T_m^{(0)} = vec\left(Conv_{1\times1\times1}\left(F_m^{local}\right)\right), T_m^{(0)} \in \mathbb{R}^{N \times C_t}, \tag{3}$$

where $N = D\prime H\prime W\prime$, and C_t is embedding size. A fixed sinusoidal positional encoding $P_m \in \mathbb{R}^{N \times C_t}$ is used and added at every layer of the Transformer. At layer l, positions are added as

$$\tilde{T}_m^{(l)} = T_m^{(l-1)} + P_m. \tag{4}$$

With $Q_m^{(l)} = LN(\tilde{T}_m^{(l)})W_{Q,m}^{(l)}$, $K_m^{(l)} = LN(\tilde{T}_m^{(l)})W_{K,m}^{(l)}$, $V_m^{(l)} = LN(\tilde{T}_m^{(l)})W_{V,m}^{(l)}$, the output of MSA is

$$head_{m,i}^{(l)} = softmax\left(\frac{Q_m^{(l)}\left(K_m^{(l)}\right)^{\top}}{\sqrt{d_k}}\right)V_m^{(l)}, \tag{5}$$

$$MSA_m^{(l)} = \left[head_{m,1}^{1}; \ldots; head_{m,h}^{(l)}\right]W_{O,m}^{(l)}, \tag{6}$$

where $LN(\bullet)$ represents layer normalization and $h = 4$ denotes the number of attention heads. Each layer stacks MSA and FFN with residual connections and the token sequence with long-range dependencies from intra-modality Transformer is shown as

$$Z_m^{(l)} = MSA_m^{(l)}\left(\tilde{T}_m^{(l)}\right) + \tilde{T}_m^{(l)}, \tag{7}$$

$$T_m^{(L)} = FFN_m^{(l)}\left(LN\left(Z_m^{(l)}\right)\right) + Z_m^{(l)}, \tag{8}$$

where FFN is a two-layer position-wise perceptron with GELU activation and dropout. All parameters are modality-specific and not shared across modalities, enabling each Transformer to enhance modality-unique textures and lesion edges. It also produces stable, global-context features for the later cross-modal fusion and the classifier [7].

2.4 Delta Function

Modality Mask. We construct a binary modality-availability mask for each sample, where 1 indicates that the modality is present and participates in computation, and 0 indicates it is missing. When the modality branch is deemed "missing," the subsequent compensation module synthesizes proxy features to replace the missing modality [14].

Delta Calibration. To address cross-modality distribution mismatch in multimodal MRI, we are inspired by Feature-wise Linear Modulation (FiLM) and Adaptive Instance Normalization (AdaIN) and apply a learnable affine calibration to each modality's token sequence, which performs learnable mean-variance alignment and reliability-aware reweighting [15, 16]. The formula can be shown as:

$$\widehat{T}_m = \frac{T_m - \mu_m}{\sigma_m + \epsilon} \odot w_m, \tag{9}$$

where μ_m, σ_m, w_m are learnable per-channel mean, scale, and reliability weights, respectively. $\epsilon = 1 \times 10^{-8}$ ensures numerical stability. This approach maps different modality features to a shared space, improving cross-modal fusion and enabling better multimodal processing. After calibration, the modality-wise tokens have two purposes:

1. Calibrated tokens as valid modality are fed into the subsequent cross-modal fusion.
2. Calibrated tokens are aggregated as reference tokens to synthesize proxy features.

Reference Token Averager. To create a unified representation for missing modality compensation, we build a reference token by averaging features from all available modalities. The reference token is computed as:

$$\overline{T}_{ref,m} = \frac{1}{M}\sum_{i=1}^{M} \widehat{T}_{m,i}, \tag{10}$$

where M is the number of available modalities.

Proxy Feature Compensation. After generating the reference sequence, we apply another MSA to it to capture global context; therefore $\overline{T}_{ref,m} = Q_{ref} = K_{ref} = V_{ref}$ and preliminary proxy features $\mathcal{P}_m$ can be expressed as

$$\mathcal{P}_m = MSA\left(\overline{T}_{ref,m}, \overline{T}_{ref,m}, \overline{T}_{ref,m}\right). \tag{11}$$

Subsequently, preliminary proxy features are passed through affine calibration again to obtain

$$\widehat{\mathcal{P}}_m = \frac{\mathcal{P}_m - \mu_m}{\sigma_m + \epsilon} \odot w_m, \tag{12}$$

ensuring the resulting target-modality proxy features are more robust [15]. Finally, the preliminary proxy features are refined by FFN, and a fixed attenuation factor $\alpha = 0.3$ is applied to attenuate their relative contribution and suppress noise from synthesized information during subsequent fusion [17]. The final proxy feature is obtained as

$$T_{proxy,m} = \alpha \times FFN(\widehat{\mathcal{P}}_m). \tag{13}$$

2.5 Modality-Correlated Encoder

Given the valid and proxy token sequences, we apply spatial alignment and standardize the token length by truncating longer sequences to the shortest length. All tokens are subsequently concatenated along token axis in a fixed order to yield the final sequence

$$T_c^{(0)} = [T_1, T_2, \cdots, T_M], T_c \in \mathbb{R}^{(M \times N_t) \times C_t}, \tag{14}$$

where M is the number of available modalities, T_c is concatenated token, and N_t is the number of tokens per modality after alignment. This encoder stacks 4 Transformer blocks. At each layer, we add a fixed sinusoidal positional encoding

$$\tilde{T}_c^{(l)} = T_c^{(l-1)} + P_c, \tag{15}$$

and apply MSA and FFN with residual connections again [7]:

$$Z_c^{(l)} = MSA^{(l)}\left(\tilde{T}_c^{(l)}\right) + \tilde{T}_c^{(l)}, \tag{16}$$

$$T_c^{(L)} = FFN^{(l)}\left(LN\left(Z_c^{(l)}\right)\right) + Z_c^{(l)}. \tag{17}$$

2.6 Classification Head

An external layer normalization is applied to the token sequence before pooling. Global average pooling (GAP) over the token yields a 256-dimensional representation, which is linearly projected with dropout to fused embedding. Also, a two-layer multi-layer perceptron (MLP) and the final linear projection layer are applied to output logits.

2.7 Model Ensemble

We employ four-fold cross-validation to train four homogeneous base models. At inference, the same sample is passed through all four models to obtain four logits, which are converted to class probabilities via SoftMax. We then perform soft voting by averaging the unweighted model probabilities for each class. Model ensemble improves robustness and generalization across splits [18].

3 Experiment and Results

Both subtasks follow the same experimental procedures and use the same equipment.

3.1 Experiment Setting

Image Preprocessing. For both training and inference, all images are reoriented to right–anterior–superior (RAS) and resampled to $1.5 \times 1.5 \times 3.0$ mm voxel spacing, improving concordance and reducing sensitivity to pixel-spacing changes [19]. Then, intensities are normalized per volume by mapping the 1st–99th percentiles to [0,1] with clipping. Volumes are resized to $200 \times 200 \times 64$ via symmetric padding or centered cropping, after which the first 20 axial slices are removed to improve target visibility, yielding a final input size of $200 \times 200 \times 44$. Missing modalities are substituted with zero-filled volumes matching the target dimensions. To accelerate training, the preprocessed modality data and corresponding modality masks are packaged into NPZ files. Finally, stage-wise data augmentations are applied to the training set: its strength scales with sample size and combines geometric (flip/rotate/zoom) and intensity perturbations (scaling, noise, contrast, smoothing, shift).

Training Hyperparameters. The training script uses the AdamW optimizer with a learning rate of 1×10^{-4} and weight decay of 1×10^{-3}, with cross-entropy loss. A cosine-annealing schedule is applied for up to 100 epochs with a minimum learning rate of 1×10^{-6}. Early stopping is triggered by validation loss with a patience of 30 epochs while continually saving the best checkpoint. Data are loaded with a batch size of 8. Training and inference are conducted on an NVIDIA A100 GPU with 40 GB VRAM.

3.2 Evaluation Metrics

We report results under the official metrics defined by the organizers, including accuracy (ACC) and AUC. Concretely, accuracy is the proportion of correct predictions among all evaluated samples [20]. As the decision threshold varies, the receiver operating characteristics (ROC) curve maps sensitivity against the false-positive rate; the area under receiver operating characteristics (AUROC) yields a threshold-independent discrimination score [21].

3.3 Model Evaluation

Table 1. Comparison between prior models and proposed model on in-distribution (ID) vendors.

Method	Cirrhosis detection (S1–S3 vs. S4)		Substantial Fibrosis detection (S1 vs. S2–S4)	
	ACC (%)	AUC (%)	ACC (%)	AUC (%)
CE	60.00	74.98	73.33	61.11

(continued)

Table 1. *(continued)*

Method	Cirrhosis detection (S1–S3 vs. S4)		Substantial Fibrosis detection (S1 vs. S2–S4)	
	ACC (%)	AUC (%)	ACC (%)	AUC (%)
BCE	**70.00**	77.90	70.00	66.67
BCE with CSL	63.33	**80.83**	73.33	68.52
Reg	**70.00**	71.81	70.00	**76.39**
CE with CSL	**70.00**	76.83	**80.00**	75.23
Proposed model (ID)	66.67	71.73	74.17	68.48

As shown in Table 1, we compare our model against the as-reported external baselines from the LiFS task of CARE 2024, including CE, BCE, Reg, BCE with CSL, and CE with CSL[1] [22]. Without using any external data or relying on pre-segmentation or lesion localization, our approach maintains competitive performance overall. For Cirrhosis Detection, the model achieves accuracy of 66.67% and AUC of 71.73%; these are 3.33% and 9.10% lower than the best results, respectively, but improved 6.67% in accuracy over the CE baseline. For Substantial Fibrosis Detection, the model achieves accuracy of 74.17% and AUC of 68.48%, ranking second in accuracy and fourth in AUC, but only 0.04% behind the third-place method (68.52%). Compared to the CE baseline, this method improves accuracy by 0.84% and AUC by 7.37% on this task. Overall, without the need for additional segmentation or external data, this method demonstrates stable discriminative ability and good robustness on both tasks.

Table 2. Comparison of proposed model on ID vendors and out-of-distribution (OOD) vendors.

Method	Cirrhosis detection (S1–S3 vs. S4)		Substantial fibrosis detection (S1 vs. S2–S4)	
	ACC (%)	AUC (%)	ACC (%)	AUC (%)
Proposed model (ID)	**66.67**	**71.73**	74.17	68.48
Proposed model (OOD)	64.29	68.83	**91.43**	**71.38**

Under an OOD vendor, Table 2 shows that Cirrhosis Detection achieves accuracy of 64.29% and AUC of 68.83%, which are 2.38% and 2.90% lower than the in-distribution results, while Substantial Fibrosis Detection improves markedly to accuracy of 91.43% and AUC of 71.38%, gains of 17.26% and 2.90%, respectively, with 91.43% being the best among all evaluated methods.

[1] Abbreviations: CE for cross-entropy; BCE for binary cross-entropy; CSL for class activation map–segmentation map loss; Reg for regression [22].

4 Conclusion

Our study presents a multimodal Transformer based on mmFormer that integrates Delta-based missing-modality compensation, an improved classification head, and a four-fold ensembling strategy. The model shows strong adaptability to missing-modality scenarios in the LiFS task. On the in-distribution vendor split, it achieved accuracies of 66.67 and 74.17% for cirrhosis and substantial fibrosis detection, with corresponding AUCs of 71.73 and 68.48%, indicating competitive discrimination and robustness. Future work will focus on enhancing cross-center and cross-vendor generalization, with systematic external validation.

Acknowledgments. We thank the CARE 2025 organizers for providing access to the LiQA dataset used in this study [10–12].

Disclosure of Interests. The authors declare that they have no competing interests.

References

1. Bataller, R., Brenner, D.A.: Liver fibrosis. J. Clin. Investig. **115**(2), 209–218 (2005)
2. Toosi, A.E.: Liver fibrosis: causes and methods of assessment, a review. Rom. J. Intern. Med. **53**(4), 304–314 (2015)
3. Tapper, E.B., Lok, A.S.F.: Use of liver imaging and biopsy in clinical practice. N. Engl. J. Med. **377**(8), 756–768 (2017)
4. Bravo, A.A., Sheth, S.G., Chopra, S.: Liver biopsy. N. Engl. J. Med. **344**(7), 495–500 (2001)
5. Azad, R., Khosravi, N., Dehghanmanshadi, M., Cohen-Adad, J., Merhof, D.: Medical image segmentation on MRI images with missing modalities: a review (2022). arXiv:2203.06217
6. Zhou, L.Q., Wang, J.Y., Yu, S.Y., et al.: Artificial intelligence in medical imaging of the liver. World J. Gastroenterol. **25**(6), 672–682 (2019)
7. Zhang, Y., et al.: MmFormer: multimodal medical transformer for incomplete multimodal learning of brain Tumor segmentation. In: Wang, L., Dou, Q., Fletcher, P.T., Speidel, S., Li, S. (eds.) Medical Image Computing and Computer Assisted Intervention – MICCAI 2022, LNCS, vol. 13435, pp. 107–117. Springer, Cham (2022)
8. Chartsias, A., Joyce, T., Dharmakumar, R., Tsaftaris, S.A.: Adversarial image synthesis for unpaired multi-modal cardiac data. In: Tsaftaris, S., Gooya, A., Frangi, A., Prince, J. (eds.) Simulation and Synthesis in Medical Imaging. SASHIMI 2017, LNCS, vol. 10557, pp. 3–13. Springer, Cham (2017)
9. Wang, H., et al.: Learnable cross-modal knowledge distillation for multi-modal learning with missing modality. In: Greenspan, H., et al. (eds.) Medical Image Computing and Computer Assisted Intervention – MICCAI 2023, LNCS, vol. 14223, pp. 216–226. Springer, Cham (2023)
10. Liu, Y., et al.: MERIT: Multi-view evidential learning for reliable and interpretable liver fibrosis staging. Med. Image Anal. **102**, 103507 (2025)
11. Gao, Z., Liu, Y., Wu, F., Shi, N., Shi, Y., Zhuang, X.: A reliable and interpretable framework of multi-view learning for liver fibrosis staging. In: Greenspan, H., et al. (eds.) Medical Image Computing and Computer Assisted Intervention – MICCAI 2023, LNCS, vol. 14224, pp. 178–188. Springer, Cham (2023)
12. Wu, F., Zhuang, X.: Minimizing estimated risks on unlabeled data: A new formulation for semi-supervised medical image segmentation. IEEE Trans. Pattern Anal. Mach. Intell. **45**(5), 6021–6036 (2023)

13. Zheng, Y., Wu, F., Papież, B.W.: An ensemble method to automatically grade diabetic retinopathy with optical coherence tomography angiography images. In: Sheng, B., Aubreville, M. (eds.) Mitosis Domain Generalization and Diabetic Retinopathy Analysis – MIDOG/DRAC 2022, LNCS, vol. 13597, pp. 46–58. Springer, Cham (2023)
14. Meng, X., Sun, K., Xu, J., He, X., Shen, D.: Multi-modal modality-masked diffusion network for brain MRI synthesis with random modality missing. IEEE Trans. Med. Imaging **43**(7), 2587–2598 (2024)
15. Perez, E., Strub, F., de Vries, H., Dumoulin, V., Courville, A.: FiLM: visual reasoning with a general conditioning layer. In: Proceedings of the AAAI Conference on Artificial Intelligence (AAAI), pp. 3942–3951. AAAI Press, New Orleans (2018)
16. Huang, X., Belongie, S.: Arbitrary style transfer in real-time with adaptive instance normalization. In: Proceedings of the IEEE International Conference on Computer Vision (ICCV), pp. 1501–1510. IEEE, Venice (2017)
17. Oktay, O., Schlemper, J., Le Folgoc, L., Lee, M., Heinrich, M., Misawa, K., et al.: Attention U-Net: learning where to look for the pancreas (2018). arXiv:1804.03999
18. Ganaie, M.A., Hu, M., Malik, A.K., Tanveer, M., Suganthan, P.N.: Ensemble deep learning: a review. Eng. Appl. Artif. Intell. **115**, 105151 (2022)
19. Park, S.H., et al.: Robustness of magnetic resonance radiomic features to pixel size resampling and interpolation in patients with cervical cancer. Cancer Imaging **21**(1), 19 (2021)
20. Grandini, M., Bagli, E., Visani, G.: Metrics for multi-class classification: an overview. arXiv: 2008.05756 (2020)
21. Huang, J., Ling, C.X.: Using AUC and accuracy in evaluating learning algorithms. IEEE Trans. Knowl. Data Eng. **17**(3), 299–310 (2005)
22. Zhang, H., Zhang, M., You, X., Gu, Y., Yang, G.-Z.: Computing assessment for liver fibrosis staging using real-world MR images. In: Zhuang, X., Ding, W., Wu, F., Gao, S., Li, L., Wang, S. (eds.) Comprehensive Analysis and Computing of Real-World Medical Images. CARE 2024, LNCS, vol. 15548, pp. 87–95. Springer, Cham (2025)

SSL-MedSAM2: A Semi-supervised Medical Image Segmentation Framework Powered by Few-Shot Learning of SAM2

Zhendi Gong(✉) and Xin Chen

School of Computer Science, University of Nottingham, Nottingham, UK
{zhendi.gong,xin.chen}@nottingham.ac.uk

Abstract. Despite the success of deep learning based models in medical image segmentation, most state-of-the-art (SOTA) methods perform fully-supervised learning, which commonly rely on large scale annotated training datasets. However, medical image annotation is highly time-consuming, hindering its clinical applications. Semi-supervised learning (SSL) has been emerged as an appealing strategy in training with limited annotations, largely reducing the labelling cost. We propose a novel SSL framework SSL-MedSAM2, which contains a training-free few-shot learning branch TFFS-MedSAM2 based on the pretrained large foundation model Segment Anything Model 2 (SAM2) for pseudo label generation, and an iterative fully-supervised learning branch FSL-nnUNet based on nnUNet for pseudo label refinement. The results on MICCAI2025 challenge CARE-LiSeg (Liver Segmentation) demonstrate an outstanding performance of SSL-MedSAM2 among other methods. The average dice scores on the test set in GED4 and T1 MRI are 0.9710 and 0.9648 respectively, and the Hausdorff distances are 20.07 and 21.97 respectively. The code is available via https://github.com/naisops/SSL-MedSAM2/tree/main.

Keywords: Medical image segmentation · Semi-supervised learning · Large foundation models

1 Introduction

Liver segmentation in MRI plays a crucial role in diagnosing and monitoring a wide range of hepatic diseases, including hepatocellular carcinoma, cirrhosis, and fatty liver disease [2]. Despite the remarkable progress facilitated by deep learning, its full potential in medical image segmentation is frequently affected by the substantial reliance on large-scale, accurately annotated training data [9]. In clinical practice, obtaining high-quality medical image annotations is an inherently difficult, time-consuming, and expensive effort [4]. This contrast has motivated semi-supervised learning (SSL) strategies, which aim to leverage abundant unlabelled data alongside a limited labelled set to train robust segmentation models.

X. Zhuang et al. (Eds.): CARE 2025, LNCS 16257, pp. 190–200, 2026.
https://doi.org/10.1007/978-3-032-16271-7_18

One common approach is **pseudo labelling**, where a model's predictions on unlabelled images are treated as pseudo ground truth to retrain the model or train a student model in an iterative manner. In this branch of approaches, pseudo labels are mostly generated directly from the predictions of the unlabelled data using a trained model followed by some post-processing methods. To increase the reliability of the pseudo labels, recent studies focus on uncertainty-aware methods. For instance, double-threshold schemes combined classification and segmentation confidences to pick reliable pixels [24]. Ssa-net [21] added a trust module to re-evaluate model outputs and retain only high-confidence predictions. Additionally, pseudo labels can also be generated from label propagation by prototype learning [6] or image registration [23]. These approaches aim to transfer the knowledge from the labelled data to the unlabelled ones. As a main constraint of the pseudo labelling strategy, the overall performance relies on the robustness of the initial model for pseudo labelling, and the inaccuracy in pseudo labels can be quickly amplified during the training process.

Another widely used approach is **consistency regularization**, which encourages a segmentation model to produce invariant predictions under different perturbations of the same input, effectively pushing the decision boundary into low-density regions of the data manifold. Normally, input-level perturbation like Gaussian noise or mix-up augmentations to shift input data [1,13], or feature-level perturbation to modify intermediate feature maps [14,18] is introduced. The widely used framework in this branch of methods is mean teacher [20], which used a "teacher" network whose weights are the exponential moving average (EMA) of the "student" network weights. Consistency is enforced between the student and teacher predictions on perturbed inputs. Beyond data-level augmentations, some methods imposed consistency between related tasks, by adding auxiliary task (e.g. signed distance map regression, contour prediction, reconstruction) to leverage geometric information [3,12]. Main limitation of the consistency regularization methods is the dependency on the strength and type of perturbations. Weak perturbations may yield little benefit, while overly strong ones can confuse the model and degrade performance [8].

Most existing SSL methods train models from scratch on the small labelled set, which may limit their ability to quickly capture generalizable features from the outset. Recently, the emergence of large foundation models for image segmentation offers a new opportunity to address these challenges due to their impressive zero-shot and few-shot segmentation capabilities [17]. In particular, the Segment Anything Model (SAM) [10] has garnered attention as a promotable segmentation model trained on billions of 2D natural image segmentation tasks, capable of generalizing to a wide range of objects with minimal user input (e.g. points or bounding boxes).

Building on SAM, Segment Anything Model 2 (SAM2) [19] extended its capabilities to video segmentation, by treating 2D images as video frames, and proposing a streaming memory mechanism to transfer knowledge between frames. The spatial continuity between adjacent slices in a 3D medical image parallels the temporal coherence of successive video frames. By treating a 3D volume data as a video, the adaption of SAM2 on medical images domain is more robust than SAM [27]. By fine-tuning SAM2 on large-scale medical datasets, MedSAM2 [16] had shown superior performance on plenty of medical segmentation tasks.

Deploying such a foundation model in medical imaging could allow rapid learning from very limited labelled data due to its reliable predictions from few-shot segmentation, potentially alleviating the need for large annotated datasets [11]. In the branch of **pseudo labelling** approaches in SSL methods, based on the prompts generated by SSL models, SAM and SAM2 can be applied to select reliable pseudo-labels, showing a superior performance compared with existing SSL algorithms. SAMDSK [26] used SAM with empty prompt on unlabelled data and selected the reliable predictions by a CNN trained on the labelled dataset. Li et al. [11] first applied CNN to generate a rough prediction on an unlabelled image, then converted the prediction into point prompts for SAM to produce reliable pseudo masks. To modify the prompt generation process, CPC-SAM [17] proposed a cross prompting consistency method to automatically generate reliable prompts for unlabelled data across two decoder branches. Furthermore, in **consistency regularization** branch, SemiSAM [25] used a trainable mean teacher framework to produce prompts for SAM, and the predictions from SAM assist in the mean teacher training.

All the above SAM-based SSL methods cannot directly transfer the valuable knowledge from the labelled data to unlabelled ones by the impressive zero-shot and few-shot segmentation capabilities of SAM or SAM2 without any training. In our method, we propose SSL-MedSAM2, an iterative **pseudo labelling** approach. Specifically, we first propose a training-free few-shot learning branch TFFS-MedSAM2 based on MedSAM2 [16], which adapted SAM2 in medical imaging, to produce initial pseudo labels for the unlabelled data in an ensemble manner. It is then followed by an iterative fully-supervised training branch FSL-nnUNet to refine the pseudo masks. In TFFS-MedSAM2, we leverage SAM2's promptable interface to perform segmentation on unlabelled images in a few-shot manner. Our proposed method was evaluated using MICCAI 2025 challenge CARELiSeg dataset [5,15,22] for both the non-contrast and contrast-enhanced subtasks. The contributions of this work are summarized as follows:

1. We propose SSL-MedSAM2, a novel semi-supervised medical image segmentation framework. To our knowledge, this is one of the first frameworks to uniquely combine a large foundation segmentation model adapted on medical images (MedSAM2) in a training-free manner with a task-specific segmentation network (nnU-Net) into a SSL pipeline.
2. We introduce TFFS-MedSAM2, a novel training-free few-shot learning branch in an ensemble predicting manner that harnesses the pre-trained MedSAM2 model for efficient and high-quality pseudo-label generation on unlabelled volumetric data without requiring of any user prompts.
3. Our framework achieves outstanding performance on the CARE-LiSeg challenge for both GED4 and T1 MRI, where only a few GED4 MRI is annotated, demonstrating its generalizability and robustness across different scans and

its efficacy and potential for clinical applications by achieving superior performance while significantly reducing labelling costs.

2 Method

2.1 Preliminaries

SSL aims to train high-performing models based on the combination of limited labelled data and a large amount of unlabelled data. We formulate the SSL task as following. Given a dataset $\mathcal{D}$, it consists of two subsets $\mathcal{D}^l$ and $\mathcal{D}^u$, i.e. $\mathcal{D} = \{\mathcal{D}^l, \mathcal{D}^u\}$. M fully annotated cases constitute the labelled subset $\mathcal{D}^l = \{x_i^l, y_i^l\}_{i=1}^M$, and N unlabelled cases constitute the unlabelled subset $\mathcal{D}^u = \{x_i^u\}_{i=1}^N$ $(M \ll N)$. x_i^l and x_i^u denote the labelled and unlabelled input images, respectively, and y_i^l denotes the corresponding ground truth mask of x_i^l. Our SSL-MedSAM2 framework aims to generate reliable pseudo masks $\hat{y}_i^u$ for $\mathcal{D}^u$ to build-up $\mathcal{D}_p^u = \{x_i^u, \hat{y}_i^u\}_{i=1}^N$ by TFFS-MedSAM2, then $\{\mathcal{D}^l, \mathcal{D}_p^u\}$ can be used for fully-supervised learning to refine $\hat{y}_i^u$ iteratively by FSL-nnUNet.

2.2 SSL-MedSAM2 Framework

SSL-MedSAM2 contains a few-shot learning branch TFFS-MedSAM2 based on the pretrained large foundation model MedSAM2 [16] and an iterative fully-supervised learning branch FSL-nnUNet based on nnUNet structure [7]. The overall workflow of SSL-MedSAM2 is shown in Algorithm 1, where f_θ indicates MedSAM2 and g_θ indicates nnUNet. The first step (Pseudo Label Initialization) is completed by TFFS-MedSAM2, while the remaining steps are performed in FSL-nnUNet. MedSAM2 is used to generate the initial pseudo masks for the unlabelled data with the assistance of the prompts from the labelled data, and nnUNet is used to iteratively refine the pseudo masks from TFFS-MedSAM2. In model inference, only the refined nnUNet (g_θ) is used. Details of TFFS-MedSAM2 and FSL-nnUNet are explained in the following sections.

TFFS-MedSAM2 SAM2 employs a transformer-based backbone augmented with a streaming memory module, enabling it to process sequences of frames. While SAM supports point, box, and mask prompts on single images, SAM2

Algorithm 1 Training procedure of SSL-MedSAM2.

1: $\hat{Y}^u \leftarrow f_\theta(X^u \mid \mathcal{D}^l = (X^l, Y^l))$ ▷ Pseudo Label Initialization
2: **while** not converge **do**
3: $\quad \mathcal{D} \leftarrow \{\mathcal{D}^l, (X^u, \hat{Y}^u)\}$ ▷ Training Set Building
4: $\quad g_\theta \leftarrow$ train on $\mathcal{D}$ ▷ Model Refinement
5: $\quad \hat{Y}^u \leftarrow g_\theta(X^u)$ ▷ Pseudo Label Updating
6: **end while**
7: **return** Refined model g_θ

extends these prompts across frame sequences, propagating and refining segmentation masks automatically as the object moves or deforms [19]. The core innovation of SAM2 is a lightweight memory bank that stores embeddings from previous frames, enabling the model to reference past context when segmenting the current frame. SAM2's streaming memory naturally propagates segmentations across 3D medical volume slices, reducing the need for per-slice prompts. By leveraging the temporal coherence, SAM2 can produce high-quality masks for the entire volumes from a minimal input. Thus, we combine the labelled and unlabelled slices together and treat them as a whole video sequence, and use the limited labelled frames as guidance (mask prompts) for SAM2 to predict on the unlabelled frames. Specifically, we use MedSAM2 [16] that was fine-tuned on the large-scale medical image segmentation tasks instead of the original SAM2 to fully utilize the domain knowledge in the pretrained large foundation model.

As shown in Fig. 1, by treating the input 3D volume data as video frames, a whole labelled 3D volume is inserted to an unlabelled volume at random slice locations. The combined frames are then input to the pretrained and frozen MedSAM2 to generate pseudo masks for the unlabelled frames, with the mask prompt provided by the labelled frames (no prompt on the unlabelled frames). With the memory attention that stores the knowledge of the prompt from the labelled frames and the predictions from the adjacent frames, MedSAM2 can detect similar image features of the unlabelled object to the predicted frames and generate predictions through the mask decoder.

The process of ensemble pseudo labelling of each unlabelled volume by TFFS-MedSAM2 is shown in Algorithm 2, where R denotes the number of random inserting locations in each unlabelled data, x_i^c denotes the labelled-unlabelled combined data (purple box in Fig. 1), and p_i^u denotes the probability map of x_i^u, generated by f_θ (MedSAM2). In TFFS-MedSAM2, each of the M labelled data is inserted to each unlabelled data at R random locations. Thus, $R \times M$ probability

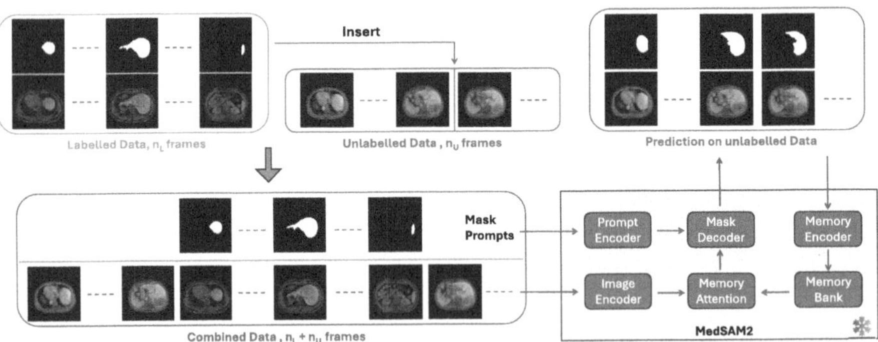

Fig. 1. The workflow of the composition of labelled data and unlabelled data, and the prediction on the unlabelled data from the composition. The inserting location is denoted by the red line in the unlabelled data. MedSAM2 is frozen in the whole process.

Algorithm 2 Pseudo-Labelling of unlabelled data x_j^u by TFFS-MedSAM2.

Input: Unlabelled data x_j^u and labelled dataset $\mathcal{D}^l = \{(x_i^l, y_i^l)\}_{i=1}^M$
Output: Pseudo-label $\hat{y}_j^u$ for x_j^u
1: $\hat{p}_j^u \leftarrow 0$ ▷ Zero Initialization
2: **for** $i \leftarrow 1$ to M **do**
3: Randomly generate R inserting locations on the unlabelled frames
4: **for** $r \leftarrow 1$ to R **do**
5: $\{x_i^c, y_i^l\} \leftarrow$ Insert $\{x_i^l, y_i^l\}$ to x_j^u between the frame index $F^{(r)}$ and $F^{(r)} + 1$
6: $\hat{p}_j^u \leftarrow \hat{p}_j^u + Sigmoid(f_\theta(x_j^u \mid \{x_i^c, y_i^l\}))$
7: **end for**
8: **end for**
9: $\hat{p}_j^u \leftarrow \hat{p}_j^u/(R \times M)$ ▷ Get Average
10: $\hat{y}_j^u \leftarrow threshould(\hat{p}_j^u)$ ▷ Get Binary Mask

maps are generated for each unlabelled data, the average of the probability maps is used to generate the pseudo mask, improving robustness through prediction ensembling. The whole process is training-free, and the pseudo-labelling of each unlabelled data is independent, requiring no user prompts and no assistance from other unlabelled data, yielding a robust and effective few-shot learning capability.

FSL-NnUNet After generating the pseudo masks for the unlabelled dataset using TFFS-MedSAM2, the second branch of our framework is an iterative fully-supervised learning process FSL-nnUNet using nnU-Net on $\mathcal{D} = \{\mathcal{D}^l, (X^u, \hat{Y}^u)\}$ to iteratively refine the pseudo masks $\hat{Y}^u$. Specifically, to avoid over-estimation when performing model inference on the unlabelled data for updating pseudo labels, the unlabelled dataset is split into 5 folds, and we perform 5-folds cross-validation using nnUNet. In each fold of training, the validation set is from one fold of the unlabelled dataset, and the remaining part of the unlabelled dataset along with the labelled dataset form the training set. After training, 5 folds predictions on the different validation sets constitute the updated pseudo masks for the whole unlabelled dataset.

Initially, the nnU-Net model is trained on the small set of labelled images together with the MedSAM2-generated pseudo-labels for the unlabelled images. Although the pseudo-labels may be imperfect, the foundation model provides a strong starting point that guides the segmentation network. The newly trained nnU-Net is used to re-predict segmentation masks for the unlabelled data, which results in more refined masks than the original MedSAM2 output due to the network's adaptation to the specific task. These refined predictions are treated as updated pseudo-labels, and we retrain the nnU-Net using the improved labels. This iterative self-training cycle can be repeated multiple times, continually improving the quality of the pseudo labels and the performance of the segmentation model. All of the final refined 5-folds models are used for model inference on the unseen testing data by taking the average of 5 different predictions. FSL-

Table 1. The data distribution of the CARE-LiSeg dataset. The value in brackets indicates the amount of annotated data in that subset.

	Vendor A	Vendor B1	Vendor B2	Vendor C
Training	130 (10)	170 (10)	60 (10)	0
Validation	20	20	20	0
Testing	40	40	40	70

nnUNet is a flexible framework, where nnUNet can be easily replaced by another fully-supervised medical segmentation method.

3 Experiments and Results

3.1 Dataset and Experimental Settings

CARE-LiSeg [5,15,22] dataset consists of T2-weighted imaging (T2WI), diffusion-weighted imaging (DWI), and Gadolinium ethoxybenzyl diethylenetriamine pentaacetic acid (Gd-EOB-DTPA)-enhanced dynamic MRIs. The Gd-EOB-DTPA-enhanced dynamic MRIs cover the non-contrast phase (T1), arterial phase, venous phase, delayed phase, and hepatobiliary phase (GED4) respectively. In the whole dataset, only limited ground truth of GED4 MRI is available. The **Contrast-Enhanced** subtask focus on the segmentation of GED4, while the **Non-Contrast** subtask focus on T1, T2WI, and DWI. The whole dataset contains 610 patients diagnosed with liver fibrosis, all of whom underwent multiphase MRI scans using three different scanners, which are Philips Ingenia3.0T, Siemens Skyra 3.0T, and Siemens Aera 1.5T (Vendor A, B1, and B2) respectively, resulting in a multi-phase and multi-center dataset. Different from the training and validation sets, the testing set also includes cases from an unseen vendor (denoted by Vendor C), evaluating the out-of-distribution (OOD) performance, additional to the in-distribution (ID) performance. The details of the dataset is shown in Table 1.

In TFFS-MedSAM2, all input frames to the pretained MedSAM2 were resized to 512×512 due to the default setting. After the model inference of MedSAM2, the predictions were resized back to the original image size for pseudo label generation. In FSL-nnUNet, the training settings were automatically defined by nnUNet. Particularly, all nnUNet models were trained for 1000 epochs, and we ran FSL-nnUNet 3 times for the **Contrast-Enhanced** subtask and twice for the **Non-Contrast** subtask. Specifically, when generating the pseudo masks for the data in non-contrast sequences by TFFS-MedSAM2, we still combined them with the labelled GED4 data (although they are in different MRI sequences). All experiments were deployed on a GPU instance with about 10 GB memory from a Nvidia A100 GPU. During evaluation, the mean value of dice coefficient (DC) and Hausdorff distance (HD) were reported.

Table 2. Evaluation results of the validation set in terms of GED4 and T1 reported on leaderboard. Top 5 teams are shown.

Team	Dice	HD	Team	Dice	HD
TanglangSled	97.30	31.01	Ours	95.74	41.14
MHIL	97.05	19.55	Ours-TFFS	95.46	40.65
Ours	97.04	21.28	LidaYang	94.88	49.10
Monster	97.04	19.28	MHIL	94.65	62.84
InteliLiver	97.00	21.34	Sigma	94.19	59.32
Ours-TFFS	95.92	24.71	CitySJTU	93.81	44.98
(a) GED4.			(b) T1.		

3.2 Results and Discussion

For the Non-Contrast subtask of the CARE 2025 challenge, results were submitted only for the T1 sequence, as the initial pseudo masks generated by TFFS-MedSAM2 for T2WI and DWI sequences were of insufficient quality for direct use in FSL-nnUNet training. This limitation likely arises from the larger appearance discrepancy between GED4 and T2WI/DWI compared to GED4 and T1, given that T1 and GED4 represent two distinct phases of the same Gd-EOB-DTPA-enhanced acquisition, thus sharing more consistent intensity and structural patterns.

The average Dice coefficient and HD on the validation datasets, as reported on the official leaderboard, are summarized in Table 2. For comparison, we also report the performance of the initial pseudo masks generated directly by TFFS-MedSAM2 (denoted as OursTFFS), prior to any refinement by FSL-nnUNet. The corresponding results on the testing datasets are presented in Table 3. Compared to the validation results, the testing phase also reported the In-Distribution (ID) and Out-Of-Distribution (OOD) performance separately to evaluate the robustness of the methods on the unseen vendor data. However, due to restrictions on the number of submissions permitted during the testing phase, the results of OursTFFS were not evaluated on the test server.

As shown in Table 2, our method ranks third in both Dice and HD for the GED4 validation data, while achieving the best overall performance for the T1 validation data. Notably, the OursTFFS results indicate that even without the iterative refinement stage, TFFS-MedSAM2 alone can generate high-quality pseudo masks through its training-free few-shot segmentation mechanism – even outperforming other participants on the T1 data. This demonstrates the strong initialization capability of the few-shot branch and its effectiveness in transferring structural priors from limited annotated volumes. Furthermore, the inclusion of FSL-nnUNet refinement substantially improves segmentation accuracy for the GED4 sequence, whereas the gain is less pronounced for T1.

On the testing datasets, our method consistently ranks among the top three approaches across all leaderboard categories. As shown in Table 3a, b, SSL-

Table 3. Evaluation results of the test set in terms of GED4 and T1 reported on leaderboard. "In-Distribution" contains data from vendor A, B1, B2. "Out-Of-Distribution" contains data from vendor C. Top 5 teams are shown.

Team	Dice	HD	Team	Dice	HD
Monster	97.03	21.40	SuperIdols	97.70	14.65
Ours	96.84	22.97	Monster	97.65	15.17
xcj	96.47	25.03	Ours	97.54	15.11
BI	96.44	22.63	BI	97.54	14.37
TeamSpace	96.41	24.32	TeamSpace	97.53	15.72

(a) In-Distribution GED4. (b) Out-Of-Distribution GED4.

Team	Dice	HD	Team	Dice	HD
Ours	96.08	19.87	Ours	97.16	25.58
BIGS2	94.34	38.06	BIGS2	95.48	22.11
Sigma	93.18	58.99	Sigma	95.03	29.04
CitySJTU	92.62	27.80	CitySJTU	94.44	25.54
BioDreamer	91.96	31.83	BioDreamer	94.18	28.24

(c) In-Distribution T1. (d) Out-Of-Distribution T1.

MedSAM2 achieves top-three performance on the GED4 data in both ID and OOD settings with respect to both Dice and HD metrics. More notably, Table 3c, d show that our method obtains the highest Dice score and lowest HD among all participants for most cases on the T1 testing data, except for the OOD HD metric, where it ranks third.

Overall, these results confirm that SSL-MedSAM2 delivers SOTA performance across both validation and testing datasets. In particular, its superior accuracy on the T1 sequence demonstrates excellent knowledge transfer between MRI sequences captured in different acquisition phases of the same contrast agent (Gd-EOB-DTPA-enhanced). Moreover, the model exhibits strong OOD generalization, often performing better on unseen vendor data than on the training-domain data. This robustness to domain shifts highlights the effectiveness of combining a foundation segmentation model (MedSAM2) with iterative semi-supervised refinement, making SSL-MedSAM2 a promising solution for practical clinical applications where data heterogeneity is inevitable.

4 Conclusion

In summary, we propose a novel semi-supervised learning medical image segmentation framework SSL-MedSAM2 containing a training-free few-shot learning branch TFFS-MedSAM2 and an iterative fully-supervised learning branch FSL-nnUNet. The evaluation results demonstrate the generalizability and robustness of our method even when labelled dataset and the unlabelled dataset are in different phases (e.g., GED4 and T1). However, when the data distribution of the support labelled data and query unlabelled data differs too much (e.g., GED4 and T2WI), TFFS-MedSAM2 tends to generate low-quality pseudo masks. Thus, in the future, we will focus on cross-domain reliable pseudo mask generation and selection in TFFS-MedSAM2 to further enhance the generalizability and robustness of our method.

References

1. Basak, H., Bhattacharya, R., Hussain, R., Chatterjee, A.: An exceedingly simple consistency regularization method for semi-supervised medical image segmentation. In: 2022 IEEE 19th International Symposium on Biomedical Imaging (ISBI), pp. 1–4. IEEE (2022)
2. Bilic, P., Christ, P., Li, H.B., Vorontsov, E., Ben-Cohen, A., Kaissis, G., Szeskin, A., Jacobs, C., Mamani, G.E.H., Chartrand, G., et al.: The liver tumor segmentation benchmark (lits). Med. Image Anal. **84**, 102680 (2023)
3. Chen, Q.Q., Sun, Z.H., Wei, C.F., Wu, E.Q., Ming, D.: Semi-supervised 3d medical image segmentation based on dual-task consistent joint learning and task-level regularization. IEEE/ACM Trans. Comput. Biol. Bioinf. **20**(4), 2457–2467 (2022)
4. Gao, Y., Jiang, Y., Peng, Y., Yuan, F., Zhang, X., Wang, J.: Medical image segmentation: a comprehensive review of deep learning-based methods. Tomography **11**(5), 52 (2025)
5. Gao, Z., Liu, Y., Wu, F., Shi, N., Shi, Y., Zhuang, X.: A reliable and interpretable framework of multi-view learning for liver fibrosis staging. In: International Conference on Medical Image Computing and Computer-Assisted Intervention, pp. 178–188 (2023)
6. Han, K., Liu, L., Song, Y., Liu, Y., Qiu, C., Tang, Y., Teng, Q., Liu, Z.: An effective semi-supervised approach for liver ct image segmentation. IEEE J. Biomed. Health Inform. **26**(8), 3999–4007 (2022)
7. Isensee, F., Jaeger, P.F., Kohl, S.A., Petersen, J., Maier-Hein, K.H.: nnu-net: a self-configuring method for deep learning-based biomedical image segmentation. Nat. Methods **18**(2), 203–211 (2021)
8. Jiao, R., Zhang, Y., Ding, L., Xue, B., Zhang, J., Cai, R., Jin, C.: Learning with limited annotations: a survey on deep semi-supervised learning for medical image segmentation. Comput. Biol. Med. **169**, 107840 (2024)
9. Jin, C., Guo, Z., Lin, Y., Luo, L., Chen, H.: Label-efficient deep learning in medical image analysis: Challenges and future directions (2023). arXiv:2303.12484
10. Kirillov, A., Mintun, E., Ravi, N., Mao, H., Rolland, C., Gustafson, L., Xiao, T., Whitehead, S., Berg, A.C., Lo, W.Y., et al.: Segment anything. In: Proceedings of the IEEE/CVF International Conference on Computer Vision, pp. 4015–4026 (2023)
11. Li, N., Xiong, L., Qiu, W., Pan, Y., Luo, Y., Zhang, Y.: Segment anything model for semi-supervised medical image segmentation via selecting reliable pseudo-labels. In: International Conference on Neural Information Processing, pp. 138–149. Springer (2023)
12. Li, S., Zhang, C., He, X.: Shape-aware semi-supervised 3d semantic segmentation for medical images. In: International Conference on Medical Image Computing and Computer-Assisted Intervention, pp. 552–561. Springer (2020)
13. Li, X., Yu, L., Chen, H., Fu, C.W., Xing, L., Heng, P.A.: Transformation-consistent self-ensembling model for semisupervised medical image segmentation. IEEE Trans. Neural Netw. Learn. Syst. **32**(2), 523–534 (2020)

14. Li, Y., Luo, L., Lin, H., Chen, H., Heng, P.A.: Dual-consistency semi-supervised learning with uncertainty quantification for covid-19 lesion segmentation from ct images. In: International Conference on Medical Image Computing and Computer-Assisted Intervention, pp. 199–209. Springer (2021)
15. Liu, Y., Gao, Z., Shi, N., Wu, F., Shi, Y., Chen, Q., Zhuang, X.: Merit: multi-view evidential learning for reliable and interpretable liver fibrosis staging. Med. Image Anal. **102**, 103507 (2025)
16. Ma, J., Yang, Z., Kim, S., Chen, B., Baharoon, M., Fallahpour, A., Asakereh, R., Lyu, H., Wang, B.: Medsam2: segment anything in 3d medical images and videos (2025). arXiv:2504.03600
17. Miao, J., Chen, C., Zhang, K., Chuai, J., Li, Q., Heng, P.A.: Cross prompting consistency with segment anything model for semi-supervised medical image segmentation. In: International Conference on Medical Image Computing and Computer-Assisted Intervention, pp. 167–177. Springer (2024)
18. Ouali, Y., Hudelot, C., Tami, M.: Semi-supervised semantic segmentation with cross-consistency training. In: Proceedings of the IEEE/CVF Conference on Computer Vision and Pattern Recognition, pp. 12674–12684 (2020)
19. Ravi, N., Gabeur, V., Hu, Y.T., Hu, R., Ryali, C., Ma, T., Khedr, H., Rädle, R., Rolland, C., Gustafson, L., et al.: Sam 2: Segment Anything in Images and Videos (2024). arXiv:2408.00714
20. Tarvainen, A., Valpola, H.: Mean teachers are better role models: Weight-averaged consistency targets improve semi-supervised deep learning results. Adv. Neural Inf. Proc. Syst. **30** (2017)
21. Wang, X., Yuan, Y., Guo, D., Huang, X., Cui, Y., Xia, M., Wang, Z., Bai, C., Chen, S.: Ssa-net: Spatial self-attention network for covid-19 pneumonia infection segmentation with semi-supervised few-shot learning. Med. Image Anal. **79**, 102459 (2022)
22. Wu, F., Zhuang, X.: Minimizing estimated risks on unlabeled data: A new formulation for semi-supervised medical image segmentation. IEEE Trans. Pattern Anal. Mach. Intell. **45**(5), 6021–6036 (2023)
23. Xu, Z., Niethammer, M.: Deepatlas: Joint semi-supervised learning of image registration and segmentation. In: International Conference on Medical Image Computing and Computer-Assisted Intervention, pp. 420–429. Springer (2019)
24. Zeng, L.L., Gao, K., Hu, D., Feng, Z., Hou, C., Rong, P., Wang, W.: Ss-tbn: a semi-supervised tri-branch network for covid-19 screening and lesion segmentation. IEEE Trans. Pattern Anal. Mach. Intell. **45**(8), 10427–10442 (2023)
25. Zhang, Y., Yang, J., Liu, Y., Cheng, Y., Qi, Y.: Semisam: enhancing semi-supervised medical image segmentation via sam-assisted consistency regularization. In: 2024 IEEE International Conference on Bioinformatics and Biomedicine (BIBM), pp. 3982–3986. IEEE (2024)
26. Zhang, Y., Zhou, T., Wang, S., Wu, Y., Gu, P., Chen, D.Z.: Samdsk: combining segment anything model with domain-specific knowledge for semi-supervised learning in medical image segmentation (2023). arXiv:2308.13759
27. Zhu, J., Hamdi, A., Qi, Y., Jin, Y., Wu, J.: Medical sam 2: segment medical images as video via segment anything model 2 (2024). arXiv:2408.00874

Early Fusion-Based Multimodal Cardiac MRI Segmentation with Domain-Aware Augmentation

Xin Lin(✉)

Instituto Tecnológico de Galicia, 15003 A Coruña, Spain
xlin@itg.es

Abstract. Accurate segmentation of myocardial lesions, such as edema and scar, is essential for the diagnosis and assessment of patients with myocardial infarction. However, automatic segmentation remains challenging due to inter-subject anatomical variability, domain shifts across scanners, and modality inconsistencies, including missing or misaligned inputs. In this work, we implement a segmentation pipeline that utilizes early fusion of multimodal cardiac MRI inputs, addressing misalignments with an Affine Spatial Transformer Network (STN) per modality before the encoder. Our method leverages domain-aware augmentation through Histogram Matching (HM) or Fourier Domain Augmentation (FDA), and integrates a modality dropout module to enhance robustness to multi-center data variability. The segmentation model builds upon a pre-trained Pyramid Vision Transformer (PVTv2) as the encoder, combined with the Efficient Multi-Scale Convolutional Attention Decoder (EMCAD). The evaluation is performed on the CARE-MyoPS 2025 challenge dataset, which contains multimodal CMR sequences from eight different centers. We evaluate our method using a leave-one-center-out strategy on the fully labeled data, treating the remaining centers as out-of-domain references.

Keywords: Multimodal cardiac MRI segmentation · Early fusion segmentation · Domain augmentation

1 Introduction

Cardiac magnetic resonance (CMR) imaging is a technique used by clinicians to obtain images of the heart for diagnosis and assessment of myocardial conditions, where the segmentation of myocardial lesions is a crucial step. Different modalities highlight different structures, such as late gadolinium enhancement (LGE) for scar tissue, T2-weighted imaging for edema, and balanced steady-state free precession (bSSFP), which provides clear anatomical boundaries [1,17]. Automatic segmentation methods are challenging due to inter-subject variability, missing modalities, misaligned sequences, and domain shifts across scanners.

X. Zhuang et al. (Eds.): CARE 2025, LNCS 16257, pp. 201–213, 2026.
https://doi.org/10.1007/978-3-032-16271-7_19

In the context of the CARE-MyoPS 2025 challenge, a real-world scenario is introduced with multi-center data, missing modalities, and misalignments in multisequence CMR [5,18].

We propose a segmentation pipeline that uses early fusion of LGE, T2, and bSSFP data with automatic misalignment handling [8]. The data with missing modalities are kept out of the main training process and used as out-of-domain references for our domain-aware augmentation approach, without hindering the robustness to missing modalities by training with a dropout technique [20]. We address the CARE-MyoPS 2025 challenge by designing a pipeline that integrates existing techniques. In the following sections, we explain the data preprocessing and the training methodology, as well as describe the architecture and the data augmentation procedure.

2 Methods

In this section, we describe the employed dataset, the preprocessing step, and the domain augmentation procedure. Then, we define the model architecture, the evaluation metrics, and the experimental setup.[1]

2.1 Data

We only used the dataset provided by the CARE-MyoPS 2025 challenge [5,18, 26]. The dataset contains 3D MRI scans divided into eight centers, namely center A to center H; center D is a hold-out data for out-of-distribution performance analysis. There are three available modalities: LGE, T2, and bSSFP; some of them are missing between centers. There are five labels: Myocardium, Left ventricle, Right ventricle, Edema, and Scar. The centers that contain all labels and have all modalities available are centers B and C. Therefore, we use the data from centers B and C as the main dataset (corresponding to approximately 40% of the total available training data, i.e., 95 of 235 patients), and leverage selected representatives from the remaining centers as references for the domain-aware augmentation methodology during the training step. In Sect. 2.3, we provide a detailed explanation of this procedure and how the samples are selected.

2.2 Preprocessing

The data has different spacing between the slices, so we normalize the scans by resampling the X and Y dimensions to 1×1 mm. We leave the Z dimension (slice dimension) untouched to preserve the original number of slices. This avoids the generation of interpolated segmentation maps. As our model will treat each slice independently, leaving the original Z dimension has no influence.

Then, each 3D scan is split into 2D slices. For each slice, we remove the ones that do not have any label in the corresponding segmentation map. Then we

[1] Our implementation is available at: https://github.com/xlinzh/rc-care-myops-2025.

apply spatial padding to smaller slices to increase their size to 256×256, the larger slices remain unchanged (except for the validation set, where the slices are center cropped to the mentioned size to ensure the same crops during all the validation process). The rest of the processing is done dynamically in the data pipeline explained in Sect. 2.4.

2.3 Domain-Aware Augmentation

We have five centers to use for domain-aware augmentation: A, E, F, G, and H. The E, F, and G centers have fewer than 10 patients each, while A and H have more than 30. To avoid imbalances in the reference representatives for domain-aware augmentation, we use K-means [12] for the centers A and H, and use farthest point sampling for centers E, F, and G. We employ a pre-trained ResNet-50 [7], initialized with MedicalNet [3] weights, to extract features for this procedure.[2]

We flatten the encoded features from the second layer onward. We leverage scikit-learn [16] for K-means and use $N = 3$ as the number of clusters (i.e., select three representatives). For the farthest point sampling, we start by randomly choosing a sample, then select iteratively the farthest point by Euclidean distance from the first sample until we get three samples in total.

In total, we get 15 (three from each center) patients as out-of-domain representatives. To further avoid imbalances due to the number of slices each patient can have, we extract the basal, mid, and apical slices from each patient. Thus, 45 slices were obtained for domain-aware augmentation. We use two techniques for the application of the reference-based augmentation: Histogram Matching (HM) [11] and Fourier Domain Adaptation (FDA) [23].

Histogram Matching. This method adjusts the overall intensity distribution of the reference image to the source image, thereby simulating a domain shift. We use the SimpleITK [24] image filter to apply this transform, with 256 histogram levels and 15 matching points.

Fourier Domain Adaptation. Let $f_\beta(x) = \hat{x}$ be the function for FDA that replaces low frequencies from the source image with low frequencies from the reference image. The parameter β is used to specify how much of the source image will be replaced with the reference low frequencies [23], where $\beta = 0$ represents the identity function $f_0(x) = x$. We draw the parameter β from the uniform distribution $\mathcal{U}([0.008, 0.02))$.

2.4 Data Pipeline

The data pipeline consists of four steps: (a) Nyúl standardization [15], (b) domain-aware augmentation, (c) data augmentation, and (d) Z-score normalization. For the validation and inference, only steps (a) and (d) are used.

[2] Model from: https://monai.readthedocs.io/en/1.5.0/networks.html#resnetfeatures.

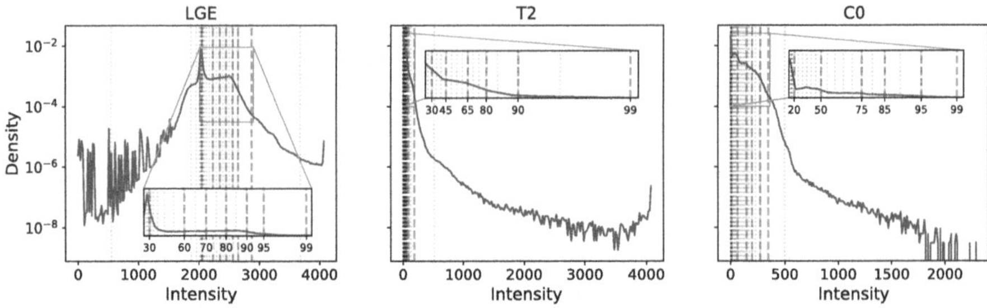

Fig. 1. Mean histogram density for each modality of center B data. Dotted lines indicate 0 to 100 percentiles every 5 steps. Insets show selected percentiles (dashed lines).

Nyúl Standardization. This method uses a piecewise linear transformation to match an input image to a standard scaled space, typically calculated with landmarks at specific percentiles. We analyze the global histogram from the training dataset for each modality to establish our landmarks. We plotted the histogram with percentiles from 0 to 100 in increments of 5 and manually selected the percentiles. In some cases, the percentiles appear very close to each other. In such cases, we empirically choose the ones that avoid the need to add a small jitter (1×10^{-5}) due to overlapping landmarks during standardization. We selected the percentiles based on the statistics of center B, as illustrated in Fig. 1. We also validated the selected percentiles on center C, checking that the spacing between them is correct and that the produced landmarks do not overlap.

Domain-Aware Augmentation. This method was detailed in Sect. 2.3. During the training, we use a probability of 50% to apply HM or FDA, which is mutually exclusive in the sense that only one of the two will be applied to the input. Since some references have missing modalities *per se*, we handle them in one of two ways during augmentation: either by zeroing the input modality channel or bypassing it, letting the original non-augmented modality channel continue through the pipeline.

Data Augmentation. To address the scarcity of available data and incorporate more variability into the input data during the training phase, we apply random spatial transformations common to all modalities and specific intensity transformations for each modality. The augmentation operations can be compounded such that any combination may be simultaneously used at a given instance.

- *Spatial Transformations*: We apply random elastic deformations with spatially varying parameters sampled from $\mathcal{U}([5, 10))$, combined with affine transformations including rotation ($\pm 0.3\,\text{rad} \approx \pm 17°$), scaling ($\pm 10\%$), and translation ($\pm 10$ pixels). Additionally, random flips along vertical and hori-

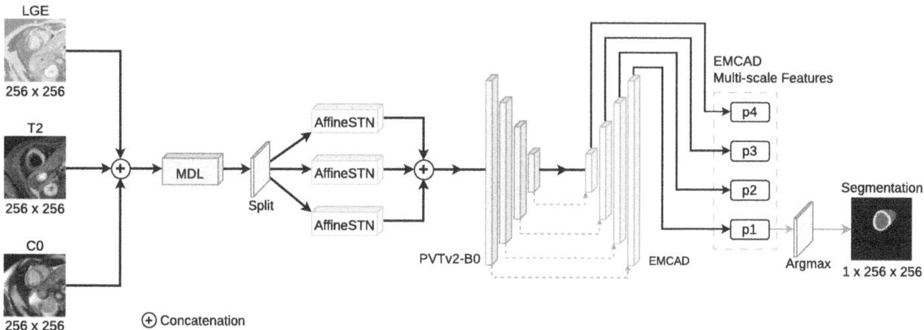

Fig. 2. The proposed model architecture. The diagram presents an example of input and segmentation, obtained from slice 3 of case 2025 of the center B.

zontal axes are performed with equal probability.[3] We include random cropping based on positive label sampling with a spatial size of 256 × 256. The probabilities are 50% for all transformations, except the elastic deformations, which have 30%, and the random cropping that is always performed.

- *Intensity Transformations*: For intensity-related transformations, we treat each modality individually. The probabilities are 50% for every transformation, except Gaussian smoothing, which has 30%.
  - LGE: Random bias field, Gaussian noise, and contrast adjustments simulate realistic intensity variations.
  - T2: Similar bias field and noise augmentations are used with slightly different parameters.
  - C0: Gaussian smoothing and noise augmentations are applied to model potential blur and acquisition noise.

Z-score Normalization. We opted for a per-sample Z-score normalization. This method transforms each data point x_i in a sample by subtracting the sample mean μ and dividing by the sample standard deviation σ, i.e., $x_i \to (x_i - \mu)/\sigma$, which normalizes the data to have zero mean and unit variance.

2.5 Model Architecture

We employ the proposed Efficient Multi-Scale Convolutional Attention Decoder (EMCAD) with the Pyramid Vision Transformer version 2 (PVTv2) [19,21] as the encoder for the segmentation model to handle multimodal and multi-center multi-sequence cardiac magnetic resonance images. Before the encoder, we include a Modality Dropout Layer (MDL) [14,20] followed by an Affine Spatial

[3] We attempted to standardize the data orientation (e.g., RAS) using the available metadata without success. Instead of trying an automatic method such as [25], we decided to add both flips to enhance model robustness. There are no major implications because our model treats each slice individually.

Transformer Network (STN) [8] for each modality. In Fig. 2, we present a diagram of the architecture. Aside from the mentioned components, the figure illustrates the multi-scale features from the EMCAD decoder and highlights that the latest decoder output (p1) is used as the final segmentation map. All outputs are used in the optimization process explained in Sect. 2.7. This architecture has 3.9M parameters (of which 3.4 M parameters are from the encoder).

Modality Dropout Layer. We use a simple approach for Modality Dropout; the core idea is to drop entire input modalities during training to improve robustness. Let MDL be defined as a function $g(x) = \hat{x}$, where the input is $x = (x_{\mathrm{LGE}}, x_{\mathrm{T2}}, x_{\mathrm{C0}})$, a three-channel 2D image with each modality in one channel. Every modality is independently retained by sampling from Bernoulli distributions:

$$m_{\mathrm{LGE}} \sim \mathrm{Bernoulli}(p_{\mathrm{LGE}}), \quad m_{\mathrm{T2}} \sim \mathrm{Bernoulli}(p_{\mathrm{T2}}), \quad m_{\mathrm{C0}} \sim \mathrm{Bernoulli}(p_{\mathrm{C0}}),$$

where $p_{\mathrm{LGE}}, p_{\mathrm{T2}}, p_{\mathrm{C0}} \in [0,1]$ denote the retention probabilities. The output of the MDL is $\hat{x} = (m_{\mathrm{LGE}} x_{\mathrm{LGE}}, \quad m_{\mathrm{T2}} x_{\mathrm{T2}}, \quad m_{\mathrm{C0}} x_{\mathrm{C0}})$. The used probabilities are $p_{\mathrm{LGE}} = 0.95$ and $p_{\mathrm{T2}} = p_{\mathrm{C0}} = 0.7$. We prioritized maximizing retention of the LGE modality, as it is consistently available across all centers in the dataset.

Affine Spatial Transformer Layer. The AffineSTN is composed of a localization network and a regression head. The network has three of these layers, one for each modality. Afterwards, the spatially transformed outputs are concatenated to form a single input for subsequent processing (hence, the modalities are early-fused).

- *Localization Network*: Consists of three convolutional layers with increasing filter sizes (4, 8, and 10) and kernel sizes (7×7, 5×5, and 3×3), each followed by a GroupNorm layer (2, 4, and 5 groups), a ReLU activation, and Max Pooling to reduce the dimensions. It ends with adaptive average pooling to generate a vector of 10 features.
- *Regression Head*: It is a Fully Connected layer that outputs six parameters that define the 2D affine transformation matrix. It is initialized to the identity transform for stable training.

EMCAD and PVTv2. We used the original EMCAD [19] and the PVTv2-B0 [21]. We replaced the BatchNorm (BN) layers from the EMCAD with GroupNorm (GN) layers to improve the effectiveness of the normalization layer when training with a small batch size [22], where we halved the number of features of the original BN to use it as the number of groups in the GN, with a minimum of 8 groups, except for the last BN in the Large-kernel Grouped Attention Gate (LGAG) of the EMCAD, which follows a 1×1 convolution. For that GN, we use a group number of one (making it equivalent to using a LayerNorm [2]).

2.6 Evaluation Metrics

Following the challenge directives, we evaluate the performance of our model using the Dice Similarity Coefficient (DSC), Sensitivity (SEN), Precision (PRE), and Hausdorff Distance (HD). Our model is trained slice-wise, so the training process uses 2D variants of these metrics. For evaluation, we report the 3D variant of the metrics, where we treat compounded slices from the same patient as a single 3D volume, as the original data. This allows fair comparison with other methods.

2.7 Experimental Setup

We leverage MONAI [4] and PyTorch Lightning [6] frameworks for our experiments. We trained our model using a batch size of 2 for 200 epochs with an NVIDIA RTX 4060 Laptop GPU with 8 GB of memory. We train using a cosine annealing schedule without restarts (i.e., $T_{max} = 200$, where T_{max} is the maximum number of epochs per cycle), combined with an initial linear warm-up of 10 epochs, starting with a factor of 0.1. The optimization is performed via AdamW [10] with a learning rate of 3×10^{-4} and a weight decay of 3×10^{-5}. The training objective combines the Dice and Focal losses [9,13] using equal weights, with the weighting value λ set to 1, to emphasize spatial overlap and address class imbalance. The focusing parameter in the Focal loss (γ) is set to 2.0. The task is a multi-class segmentation, so we use the softmax activation function.

Label Weights at Loss Computation. To further enhance data imbalance handling, we use label-wise weights based on the inverse pixel frequency of each class across all segmentation maps in the training set.

Deep Supervision. We use deep supervision as in [19] to fully utilize the multi-scale nature of the decoder. Each scale is bilinearly interpolated to the input size (256×256) and used individually in the loss function. The final loss is the sum of the values obtained at each scale.

Pre-trained Weights and Unfreezing. At the start of the training, we load a pre-trained set of ImageNet weights for the PVTv2-B0 encoder.[4] The encoder is initially frozen and remains so until epoch 15, when it is unfrozen to begin joint training with the decoder after the latter has stabilized.

Hyperparameter Selection. The hyperparameters were selected through exploratory runs rather than using a cross-validation methodology, so the final results may be biased.

[4] Pre-trained PVT weights from: https://github.com/whai362/PVT/releases/tag/v2.

2.8 Experiments and Final Training

We employ a leave-one-center-out (LOCO) strategy to refine our methodology using centers B and C. The dataset is split with a ratio of 80/20 for training and validation, ensuring all scans of the same patient appear exclusively in one of the two sets. This avoids cross-patient overlap, which we consider a form of data leak. We trained three versions of the model: without augmentations (baseline), with augmentations keeping modalities when the reference does not have them (DAA), and with augmentations enforcing the modalities' circumstances of the reference (DAA-force). For the submission, we train using the data from both centers, applying the same splitting strategy where the validation set is kept to monitor the training. We trained using the DAA-force method.

3 Results

In this section, we present the leave-one-center-out (LOCO) results applied to center B and center C. The inference is made using the original data with actual modality presence/absence; we did not evaluate performance with missing modalities. We report the metrics mentioned in Sect. 2.6 via mean and standard deviation. We exclude NaN and Inf values for the Hausdorff Distance (HD), while for the other metrics, NaN values are excluded. An additional pseudo-label is included in the reported results, the S+E, where the segmentation maps of Scar and Edema are merged as one single target. Table 1 shows the real-world (RW) results based on the scores of the dataset from both the validation set and the left-out center, while Table 2 shows the results disaggregated from in-distribution (ID) and out-of-distribution (OOD) data. Finally, Table 3 displays the metrics obtained from the final CARE2025-MyoPS test submission.

4 Discussion and Conclusion

In Table 1, we can see that domain-augmented models have improvements over the Scar target in both settings, LOCO-C and LOCO-B. Meanwhile, Edema performance is slightly worse in LOCO-C, and has modest gains in LOCO-B. In Table 2, the results are disaggregated between ID and OOD data, allowing a more detailed view of performance across different distributions. We can see that the OOD performance in the baseline model is especially low in LOCO-B, even though HD appears to be on par (due to the omission of NaN and Inf values).[5] In contrast, the LOCO-C OOD baseline performance is acceptable for Scar, while for Edema is also low. With these observations, we hypothesize that the inferior baseline performance on OOD data at LOCO-B is due to that center C data may be less heterogeneous than center B, making the basic augmentations less efficient for out-of-domain generalization and also making the effects

[5] The OOD data in LOCO-B (i.e., center B data) has 50 cases. Out of those, the baseline model has 40 missing values, DAA has 2, and DAA-force has 1.

Table 1. Real-world leave-one-center-out (LOCO) results. Values are represented as mean ± standard deviation. Metrics: DSC = Dice similarity coefficient, SEN = Sensitivity, PRE = Precision, HD = Hausdorff distance. Results for S (Scar), E (Edema), and their union (S + E). Distributions: RW = Real-world. The RW consists of the validation set used during training and the complete left-out center. Best values are underlined.

Model	Target	Dist.	DSC (↑)	SEN (↑)	PRE (↑)	HD (↓)
LOCO-C: train/val (center B), left out (center C)						
Baseline	S	RW	0.508 ± 0.206	0.503 ± 0.192	0.562 ± 0.232	28.259 ± 31.418
	E	RW	0.331 ± 0.183	0.425 ± 0.182	0.315 ± 0.217	29.574 ± 17.046
	S+E	RW	0.641 ± 0.145	0.696 ± 0.181	0.615 ± 0.155	29.826 ± 29.117
DAA	S	RW	0.544 ± 0.204	0.559 ± 0.202	0.578 ± 0.228	23.633 ± 16.040
	E	RW	0.323 ± 0.183	0.396 ± 0.196	0.343 ± 0.242	46.693 ± 50.709
	S+E	RW	0.653 ± 0.142	0.691 ± 0.189	0.657 ± 0.158	43.105 ± 49.625
DAA-force	S	RW	0.575 ± 0.198	0.599 ± 0.175	0.597 ± 0.225	23.481 ± 15.920
	E	RW	0.314 ± 0.198	0.378 ± 0.205	0.323 ± 0.231	43.437 ± 45.318
	S+E	RW	0.656 ± 0.144	0.699 ± 0.175	0.642 ± 0.156	39.963 ± 44.754
LOCO-B: train/val (center C), left out (center B)						
Baseline	S	RW	0.156 ± 0.293	0.138 ± 0.285	0.568 ± 0.299	22.056 ± 15.193
	E	RW	0.063 ± 0.131	0.072 ± 0.149	0.198 ± 0.233	26.560 ± 11.448
	S+E	RW	0.144 ± 0.257	0.144 ± 0.276	0.510 ± 0.267	25.409 ± 12.004
DAA	S	RW	0.376 ± 0.268	0.422 ± 0.311	0.388 ± 0.270	23.934 ± 15.412
	E	RW	0.196 ± 0.125	0.225 ± 0.167	0.203 ± 0.138	23.385 ± 14.233
	S+E	RW	0.455 ± 0.200	0.492 ± 0.249	0.464 ± 0.200	22.416 ± 14.460
DAA-force	S	RW	0.408 ± 0.245	0.431 ± 0.257	0.419 ± 0.250	22.640 ± 15.175
	E	RW	0.190 ± 0.117	0.193 ± 0.126	0.217 ± 0.147	22.821 ± 13.721
	S+E	RW	0.443 ± 0.185	0.448 ± 0.199	0.467 ± 0.200	21.330 ± 14.458

of domain-aware augmentation more visible; and that the lower retention rate of the T2 weighted modality (the one that highlights edema) during training has a negative influence in this target. Nevertheless, we applied the Wilcoxon signed-rank test with Holm–Bonferroni correction on both ID and OOD data, across all metrics and for Scar and Edema targets (excluding the Scar+Edema to avoid inflated values), comparing domain-augmented models against the baseline. We observe that for the OOD data, the domain-augmented models have significant improvements in the Dice score.

The results obtained from the official CARE-MyoPS 2025 test set are presented in Table 3. In this case, we see an overall higher performance on Edema segmentation than on Scar segmentation, in contrast to what was observed in the LOCO metrics (in Tables 1 and 2). This difference can be attributed to the fact that the submitted model was trained using a combination of data from centers B and C, while the LOCO-C and LOCO-B models were trained with data from

Table 2. Disaggregated leave-one-center-out (LOCO) results. Values are represented as mean ± standard deviation. Metrics: DSC = Dice similarity coefficient, SEN = Sensitivity, PRE = Precision, HD = Hausdorff distance. Results for S (Scar), E (Edema), and their union (S + E). Distributions: ID = In-distribution, OOD = Out-of-distribution. The ID is the validation set, and the OOD is the whole left-out center. Asterisk (*) indicates statistically significant improvement over the baseline model after Holm–Bonferroni correction with $p \leq 0.05$, calculated for S and E. Best values are underlined.

Model	Target	Dist.	DSC (↑)	SEN (↑)	PRE (↑)	HD (↓)
LOCO-C: train/val (center B), left out (center C)						
Baseline	S	ID	0.673 ± 0.123	0.679 ± 0.105	0.674 ± 0.146	10.473 ± 8.180
		OOD	0.471 ± 0.203	0.463 ± 0.185	0.537 ± 0.240	32.301 ± 33.287
	E	ID	0.541 ± 0.156	0.581 ± 0.172	0.546 ± 0.185	10.428 ± 4.489
		OOD	0.285 ± 0.153	0.390 ± 0.165	0.264 ± 0.189	33.829 ± 15.845
	S+E	ID	0.718 ± 0.129	0.746 ± 0.161	0.715 ± 0.152	9.895 ± 4.581
		OOD	0.624 ± 0.143	0.685 ± 0.183	0.593 ± 0.147	34.255 ± 30.391
DAA	S	ID	0.670 ± 0.123	0.712 ± 0.118	0.638 ± 0.137	13.587 ± 10.511
		OOD	0.516 ± 0.208 *	0.524 ± 0.201*	0.565 ± 0.241	25.916 ± 16.202
	E	ID	0.525 ± 0.175	0.547 ± 0.192	0.552 ± 0.188	11.586 ± 5.223
		OOD	0.278 ± 0.151	0.362 ± 0.181	0.297 ± 0.228	54.494 ± 52.935
	S+E	ID	0.720 ± 0.122	0.743 ± 0.165	0.723 ± 0.138	11.270 ± 6.433
		OOD	0.638 ± 0.142	0.679 ± 0.191	0.642 ± 0.158	50.180 ± 52.206
DAA-force	S	ID	0.673 ± 0.116	0.713 ± 0.111	0.642 ± 0.130	13.863 ± 11.091
		OOD	0.553 ± 0.206 *	0.574 ± 0.177 *	0.587 ± 0.240 *	25.667 ± 16.040
	E	ID	0.549 ± 0.184	0.581 ± 0.198	0.553 ± 0.193	11.497 ± 10.431
		OOD	0.262 ± 0.159	0.333 ± 0.178	0.271 ± 0.206	50.535 ± 46.998
	S+E	ID	0.727 ± 0.129	0.763 ± 0.161	0.714 ± 0.138	11.364 ± 10.314
		OOD	0.640 ± 0.142	0.685 ± 0.175	0.627 ± 0.156	46.318 ± 46.928
LOCO-B: train/val (center C), left out (center B)						
Baseline	S	ID	0.737 ± 0.167	0.767 ± 0.198	0.728 ± 0.186	19.195 ± 21.042
		OOD	0.052 ± 0.157	0.022 ± 0.056	0.424 ± 0.307	24.631 ± 5.108
	E	ID	0.293 ± 0.165	0.366 ± 0.148	0.276 ± 0.189	32.167 ± 15.070
		OOD	0.022 ± 0.065	0.019 ± 0.062	0.154 ± 0.244	23.407 ± 7.031
	S+E	ID	0.674 ± 0.173	0.742 ± 0.165	0.635 ± 0.204	29.958 ± 16.406
		OOD	0.048 ± 0.113	0.037 ± 0.095	0.440 ± 0.273	22.850 ± 7.453
DAA	S	ID	0.751 ± 0.120	0.788 ± 0.154	0.735 ± 0.144	22.919 ± 17.928
		OOD	0.308 ± 0.228 *	0.354 ± 0.285 *	0.325 ± 0.237	24.124 ± 14.886
	E	ID	0.289 ± 0.180	0.350 ± 0.169	0.270 ± 0.197	30.135 ± 16.782
		OOD	0.179 ± 0.103 *	0.202 ± 0.157 *	0.191 ± 0.121	22.170 ± 13.366
	S+E	ID	0.687 ± 0.137	0.760 ± 0.135	0.641 ± 0.170	27.298 ± 16.671
		OOD	0.413 ± 0.180	0.444 ± 0.233	0.432 ± 0.188	21.538 ± 13.843
DAA-force	S	ID	0.719 ± 0.169	0.748 ± 0.196	0.711 ± 0.191	21.918 ± 17.608
		OOD	0.352 ± 0.213 *	0.373 ± 0.222 *	0.367 ± 0.221	22.772 ± 14.680
	E	ID	0.265 ± 0.155	0.340 ± 0.164	0.249 ± 0.174	35.194 ± 16.060
		OOD	0.176 ± 0.104 *	0.167 ± 0.096 *	0.211 ± 0.141	20.593 ± 11.967
	S+E	ID	0.654 ± 0.177	0.723 ± 0.182	0.617 ± 0.210	31.062 ± 16.459
		OOD	0.405 ± 0.159	0.398 ± 0.157	0.440 ± 0.185	19.578 ± 13.334

Table 3. CARE-MyoPS 2025 test submission results. Values are represented as mean ± standard deviation. Metrics: DSC = Dice similarity coefficient, SEN = Sensitivity, PRE = Precision, HD = Hausdorff distance. Results for S (Scar), E (Edema), and their union (S + E). Distributions: ID = In-distribution, OOD = Out-of-distribution, RW = Real-world. The ID has 15 patients of center B, the OOD has 25 patients of center D, and the RW is the combination of the previous two.

Team	Target	Dist.	DSC (↑)	SEN (↑)	PRE (↑)	HD (↓)
fpt	S	ID	0.493 ± 0.185	0.608 ± 0.191	0.439 ± 0.201	28.796 ± 15.622
		OOD	0.646 ± 0.095	0.577 ± 0.112	0.755 ± 0.114	24.150 ± 16.202
		RW	0.589 ± 0.155	0.588 ± 0.147	0.637 ± 0.216	25.892 ± 16.144
	E	ID	0.618 ± 0.116	0.625 ± 0.111	0.660 ± 0.182	32.783 ± 12.231
		OOD	0.640 ± 0.103	0.555 ± 0.142	0.793 ± 0.080	27.045 ± 15.465
		RW	0.632 ± 0.109	0.581 ± 0.135	0.743 ± 0.143	29.197 ± 14.605
	S+E	ID	0.556 ± 0.139	0.616 ± 0.131	0.549 ± 0.173	30.789 ± 12.495
		OOD	0.643 ± 0.089	0.566 ± 0.114	0.774 ± 0.074	25.597 ± 14.758
		RW	0.610 ± 0.118	0.585 ± 0.123	0.690 ± 0.163	27.544 ± 14.177

centers B and C, respectively. As observed in the LOCO results, adding data variability with domain-aware augmentation techniques improves overall performance. Therefore, we hypothesize that using actual diverse data in training leads to the observed performance discrepancies. A further comparison is needed to see how the model would perform on the test set when it is trained using the data of one of the two centers.

In conclusion, we successfully explored the usefulness of domain-aware augmentation techniques, key to improving model performance on out-of-domain data. For future work, we plan to investigate how different modality-dropping probabilities affect model performance and explore the usage of test-time augmentation at inference, as augmentations are highly used at the training step.

Disclosure of Interests. The authors have no competing interests to declare that are relevant to the content of this article.

Acknowledgments. We thank the organizers of the CARE2025 for hosting this competition and for providing the dataset. We are grateful to David Rivas-Villar for their constructive feedback. No external funding was received for this work.

References

1. Abdel-Aty, H., Zagrosek, A., Schulz-Menger, J., Taylor, A.J., Messroghli, D., Kumar, A., Gross, M., Dietz, R., Friedrich, M.G.: Delayed enhancement and t2-weighted cardiovascular magnetic resonance imaging differentiate acute from chronic myocardial infarction. Circulation **109**(20), 2411–2416 (2004)

2. Ba, J.L., Kiros, J.R., Hinton, G.E.: Layer normalization (2016). arXiv:1607.06450
3. Chen, S., Ma, K., Zheng, Y.: Med3d: transfer learning for 3D medical image analysis (2019). arXiv:1904.00625
4. Consortium, M.: MONAI: medical open network for ai (2025). https://doi.org/10.5281/zenodo.15661201
5. Ding, W., Li, L., Qiu, J., Wang, S., Huang, L., Chen, Y., Yang, S., Zhuang, X.: Aligning multi-sequence CMR towards fully automated myocardial pathology segmentation. IEEE Trans. Med. Imaging (2023)
6. Falcon, W.: The PyTorch Lightning team: PyTorch Lightning (2019). https://doi.org/10.5281/zenodo.3828935
7. He, K., Zhang, X., Ren, S., Sun, J.: Deep residual learning for image recognition. In: 2016 IEEE Conference on Computer Vision and Pattern Recognition (CVPR), pp. 770–778 (2016). https://doi.org/10.1109/CVPR.2016.90
8. Jaderberg, M., Simonyan, K., Zisserman, A., kavukcuoglu, k.: Spatial transformer networks. In: Cortes, C., Lawrence, N., Lee, D., Sugiyama, M., Garnett, R. (eds.) Advances in Neural Information Processing Systems. vol. 28. Curran Associates, Inc. (2015)
9. Lin, T.Y., Goyal, P., Girshick, R., He, K., Dollár, P.: Focal loss for dense object detection. IEEE Trans. Pattern Anal. Mach. Intell. **42**(2), 318–327 (2020). https://doi.org/10.1109/TPAMI.2018.2858826
10. Loshchilov, I., Hutter, F.: Decoupled weight decay regularization. In: International Conference on Learning Representations (2019)
11. Ma, J.: Histogram matching augmentation for domain adaptation with application to multi-centre, multi-vendor and multi-disease cardiac image segmentation (2020). arXiv:2012.13871
12. MacQueen, J.: Multivariate observations. In: Proceedings of the 5th Berkeley Symposium on Mathematical Statisticsand Probability, vol. 1, pp. 281–297 (1967)
13. Milletari, F., Navab, N., Ahmadi, S.A.: V-net: fully convolutional neural networks for volumetric medical image segmentation. In: 2016 Fourth International Conference on 3D Vision (3DV), pp. 565–571 (2016)
14. Neverova, N., Wolf, C., Taylor, G., Nebout, F.: ModDrop: adaptive multi-modal gesture recognition. IEEE Trans. Pattern Anal. Mach. Intell. **38**(8), 1692–1706 (2016). https://doi.org/10.1109/TPAMI.2015.2461544
15. Nyúl, L.G., Udupa, J.K.: On standardizing the MR image intensity scale. Magn. Reson. Med. **42**(6), 1072–1081 (1999)
16. Pedregosa, F., Varoquaux, G., Gramfort, A., Michel, V., Thirion, B., Grisel, O., Blondel, M., Prettenhofer, P., Weiss, R., Dubourg, V., Vanderplas, J., Passos, A., Cournapeau, D., Brucher, M., Perrot, M., Duchesnay, E.: Scikit-learn: machine learning in Python. J. Mach. Learn. Res. **12**, 2825–2830 (2011)
17. Plein, S., Bloomer, T.N., Ridgway, J.P., Jones, T.R., Bainbridge, G.J., Sivananthan, M.U.: Steady-state free precession magnetic resonance imaging of the heart: comparison with segmented k-space gradient-echo imaging. J. Magn. Reson. Imaging **14**(3), 230–236 (2001). https://doi.org/10.1002/jmri.1178
18. Qiu, J., Li, L., Wang, S., Zhang, K., Chen, Y., Yang, S., Zhuang, X.: MyoPS-Net: myocardial pathology segmentation with flexible combination of multi-sequence CMR images. Med. Image Anal. **84**, 102694 (2023)
19. Rahman, M.M., Munir, M., Marculescu, R.: EMCAD: efficient multi-scale convolutional attention decoding for medical image segmentation. In: Proceedings of the IEEE/CVF Conference on Computer Vision and Pattern Recognition (CVPR), pp. 11769–11779 (2024)

20. Srivastava, N., Hinton, G., Krizhevsky, A., Sutskever, I., Salakhutdinov, R.: Dropout: a simple way to prevent neural networks from overfitting. J. Mach. Learn. Res. **15**(56), 1929–1958 (2014)
21. Wang, W., Xie, E., Li, X., Fan, D.P., Song, K., Liang, D., Lu, T., Luo, P., Shao, L.: Pvt v2: improved baselines with pyramid vision transformer. Comput. Vis. Media **8**(3), 415–424 (2022). https://doi.org/10.1007/s41095-022-0274-8
22. Wu, Y., He, K.: Group normalization. In: Computer Vision – ECCV 2018: 15th European Conference. Munich, Germany, September 8–14, 2018, Proceedings, Part XIII, pp. 3–19. Springer, Berlin, Heidelberg (2018)
23. Yang, Y., Soatto, S.: FDA: fourier domain adaptation for semantic segmentation. In: 2020 IEEE/CVF Conference on Computer Vision and Pattern Recognition (CVPR), pp. 4084–4094 (2020). https://doi.org/10.1109/CVPR42600.2020.00414
24. Yaniv, Z., Lowekamp, B.C., Johnson, H.J., Beare, R.: Simpleitk image-analysis notebooks: a collaborative environment for education and reproducible research. J. Digit. Imaging **31**(3), 290–303 (2017). https://doi.org/10.1007/s10278-017-0037-8
25. Zhang, K., Zhuang, X.: Recognition and standardization of cardiac MRI orientation via multi-tasking learning and deep neural networks. In: Zhuang, X., Li, L. (eds.) Myocardial Pathology Segmentation Combining Multi-Sequence Cardiac Magnetic Resonance Images, pp. 167–176. Springer International Publishing, Cham (2020)
26. Zhuang, X.: Multivariate mixture model for myocardial segmentation combining multi-source images. IEEE Trans. Pattern Anal. Mach. Intell. **41**(12), 2933–2946 (2019)

Dual-Task Multi-modal 2.5D Swin Transformer for Liver Fibrosis Staging

Xin Hong(✉), Nao Wang, and Ying Shi

College of Computer Science and Technology, Huaqiao University, Xiamen, Fujian 361021, China
xinhong@hqu.edu.cn

Abstract. Liver fibrosis and cirrhosis are major complications of chronic liver disease, in which accurate staging is essential for personalized treatment and prognosis. Existing imaging methods face a trade-off between accuracy and efficiency: full-volume 3D models are computationally expensive and sensitive to resolution variations, while patch- or slice-based approaches often lose global anatomical continuity. To address these limitations, we propose a dual-task, multi-modal Swin Transformer framework for MRI-based liver fibrosis staging. The model learns compact 2.5D representations from each modality and employs task-specific residual MLP heads to independently predict cirrhosis (S4 vs. S1–S3) and fibrosis (S1 vs. S2–S4), thereby reducing cross-task interference. Evaluated on the CARE2025 Challenge dataset, our method achieved an overall 2nd-place ranking out of 7 participating teams, demonstrating its competitiveness under multi-center and multi-modal conditions. The framework attained AUCs of 72.50 and 77.22%, and accuracies of 71.67 and 78.51% for cirrhosis and substantial fibrosis detection, respectively. The code is available at https://github.com/hxpotato/CARE2025.

Keywords: Liver fibrosis staging · Multi-modal MRI network · Swin Transform

1 Introduction

Liver fibrosis staging is a critical biomarker for assessing the severity and progression of chronic liver disease, guiding both treatment planning and prognosis evaluation. The CARE2025 Challenge[1] provides a large-scale, multi-modal, multi-center MRI dataset for developing robust AI models for liver fibrosis staging (LiFS). However, substantial heterogeneity–arising from site-specific MRI protocols, variable resolutions, and missing modalities–poses major challenges to building models that remain accurate and computationally scalable across clinical environments [1,2,7] as shown in Fig. 1. Accurate differentiation between cirrhosis (S4) and non-cirrhotic fibrosis (S1–S3), as well as between early (S1)

[1] https://zmic.org.cn/care_2025/track4.

X. Zhuang et al. (Eds.): CARE 2025, LNCS 16257, pp. 214–224, 2026.
https://doi.org/10.1007/978-3-032-16271-7_20

and advanced stages (S2–S4), is clinically essential [4,11], yet remains difficult due to complex tissue alterations and the inherent limitations of current imaging techniques.

Despite substantial advances in medical image analysis, existing liver imaging methods still face a fundamental trade-off between accuracy and efficiency. Various strategies have been proposed to alleviate this dilemma. Patch-based and single-slice approaches focus on fine-grained structural details but inevitably compromise volumetric and anatomical continuity–patch-based inputs often lose global spatial context [3,8], whereas single-slice inputs fail to capture inter-slice dependencies [10,13,14]. In contrast, full-volume 3D models preserve complete anatomical structures and spatial coherence but are computationally demanding [6,15] and sensitive to cross-site resolution variations [5,9]. Overall, 2D and 3D paradigms exhibit complementary strengths and weaknesses: 2D-based methods offer higher computational efficiency and easier deployment, but they often lack volumetric context and robustness. In contrast, 3D models provide a richer spatial representation and higher accuracy at the cost of scalability and computational burden. These limitations highlight the necessity of developing a representation that harmonizes global contextual awareness, computational efficiency, and robustness to acquisition heterogeneity.

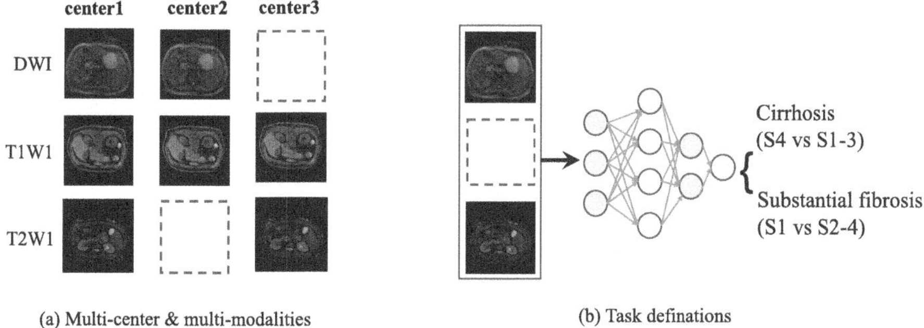

Fig. 1. (a) Modality Heterogeneity Across Centers. Imaging modalities vary by center and spatial resolution, with random modality missingness. (b) Task Objective. Perform Cirrhosis and Substantial Fibrosis Detection under these constraints.

To address these challenges, we propose a 2.5D dual-task multi-modal network that efficiently integrates cross-modality and cross-task information. By extracting ten central slices per MRI volume, the network preserves volumetric context while reducing computational overhead [17]. A Swin Transformer backbone captures multi-scale spatial dependencies, followed by task-specific heads for Cirrhosis and Substantial Fibrosis Detection, each trained with dedicated losses to minimize gradient interference [12,18]. This design leverages complementary information across modalities and tasks, achieving robust, accurate, and efficient liver fibrosis assessment suitable for clinical deployment.

2 Methods

We provide an overview of the proposed framework in Fig. 2, comprising modality-consistent 2.5D slice extraction, modality-specific Swin Transformer 3D encoders, and dual residual MLP prediction heads. Ten central slices are extracted per MRI volume to form a 2.5D representation that preserves volumetric context with reduced computational cost. Each modality is encoded through a dedicated Swin Transformer to capture multi-scale spatial features. Finally, two residual MLP heads perform Cirrhosis and Substantial Fibrosis Detection, with task-specific losses mitigating gradient interference and enabling robust multi-task predictions.

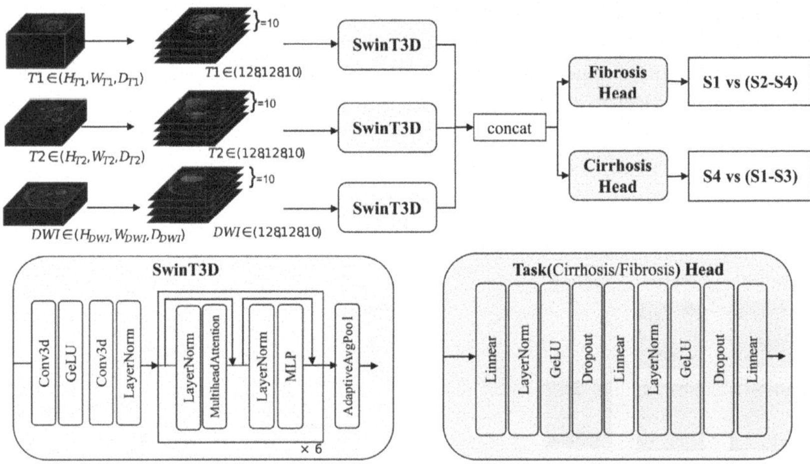

Fig. 2. Overview of the Proposed Framework. For each modality, 10 central axial slices are extracted, resized, and intensity-normalized to create a modality-consistent 2.5D representation. These stacks are processed by modality-specific Swin Transformer 3D encoders (SwinT3D Block), and the resulting features are concatenated and fed into dual residual MLP heads (Task Head) for Cirrhosis and Fibrosis regression.

2.1 Modality-Consistent 2.5D Slice Extraction

In multi-center clinical practice, liver MRI protocols exhibit substantial variability in acquisition range, spatial resolution, and slice count. Purely 2D approaches, although computationally efficient, often fail to capture global contextual information across slices, limiting their effectiveness in assessing liver pathology. Full-volume 3D analysis can preserve such spatial context, but it is computationally expensive and prone to domain shifts across centers. To balance these considerations, we adopt a 2.5D slice extraction strategy: focusing on the middle 10 slices, which contain the most critical pathological information, our approach preserves essential spatial context while remaining computationally efficient.

For each modality m of a subject, let the total number of axial slices be N_m, and denote the central slice index as $c_m = \lfloor \frac{N_m}{2} \rfloor$. We extract a set of K consecutive slices, $K = 10$ in our implementation,as defined in Eq. (1). To handle missing modalities, absent inputs are zero-padded, while available ones are independently encoded before feature-level fusion to ensure consistent input dimensionality. When the number of valid slices is fewer than K, zero-padding is applied to reach the predefined slice count, preserving a uniform spatio-temporal structure across samples. Each slice is resized to 128×128 using bilinear interpolation and normalized in intensity per modality to mitigate inter-scanner contrast variations.

$$S_m = \left\{ I_m^{(c_m - \frac{K}{2}+1)}, \ldots, I_m^{(c_m + \frac{K}{2})} \right\} \tag{1}$$

where I_m denotes a 2D axial slice of modality m, and S_m represents the stacked 2.5D slice set that serves as the model input.

2.2 Modality-Specific Swin Transformer(SwinT 3D) Backbone

To capture modality-specific 3D context from the extracted 2.5D stacks , we design a lightweight Swin Transformer-based encoder for each available MRI sequence (t1, t2, and dwi). Each encoder follows a hierarchical design consisting of a 3D patch embedding stem, multiple Swin Transformer blocks, and global average pooling. We obtain the modality-specific feature representation f_m, as formulated in Eq. (2)

$$\text{SwinT3D Block}(f_m) \tag{2}$$

To obtain a compact modality-specific vector f_m from Z_m^l, global average pooling (GAP) is applied. Given the feature map Z_m^l from modality m, this operation produces the vector representation f_m

$$f_m = \text{GAP}(Z_m^l) \in \mathbb{R}^C. \tag{3}$$

The three modality features f_{t1}, f_{t2}, and f_{dwi} are concatenated along the channel dimension to form a unified multi-modal feature vector. This unified representation is subsequently fed into the task-specific residual MLP heads for cirrhosis and fibrosis prediction.

To model hierarchical spatial dependencies from modality-specific embeddings Z_m^l, each encoder first maps the input tokens to the initial embedding Z_m^0 and then applies a series of identical transformer layers.

To extract a compact feature representation Z_m^0 from 2.5D stacks S_m, we apply two consecutive 3D convolutions with a stride of 2, which downsample and project the raw voxel intensities into an embedding space of dimension C, as shown in Eq. (4). Given an input stack $S_m \in \mathbb{R}^{1 \times D \times H \times W}$ from modality m, this process yields $Z_m^0 \in \mathbb{R}^{C \times \frac{D}{4} \times \frac{H}{4} \times \frac{W}{4}}$.

$$Z_m^0 = \text{LayerNorm}(\text{Con3d}(\text{GeLU}(\text{Conv3d}(S_m)))) \tag{4}$$

The output of the l-th layer is computed recursively as Z_m^l, with each block performing the operations defined in Eq. (5). In our implementation, each encoder comprises six layers.

$$Z_m^l = Z_m^{l-1} + \mathrm{W\!-\!MSA}(\mathrm{LN}(Z_m^{l-1})) + \mathrm{MLP}(\mathrm{LN}(Z_m^{l-1} + \mathrm{W\!-\!MSA}(\mathrm{LN}(Z_m^{l-1})))) \tag{5}$$

where $\mathrm{LN}(\cdot)$ denotes Layer Normalization, $\mathrm{W\!-\!MSA}(\cdot)$ is the window-based multi-head self-attention, and $\mathrm{MLP}(\cdot)$ is a two-layer feed-forward network with GELU activation. Residual connections are applied after both the attention and MLP modules to enhance gradient flow.

2.3 Dual-Task Optimization via Task-Specific Heads

Although both cirrhosis detection and substantial fibrosis detection derive from the same fibrosis grading system, they target distinct clinical decision boundaries and exhibit varying class distributions. To accommodate these differences, we design a dual-task architecture with two independent residual MLP heads operating on the aggregated multi-modal feature vector, each optimized with a task-specific loss.

The overall loss $\mathcal{L}_{\text{task}}$ is defined as Eq. (6)

$$\mathcal{L}_{\text{task}} = \begin{cases} \mathcal{L}_{\text{Focal}}(y, \hat{y}), & \text{if task} = \text{cirrhosis}, \\ \mathcal{L}_{\text{CE}}(y, \hat{y}), & \text{else} . \end{cases} \tag{6}$$

where y and $\hat{y}$ denote the ground-truth label and predicted probability, respectively.

For cirrhosis detection, we employ focal loss to address class imbalance, as defined in Eq. (7).

$$\mathcal{L}_{\text{Focal}}(y, \hat{y}) = -\alpha_y \, (1 - \hat{y}_k)^{\gamma} \, \log \hat{y}_k, \tag{7}$$

where $\hat{y}_k$ denotes the predicted probability of the true class k, α_y is the class-balancing factor (set to 1.0 in our implementation), and γ is the focusing parameter (set to 2.0) that controls the down-weighting of well-classified samples.

For substantial fibrosis detection, we use the standard cross-entropy (CE) loss, as shown in Eq. (8).

$$\mathcal{L}_{\text{CE}}(y, \hat{y}) = -\sum_{k=0}^{K-1} \mathbf{1}_{[y=k]} \log(\hat{y}_k), \tag{8}$$

where y_k is the predicted probability for class k, y is the ground-truth label, and K denotes the total number of classes.

2.4 Training Strategy

We train two independent models that share the same multi-modal encoder architecture but are equipped with distinct task-specific heads: one for cirrhosis detection and the other for substantial fibrosis detection. Both tasks use the same dataset with different label definitions–cirrhosis detection distinguishes stage S4 from S1–S3, whereas substantial fibrosis detection separates stage S1 from S2–S4. Accordingly, the dataset is prepared twice with task-specific label mappings.

Cirrhosis Detection Model. This network is trained end-to-end from random initialization using cirrhosis-specific labels, jointly optimizing the encoder and a residual MLP head. The checkpoint that achieves the best validation performance is selected as the final cirrhosis detection model.

Substantial Fibrosis Detection Model. A separate network with an identical architecture is trained from scratch using fibrosis-specific labels, optimizing the encoder and the corresponding residual MLP head. The best validation checkpoint is adopted as the final fibrosis detection model. This fully independent training strategy ensures that each model is optimized exclusively for its respective task, eliminating cross-task interference while maintaining a consistent architecture and preprocessing.

3 Experiments

3.1 Datasets and Evaluation Protocol

The CARE2025 Challenge[2] focuses on developing robust AI models for multi-phase liver fibrosis staging (LiFS) [4,11,16]. Using multi-center, multi-phase MRI data, participants are required to design methods capable of handling heterogeneous imaging protocols, scanner variations, and missing modalities. The LiFS task comprises two binary subtasks: cirrhosis detection (S1–S3 vs. S4) and fibrosis staging (S1 vs. S2–S4), where S denotes the stage. These tasks are based on non-contrast T1-weighted (T1WI), T2-weighted (T2WI), and diffusion-weighted (DWI) MRI sequences. The dataset includes 330 labeled and 170 unlabeled cases collected from four clinical centers, providing a benchmark for developing robust and generalizable liver analysis models under real-world variability. As summarized in Table 1, all patients underwent multi-phase MRI examinations from centers A, B1, B2, and C, each comprising the three aforementioned imaging modalities. The evaluation on the unseen dataset C highlights the strong generalization capability of the proposed models and algorithms (Table 1).

[2] https://zmic.org.cn/care_2025/track4.

Table 1. Data distribution across different centers.

Vendors	Train data			Test data			
	A	B	B	A	B	B	C
Center	A	B1	B2	A	B1	B2	C
Cases number	130	170	60	40	40	40	70

Implementation Details. The training data are randomly split (80/20) for model training and local validation. Predictions on the official validation set are evaluated by the organizers using hidden labels. The test set comprises in-distribution (ID) and out-of-distribution (OOD) subsets from known and unseen sites, respectively. Following the challenge protocol, participants submit Docker images, and results are reported in terms of ACC and AUC for both detection tasks.

Implementation Setting. All experiments are implemented in PyTorch and conducted on a workstation equipped with an NVIDIA RTX 4090 GPU (24 GB of memory). The model is trained in two stages, each using identical hyper-parameters: a batch size of 10, the AdamW optimizer with a weight decay of 1×10^{-4}, and an initial learning rate of $\eta_0 = 5 \times 10^{-4}$, decayed via a cosine annealing schedule. Each stage undergoes training for 50 epochs.

3.2 Ablation Studies

To better understand the contribution of each design choice in our framework, we conduct ablation studies on the official training/validation split, using the same training protocol described in Sect. 2.4. We analyze the impact of (1) the number of slices in the 2.5D stack and (2) different loss functions for each task.

Effect of Slice Number and 2.5D Design. We vary the number of slices $K \in \{1, 5, 10, 15\}$ in the 2.5D stack to examine the trade-off between inter-slice context and computational cost, and we compare it with a 2D baseline ($K = 1$). As shown in Table 2, performance improves with larger K up to 10, after which the gain saturates. Increasing to $K = 15$ or full 3D inputs offers no further benefit, likely due to redundant context and reduced batch sizes of 6 for $K = 15$ and 2 for 3D under GPU memory limits. **Bold** indicates the best result, and underline denotes the second best.

Loss Function Variants. We compare cross-entropy (CE) and focal loss for both detection of both cirrhosis and substantial fibrosis. As shown in Table 3. Focal loss performs comparably or slightly better for cirrhosis detection (S4 vs. S1–S3), likely due to its focus on hard examples. However, for substantial fibrosis

Table 2. Ablation study of input dimensionality on the local validation set

Number of slices	**Cirrhosis detection**		**Fibrosis detection**	
	ACC	AUC	ACC	AUC
K = 1	48.61	69.31	**79.16**	71.60
K = 5	65.27	70.58	69.44	64.81
K = 10	66.67	71.67	68.06	**72.72**
K = 15	65.27	71.67	69.44	70.66
3D	**68.05**	**77.81**	59.72	65.53

detection (S1 vs. S2–S4, imbalanced), it biases towards the majority class, providing no improvement in ACC and only marginal gains in AUC. These results indicate that focal loss benefits balanced tasks but may underperform when the minority class is clinically critical. Focal loss brings a slight improvement in cirrhosis detection. For substantial fibrosis detection, focal loss produces nearly identical predictions (biased toward the majority class); thus, its ACC/AUC values are omitted.**bold** indicates the best result.

Table 3. Comparison of loss function variants on the local set

Loss	**Cirrhosis detection**		**Fibrosis detection**	
	ACC	AUC	ACC	AUC
CE	63.88	70.41	**68.06**	**72.72**
Focal	**66.67**	**71.67**	–	–

Training Strategy. The two-stage scheme follows the protocol in Sect. 2.4, where the backbone is trained separately with each MLP head. In contrast, the end-to-end scheme optimizes both heads jointly. Results in Table 4 show the comparative performance of the two strategies; **bold** indicates the best result.

Table 4. Comparison between two-stage and end-to-end training on the local set

Train Strategy	**Cirrhosis detection**		**Fibrosis detection**	
	ACC	AUC	ACC	AUC
End-to-end	52.77	61.60	63.88	67.98
Two-stage	**66.67**	**71.67**	**68.06**	**72.72**

3.3 Evaluation Results

We report the performance of our team named 'potato', on the official *test* sets of the CARE2025 Challenge. For evaluation, the organizers executed our submitted Docker container, which contained the trained model weights. Performance was assessed using accuracy (ACC) and the area under the ROC curve (AUC) for both cirrhosis and substantial fibrosis detection. The test set includes two subsets: in-distribution (ID) data from the same sites as training/validation and out-of-distribution (OOD) data from unseen sites. Results are summarized in Tables 5 and 6.

On the ID test set in Table 5, team potato(our) achieved 72.50% ACC and 77.22% AUC for cirrhosis detection, and 71.67% ACC and 78.51% AUC for fibrosis detection, ranking 2nd out of 7 participating teams. These results indicate that our method effectively captures disease-relevant features and performs robustly within the training distribution. On the OOD test set in Table 6, performance decreased to 70.00% ACC and 71.51% AUC for cirrhosis detection, and 67.14% ACC and 33.23% AUC for fibrosis detection. While cirrhosis detection remained relatively stable, the substantial drop in the fibrosis AUC highlights the challenges posed by distribution shifts and class imbalance.

Overall, team potato(our) demonstrates competitive in-distribution performance and strong discriminative ability for clearly separable disease stages, while future work should focus on improving OOD robustness and addressing class imbalance to enhance generalization.

Table 5. Official CARE2025 challenge leaderboard on ID test set (%)

Rank	Team	**Cirrhosis detection**		**Fibrosis detection**	
		ACC	AUC	ACC	AUC
1	Team space	74.17	81.33	76.67	83.93
2	potato(Ours)	72.50	77.22	71.67	78.51
3	CitySJTU	71.67	78.61	70.00	73.70
4	BioDreamer	70.83	77.89	70.00	77.11
5	Sigma	70.00	77.22	65.00	74.28
6	TeamZhang	66.67	71.73	74.17	68.48
7	NW-Radio	47.50	79.78	65.83	67.27

Table 6. Official CARE2025 challenge leaderboard on OOD test set (%)

Rank	Team	**Cirrhosis detection**		**Fibrosis detection**	
		ACC	AUC	ACC	AUC
1	Sigma	71.43	69.47	92.86	86.31
2	potato(Ours)	70.00	71.51	67.14	33.23
3	Team space	64.29	52.73	88.57	61.23
4	TeamZhang	64.29	68.83	91.43	71.38
5	CitySJTU	42.86	49.31	70.00	31.08
6	BioDreamer	32.86	56.65	88.29	59.40
7	NW-Radio	32.86	46.25	92.86	40.31

4 Conclusion

We propose a modality-consistent 2.5D multi-modal MRI framework featuring task-specific Swin Transformer 3D encoders and dual residual MLP heads, achieving strong performance in cirrhosis detection and fibrosis staging. By decoupling tasks and applying tailored loss functions, the model effectively handles label imbalance and semantic differences while exposing challenges in out-of-distribution (OOD) generalization. Future work will explore adaptive fusion for incomplete modality inputs and enhance OOD robustness.

Competing interest statement The authors have no competing interests to declare that are relevant to the content of this article.

References

1. Babar, M., Qureshi, B., Koubaa, A.: Investigating the impact of data heterogeneity on the performance of federated learning algorithm using medical imaging. PLoS ONE **19**(5), e0302539 (2024)
2. Chang, Q., Yan, Z., Zhou, M., Qu, H., He, X., Zhang, H., Baskaran, L., Al'Aref, S., Li, H., Zhang, S., et al.: Mining multi-center heterogeneous medical data with distributed synthetic learning. Nat. Commun. **14**(1), 5510 (2023)
3. Chen, W., Han, Y., Ashraf, M.A., Liu, J., Zhang, M., Su, F., Huang, Z., Wong, K.K.: A patch-based deep learning MRI segmentation model for improving efficiency and clinical examination of the spinal tumor. J. Bone Oncol. **49**, 100649 (2024)
4. Gao, Z., Liu, Y., Wu, F., Shi, N., Shi, Y., Zhuang, X.: A reliable and interpretable framework of multi-view learning for liver fibrosis staging. In: International Conference on Medical Image Computing and Computer-Assisted Intervention, pp. 178–188 (2023)
5. Huang, Y., Khodabakhshi, Z., Gomaa, A., Schmidt, M., Fietkau, R., Guckenberger, M., Andratschke, N., Bert, C., Tanadini-Lang, S., Putz, F.: Multicenter privacy-preserving model training for deep learning brain metastases autosegmentation. Radiother. Oncol. **198**, 110419 (2024)

6. Ilesanmi, A.E., Ilesanmi, T.O., Ajayi, B.O.: Reviewing 3D convolutional neural network approaches for medical image segmentation. Heliyon **10**(6) (2024)
7. Javed, H., El-Sappagh, S., Abuhmed, T.: Robustness in deep learning models for medical diagnostics: security and adversarial challenges towards robust ai applications. Artif. Intell. Rev. **58**(1), 12 (2024)
8. Lian, T., Deng, C., Feng, Q.: Patch-based texture feature extraction towards improved clinical task performance. Bioengineering **12**(4), 404 (2025)
9. Lilhore, U.K., Sunder, R., Simaiya, S., Alsafyani, M., Monish Khan, M., Alroobaea, R., Alsufyani, H., Baqasah, A.M.: AG-MS3D-CNN multiscale attention guided 3D convolutional neural network for robust brain tumor segmentation across MRI protocols. Sci. Rep. **15**(1), 24306 (2025)
10. Lindquist, D.M., Manhard, M.K., Levoy, J., Dillman, J.R.: Feasibility of sodium and amide proton transfer-weighted magnetic resonance imaging methods in mild steatotic liver disease. Tomography **11**(8), 89 (2025)
11. Liu, Y., Gao, Z., Shi, N., Wu, F., Shi, Y., Chen, Q., Zhuang, X.: Merit: multi-view evidential learning for reliable and interpretable liver fibrosis staging. Med. Image Anal. **102**, 103507 (2025)
12. Liu, Z., Ning, J., Cao, Y., Wei, Y., Zhang, Z., Lin, S., Hu, H.: Video Swin transformer. In: Proceedings of the IEEE/CVF Conference on Computer Vision and Pattern Recognition, pp. 3202–3211 (2022)
13. Manhard, M.K., Kilpattu Ramaniharan, A., Tkach, J.A., Trout, A.T., Dillman, J.R., Pednekar, A.S.: Simultaneous multiparameter mapping of the liver in a single breath-hold or respiratory-triggered acquisition using multi-inversion spin and gradient echo MRI. J. Magn. Reson. Imaging **61**(4), 1925–1936 (2025)
14. Obmann, V.C., Ardoino, M., Klaus, J., Catucci, D., Berzigotti, A., Montani, M., Peters, A., Todorski, I., Wagner, B., Zbinden, L., et al.: MRI extracellular volume fraction in liver fibrosis-a comparison of different time points and blood pool measurements. J. Magn. Reson. Imaging **60**(4), 1678–1688 (2024)
15. Rahman, H., Khan, A.R., Sadiq, T., Farooqi, A.H., Khan, I.U., Lim, W.H.: A systematic literature review of 3D deep learning techniques in computed tomography reconstruction. Tomography **9**(6), 2158–2189 (2023)
16. Wu, F., Zhuang, X.: Minimizing estimated risks on unlabeled data: a new formulation for semi-supervised medical image segmentation. IEEE Trans. Pattern Anal. Mach. Intell. **45**(5), 6021–6036 (2023)
17. Yang, Z., Fan, T., Smedby, Ö., Moreno, R.: 3D breast ultrasound image classification using 2.5D deep learning. In: 17th International Workshop on Breast Imaging (IWBI 2024), vol. 13174, pp. 443–449. SPIE (2024)
18. Zhai, H., Chen, Z., Li, L., Tao, H., Wang, J., Li, K., Shao, M., Cheng, X., Wang, J., Wu, X., et al.: Two-stage multi-task deep learning framework for simultaneous pelvic bone segmentation and landmark detection from ct images. Int. J. Comput. Assist. Radiol. Surg. **19**(1), 97–108 (2024)

EHU-Mamba2: Enhanced U-Mamba for Multi-center Cardiac MR Segmentation with Dynamic Alignment and Adaptive Upsampling

Xiaoning Zhang, Yanjun Peng(✉), and Zengmin Zhang

Shandong University of Science and Technology, 579 Qianwan Gang Road, 266590 Huangdao, Qingdao, Shandong, China
{zhangxiaoning,yjpeng,zhangzengmin}@sdust.edu.cn

Abstract. Multi-center cardiac Magnetic Resonance (MR) segmentation aims to automati-cally delineate anatomical structures of the heart from scanned images acquired from diverse devices. However, Multi-center cardiac MR segmentation faces several challenges, e.g., cross-center intensity shifts, heterogeneous imaging pro-tocols, and ambiguous lesion boundaries, which significantly limit model general-ization in real-world clinical scenarios. To address these issues, we propose an enhanced U-Mamba framework explicitly optimized for domain generalization across multiple centers and imaging conditions. Our method incorporates three key strategies: (1) Dynamic Histogram Matching, which enables robust intensity alignment across heterogeneous centers; (2) CBAM (Convolutional Block Attention Module), which adaptively emphasizes lesion-relevant spatial and channel features to improve representation; and (3) Dynamic Upsampling (DySample), employing content-adaptive kernels for precise and fine-grained boundary refinement. Our method achieves Dice scores of 67.45% for edema, 63.09% for scar, and 65.27% for the combined region (scar + edema) on the multi-center MyoPS++ 2025 dataset that exhibits severe domain shifts across seven centers. These results highlight the strong cross-domain robustness, reliability, and clinical potential of our framework for multi-center cardiac MR analysis.

Keywords: Multi-center Cardiac MRI · Myocardial Pathology Segmentation · Domain Generalization · Dynamic Upsampling

1 Introduction

Myocardial infarction (MI) remains one of the leading causes of death and disability worldwide, underscoring the importance of accurately assessing myocardial viability for effective diagnosis and treatment. Multi-center cardiac MR segmentation imaging provides complementary information on myocardial pathology and plays a critical role in patient management [1]. Specifically, balanced steady-state free precession (bSSFP) cine sequences offer high-contrast anatomical delineation, late gadolinium enhancement

X. Zhuang et al. (Eds.): CARE 2025, LNCS 16257, pp. 225–234, 2026.
https://doi.org/10.1007/978-3-032-16271-7_21

(LGE) sequences reveal myocardial scar tissue, and T2-weighted (T2) sequences identify edema regions associated with MI. These modalities are widely employed in clinical practice to evaluate myocardial viability in patients with cardiomyopathy.

Accurate delineation of the myocardium into normal tissue, scar, and edema is essential for clinical decision-making. However, manual segmentation is labor-intensive, time-consuming, and subject to inter- and intra-observer variability. Automated segmentation using machine learning techniques offers a potential solution, yet differentiating between edema and scar remains challenging [2]. This difficulty arises from their small, scattered distribution and the substantial overlap in imaging characteristics. Moreover, the data are collected from multiple centers, where some centers lack specific sequences, image quality varies across institutions [3], and even within-center CMR sequences are often unregistered [4].

Recent advances in Multi-center cardiac MR segmentation, particularly in the context of the MyoPS++ 2024 challenge, have focused on leveraging complementary information across modalities to improve the delineation of myocardial scar and edema. GenSegNet [5] integrates a generative adversarial network (GAN) with a 3D U-Net to synthesize missing MRI sequences and employs a self-training strategy with pseudo labels to enhance performance on incomplete datasets, achieving notable improvements in both edema and scar segmentation accuracy. Building on modality complementarity, the Progressive Multi-channel Fusion Network [6] introduces an interactive progressive segmentation strategy that incorporates channel attention within a U-Net framework, enabling effective cross-modal feature fusion from C0, T2, and LGE sequences for more accurate myocardial pathology segmentation. More recently, ME-UNet [7] combines U-Net with state space models (SSMs) by embedding a Vision Mamba block to efficiently capture long-range dependencies while integrating enhanced 3D residual blocks to strengthen local feature extraction, achieving robust performance on multi-center, multi-sequence CMR datasets. These studies demonstrate the effectiveness of data augmentation, cross-modal fusion, and global context modeling in advancing myocardial pathology segmentation.

In this work, we propose an enhanced hybrid Upsampling Mamba2 framework for automatic myocardial pathology segmentation in multi-center, multi-sequence CMR images. Our framework is explicitly designed to address cross-center intensity variations and ambiguous lesion boundaries, which pose significant challenges for real-world clinical deployment. Specifically, we introduce Dynamic Histogram Matching to achieve robust intensity alignment across heterogeneous centers, and incorporate CBAM (Convolutional Block Attention Module) [8] to enhance lesion-relevant feature representation. Additionally, we employ Dynamic Upsampling (DySample) [9], which utilizes content-adaptive kernels to refine lesion boundaries in a fine-grained manner. Extensive experiments on the MyoPS++ 2025 dataset, encompassing seven centers with severe domain shifts, demonstrate that our framework achieves Dice scores of 67.38% for edema, 62.38% for scar, and 64.88% for the combined region (scar + edema). These results highlight the superior cross-domain robustness of our method and its potential for reliable clinical application in multi-center cardiac MR analysis.

2 Method

2.1 Overview of EHU-Mamba2 Architecture

EHU-Mamba2 takes as input multi-sequence cardiac MR images acquired from different centers, aiming to address domain variability and improve cross-center generalization. The network adopts an enhanced U-Mamba2 backbone [10], where the EHU (Enhanced Hybrid Upsampling) module is introduced to dynamically align multi-scale features and restore high-resolution spatial details with greater fidelity.

Unlike conventional upsampling strategies that rely solely on fixed interpolation or deconvolution, the EHU module adaptively integrates both local detail preservation and global structural consistency, guided by learned alignment weights. This enables the network to recover fine-grained anatomical information while mitigating artifacts and distortions caused by domain shifts.

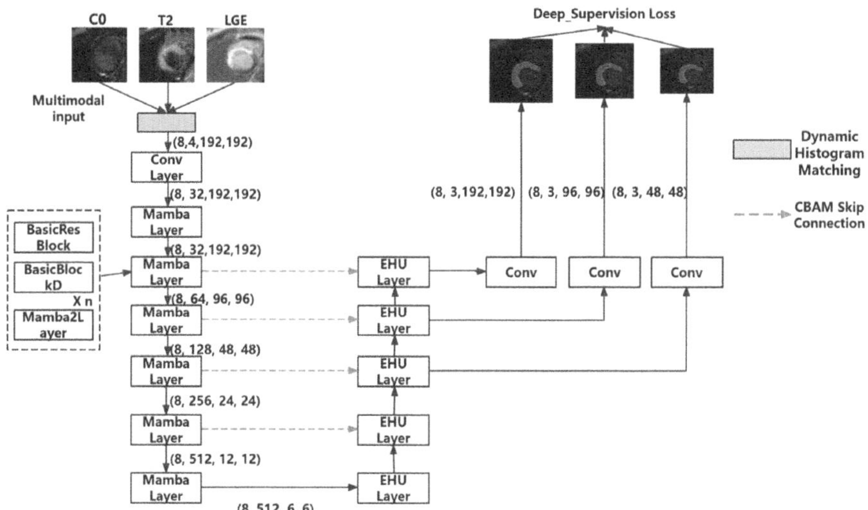

Fig. 1. Overview of the EHU-Mamba2.

In the encoder pathway, Mamba blocks extract both long-range dependencies and local contextual patterns, progressively building hierarchical feature representations. Skip connections are enhanced by dynamic alignment within the EHU module, ensuring that the fused features from encoder and decoder are spatially consistent and semantically complementary. As shown in Fig. 1, EHU-Mamba2 maintains a U-shaped encoder–decoder architecture [11], but replaces standard skip connection fusion with EHU-based adaptive alignment and hybrid upsampling.

To further boost segmentation precision in challenging multi-center scenarios, EHU-Mamba2 incorporates adaptive domain-aware normalization within its feature extraction stages, enabling the network to modulate its feature statistics according to the input domain characteristics. This, combined with deep supervision across decoder stages, facilitates stable optimization and robust performance across diverse clinical datasets.

The detailed architecture of the EHU module, as well as the integration of Mamba blocks in the encoder–decoder framework, are presented in Sects. 2.2 and 2.3, respectively.

2.2 The Enhanced Hybrid Upsampling Module

The EHU module is designed to improve the fusion of multi-scale features and the restoration of high-resolution spatial details in multi-center cardiac MR segmentation. Unlike conventional upsampling methods that rely solely on fixed interpolation or deconvolution, the EHU module dynamically integrates local detail preservation with global structural consistency using learned alignment weights.

Specifically, EHU aligns features from different encoder stages and adaptively fuses them with decoder features, as illustrated in Fig. 2, ensuring spatial consistency and semantic complementarity across scales. This hybrid upsampling strategy enables the network to recover fine-grained anatomical structures while mitigating artifacts and distortions caused by domain variability. By enhancing skip connections with dynamic alignment, EHU facilitates accurate feature propagation throughout the U-shaped encoder–decoder architecture.

Overall, the EHU module allows EHU-Mamba2 to effectively leverage multi-scale contextual information, improving segmentation precision and robustness in heterogeneous multi-center datasets.

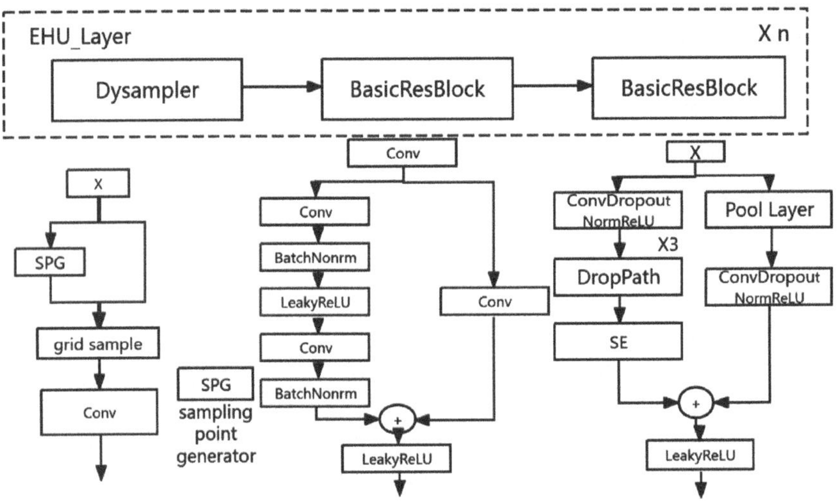

Fig. 2. The EHU layer.

2.3 Encoder and Decoder

The proposed EHU-Mamba2 architecture is built upon a U-shaped encoder–decoder backbone, integrating Enhanced Hybrid Upsampling (EHU) to achieve precise multi-center cardiac MR segmentation. The network consists of a Residual Mamba2 encoder and a residual-based decoder, symmetrically connected through skip connections enhanced by CBAM attention and dynamic feature alignment.

The encoder comprises multiple Residual Mamba2 stages, each containing a series of residual blocks and a Mamba2 layer. In each stage, the Mamba2 block captures both long-range dependencies and local contextual information, progressively building hierarchical multi-scale feature representations. Skip connections are extracted from all encoder stages and subsequently refined by CBAM modules, which apply feature-aware weighting to emphasize important spatial and channel-wise features, suppressing irrelevant responses.

In the decoder, features from corresponding encoder stages are adaptively aligned and fused with upsampled decoder representations through the Enhanced Hybrid Upsampling (EHU) module. EHU combines dynamic feature alignment with hybrid upsampling to restore high-resolution anatomical details while maintaining global structural consistency. This ensures that fused features are both spatially coherent and semantically complementary, effectively mitigating misalignment caused by domain variability.

The decoder also incorporates deep supervision, producing intermediate predictions at multiple scales to stabilize training and enhance feature refinement. Together, the encoder and decoder work synergistically: the Mamba2-enhanced encoder extracts rich hierarchical representations, CBAM selectively emphasizes informative features, and the EHU module ensures precise multi-scale feature fusion. This combination enables accurate, robust, and high-fidelity segmentation across heterogeneous multi-center cardiac MR datasets.

2.4 Dynamic Histogram Matching

Shapira [12] proposed a Generalized Histogram Matching (GHM) method to derive a unified optimal monotonic mapping across multiple pairs of histograms. In contrast to traditional histogram matching, which is limited to a single histogram pair, GHM can simultaneously account for numerous histograms and supports various additive distance metrics. Building upon this idea, we perform dynamic histogram matching for multi-modal cardiac MRI, aligning the intensity distributions of different modalities (e.g., LGE, T2) to a reference modality (e.g., C0) on a per-case basis. This strategy ensures consistent contrast and anatomical representation across modalities while preserving modality-specific characteristics. By adapting the intensity alignment for each patient, our method effectively mitigates inter-scan and inter-modality variations, thereby enhancing multi-modal fusion for subsequent segmentation tasks.

3 Experiments

3.1 Dataset and Preprocessing

Since the test data are not yet publicly available, we conducted experiments and evaluations using the training and validation sets provided in the CARE 2025 MyoPS++ challenge dataset. This dataset comprises 260 cases (with some centers missing specific sequences), including 235 training cases with ground truth annotations and 25 testing cases. The dataset contains CMR images from seven centers and has been pre-processed using the MVMM method [1]. We employed 95 cases with complete modality sequences from centers B and C for training, and 25 cases from center D for testing, applying dynamic histogram matching using the data from center D as the reference.

3.2 Implementation Details

In our experiments, the model was trained using a weighted combination of binary cross-entropy (BCE) and Dice loss, balancing pixel-level classification accuracy and structural consistency. The initial learning rate was set to 1e-3. To ensure robustness and generalization, we employed five-fold cross-validation, with each fold containing 75 training cases and 20 validation cases. Model performance was quantified using the Dice coefficient and precision. All experiments were implemented in PyTorch and conducted on an NVIDIA RTX 4090 24GB GPU, with a batch size of 8.

4 Results

4.1 Ablation Study Results

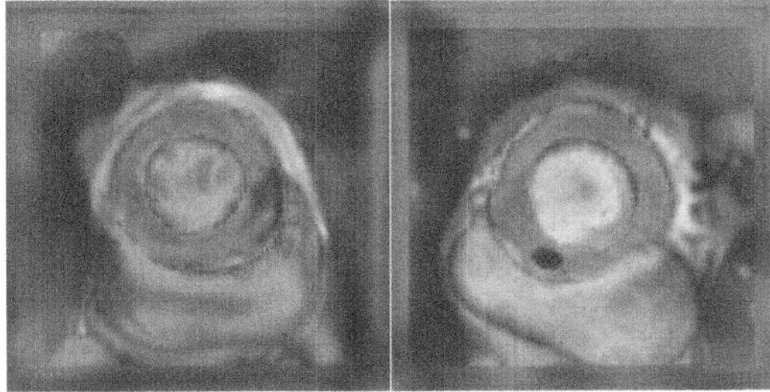

Fig. 3. Score-CAM feature heatmap of myocardial segmentation with the EHU

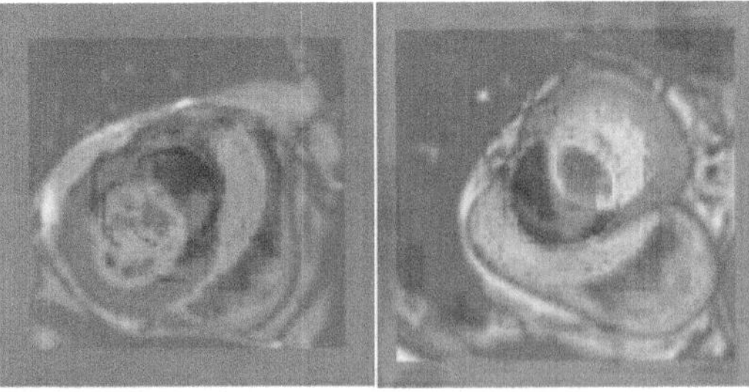

Fig. 4. Score-CAM feature heatmap of myocardial segmentation without the EHU

The experimental results indicate that the incorporation of the EHU module markedly improves both the accuracy and attentiveness of feature representation. As depicted in Fig. 3, the spatial distribution of feature attributions—highlighted as red and blue activation points—becomes more compact and better aligned with cardiac anatomical structures when the EHU module is utilized. This attentive behavior demonstrates the module's capacity to selectively amplify salient features while suppressing irrelevant responses, thereby directing the network's focus toward clinically significant regions.

In contrast, Fig. 4 shows that, in the absence of the EHU module, the contribution points are dispersed and less consistent with anatomical relevance. Such scattered responses indicate a reduced discriminative focus, which may ultimately undermine segmentation performance.

The EHU module is implemented by integrating CBAM into the skip connections and replacing conventional upsampling with dysample. This design enables adaptive modulation of multi-scale feature importance, thereby facilitating the learning of context-aware and attentive representations. Consequently, the network attains improved boundary delineation and structural fidelity, while simultaneously enhancing interpretability, as reflected in the more coherent and anatomically consistent activation patterns.

Table 1 further quantifies the impact of each component, revealing that both CBAM and EHU modules yield substantial improvements in overall performance. When integrated into the framework, their synergistic effects translate to consistent enhancements across all evaluated cardiac structures, with gains accompanied by discernible computational overhead as reflected in the Time (s) column, where "s" denotes the average training time per epoch. Specifically, relative to the baseline (both modules disabled, 57.62 s), enabling CBAM alone increases training time moderately (63.12 s), while EHU alone induces a more pronounced rise (71.55 s); concurrent deployment of both modules results in the highest demand, with training time reaching 81.09 s. Nonetheless, this augmented overhead is warranted by significant strides in segmentation accuracy, evident in improved DSC and PRE metrics for myocardial edema and scar regions. In contexts where segmentation precision is paramount, the enhanced task utility from more reliable lesion localization far outweighs the additional training time expenditure.

Table 1. Ablation study on the application of EHU blocks and boundary constraints on the Myops++ 2025 dataset.

CBAM	EHU	DSC		PRE		Time (s)
		Edema	Edema and scar	Edema	Edema and scar	
×	×	66.96	63.56	72.99	70.12	57.62
×	√	67.28	64.34	75.81	72.81	71.55
√	×	67.08	63.95	75.53	70.93	63.12
√	√	67.45	65.27	75.74	72.75	81.09

4.2 Comparison with Other Methods

To further validate the effectiveness of the proposed EHU, we compared it with three representative baselines, namely nnUNetv2 [13], Swin-UNETR [14], and U-Mamba [10], as illustrated in Fig. 5. Although nnUNetv2 achieves relatively stable myocardial segmentation, it suffers from limited capability in distinguishing scar from edema, often leading to class confusion and imprecise boundary delineation. Swin-UNETR benefits from the long-range dependency modeling of Transformers, resulting in more complete global contours. However, it tends to miss small, scattered lesions and shows blurred boundaries between scar and edema. U-Mamba, by incorporating state space modeling, produces more compact segmentations and demonstrates improved localization of scar in some cases. Nevertheless, its performance is less robust across heterogeneous modalities, and prediction misalignment is frequently observed. In contrast, EHU consistently achieves more accurate delineation of myocardial structures, with sharper boundary depiction and superior differentiation between edema (orange) and scar (green). Moreover, EHU exhibits higher sensitivity to small lesions and maintains stable responses across different modalities, underscoring its robustness and generalizability. These qualitative findings are further corroborated by quantitative metrics in Table 2.

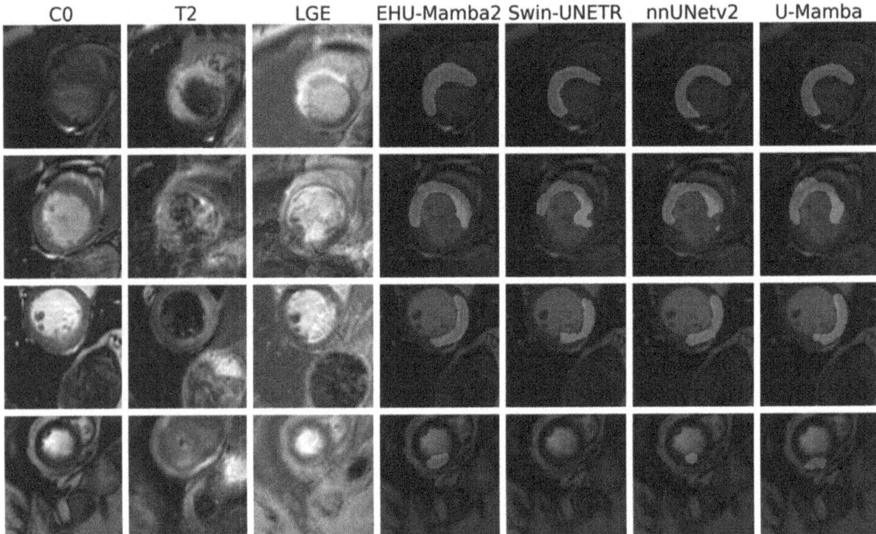

Fig. 5. Visual comparison of segmentation results on the MyoPs++ 2025 dataset between the proposed EHU-Mamba2 and Swin-UNETR, nnUNetv2, and U-Mamba. Orange and green regions represent edema and scar, respectively.

Table 2. Comparison of our method with other advanced medical image segmentation techniques on the MyoPS++ 2025 dataset.

Method	DSC		PRE	
	Edema	Edema + Scar	Edema	Edema + Scar
nnUNetv2	67.39	64.88	75.74	73.46
U-mamba	66.54	63.25	72.70	71.95
Swin-unetr	64.84	61.16	71.83	71.40
Ours	67.45	65.27	74.48	72.75

5 Discussion and Conclusion

In this paper, we propose EHU-Mamba2, an enhanced U-Mamba framework for multi-center cardiac MR segmentation. EHU-Mamba2 leverages the Enhanced Hybrid Upsampling module, Mamba2 residual feature extraction, attention-guided skip connections, and dynamic histogram matching to improve multi-scale feature alignment and mitigate inter-scan and inter-modality variations. Experiments demonstrate that the framework achieves robust, high-fidelity segmentation of myocardial scar and edema across heterogeneous datasets, highlighting its potential for reliable multi-center cardiac MR analysis. Although EHU-Mamba2 performs well on multi-modal datasets, its application to cases with missing C0 or T2 sequences remains challenging, which will be addressed in future work to improve robustness on incomplete datasets.

References

1. Zhuang, X.: Multivariate mixture model for myocardial segmentation combining multi-source images. IEEE Trans. Pattern Anal. Mach. Intell. **41**(12), 2933–2946 (2019)
2. Al'Aref, S.J. et al.: Clinical applications of machine learning in cardiovascular disease and its relevance to cardiac imaging. Eur. Heart J. **40**(24), 1975–1986 (2019)
3. Qiu, J., et al.: Myops-net: myocardial pathology segmentation with flexible com-bination of multi-sequence CMR images. Med. Image Anal. **84**, 102694 (2023)
4. Ding, W., et al.: Aligning multi-sequence CMR towards fully automated myocardial pathology segmentation. IEEE Trans. Med. Imaging (2023)
5. Lin, H. et al.: GenSegNet: leveraging synthetic sequences and pseudo labels for multi-sequence myocardial pathology segmentation. MICCAI Challenge on Comprehensive Analysis and Computing of Real-World Medical Images, pp 227–239. Springer Nature Switzerland, Cham (2024)
6. Wang, J., et al.: Progressive multi-channel fusion network for myocardial pathology segmentation on multi-modality CMR images. In: MICCAI Challenge on Comprehensive Analysis and Computing of Real-World Medical Images. Springer, Cham (2025)
7. Zhu, Z., Lin, Y., Yang, M.: ME-UNet: enhancing mamba for myocardial pathology segmentation in multi-center multi-sequence CMR images. In: MICCAI challenge on comprehensive analysis and computing of real-world medical images. Springer, Cham (2025)

8. Woo, S., et al.: CBAM: Convolutional Block Attention Module. Springer, Cham (2018)
9. Liu, W., et al.: Learning to upsample by learning to sample. In: Proceedings of the IEEE/CVF International Conference on Computer Vision (2023)
10. Ma, J., Li, F., Wang, B.: U-mamba: enhancing long-range dependency for biomedical image segmentation. arXiv:2401.04722 (2024)
11. Ronneberger, O., Fischer, P., Brox, T.:. U-net: convolutional networks for biomedical image segmentation. In: International conference on medical image computing and computer-assisted intervention. Springer international publishing, Cham (2015)
12. Shapira, D., Avidan, S., Hel-Or, Y.: Multiple histogram matching. In: 2013 IEEE Iernational Conference on Image Processing, pp. 2269–2273 (2013). https://api.semanticscholar.org/CorpusID:8298830
13. Isensee, F., et al.: nnu-net revisited: a call for rigorous validation in 3d medical image segmentation. In: International Conference on Medical Image Computing and Computer-Assisted Intervention. Springer Nature Switzerland, Cham (2024)
14. Hatamizadeh, A., et al.: Swin unetr: swin transformers for semantic segmentation of brain tumors in MRI images. International MICCAI brainlesion workshop. Springer International Publishing, Cham (2021)

Multi-modal Liver Segmentation and Fibrosis Staging Using Real-world MRI Images

Yang Zhou[1](✉), Kunhao Yuan[2](✉), Ye Wei[3], and Jishizhan Chen[1]

[1] Multiscale X-ray Imaging (MXI) Lab, Department of Mechanical Engineering, University College London, London, UK
{yang.zhou,jishizhan.chen}@ucl.ac.uk

[2] Centre for Clinical Brain Sciences, University of Edinburgh, Edinburgh, UK
kyuan3@ed.ac.uk

[3] MRC Weatherall Institute of Molecular Medicine, University of Oxford, Oxford, UK
ye.wei@imm.ox.ac.uk

Abstract. Liver fibrosis represents the accumulation of excessive extracellular matrix caused by sustained hepatic injury. It disrupts normal lobular architecture and function, increasing the chances of cirrhosis and liver failure. Precise staging of fibrosis for early diagnosis and intervention is often invasive, which carries risks and complications. To address this challenge, recent advances in artificial intelligence-based liver segmentation and fibrosis staging offer a non-invasive alternative. As a result, the CARE 2025 Challenge aimed for automated methods to quantify and analyse liver fibrosis in real-world scenarios, using multi-centre, multi-modal, and multi-phase MRI data. This challenge included tasks of precise liver segmentation (LiSeg) and fibrosis staging (LiFS). In this study, we developed an automated pipeline for both tasks across all the provided MRI modalities. This pipeline integrates pseudo-labelling based on multi-modal co-registration, liver segmentation using deep neural networks, and liver fibrosis staging based on shape, textural, appearance, and directional (STAD) features derived from segmentation masks and MRI images. By solely using the released data with limited annotations, our proposed pipeline demonstrated excellent generalisability for all MRI modalities, achieving top-tier performance across all competition subtasks. This approach provides a rapid and reproducible framework for quantitative MRI-based liver fibrosis assessment, supporting early diagnosis and clinical decision-making. Code is available at https://github.com/YangForever/care2025_liver_biodreamer.

Keywords: Liver segmentation · Fibrosis staging · Multi-modal MRI images · Machine learning · Deep learning

X. Zhuang et al. (Eds.): CARE 2025, LNCS 16257, pp. 235–246, 2026.
https://doi.org/10.1007/978-3-032-16271-7_22

1 Introduction

Liver fibrosis is a key pathological process during chronic liver disease (CLD) that represents a critical global health challenge and leads to an estimated two million deaths annually and substantial socioeconomic costs [3]. Fibrosis can progressively disrupt liver microstructures and functions, potentially resulting in cirrhosis and even liver failure [5]. Nevertheless, early fibrosis is often asymptomatic and potentially reversible with timely intervention [2], demanding the need for accurate and reproducible staging methods. The gold standard for fibrosis staging remains invasive liver biopsy [7], but it is limited in clinical scalability. Magnetic resonance imaging (MRI) offers a promising non-invasive alternative due to its superior high soft tissue contrast. Multi-modal MRI further enriches analysis by providing complementary insights from different imaging sequences of the same anatomical structures.

Effective fibrosis staging on MRI is highly dependent on accurate liver segmentation. Although recent developments in artificial intelligence (AI), especially U-Net and its variants [9,10], have greatly advanced medical segmentation tasks, clinical segmentation applications on MRI remain challenging due to its diverse sequences and protocols. Therefore, to integrate medical AI into real-world clinical practice, the Comprehensive Analysis&computing of REal-world medical images (CARE2025) proposed a Challenge track, named CARE-Liver. The track aimed to facilitate Liver Segmentation (LiSeg) and Fibrosis Staging (LiFS) on multi-centre, multi-modal, and multi-phase MRI datasets with limited single-modal annotations. The data modality involved non-contrast data: T1-weighted imaging (T1WI), T2-weighted imaging (T2WI), and diffusion-weighted imaging (DWI), and contrast-enhanced data from different phases of Gd-EOB-DTPA (GED1-4).

To address the challenge of limited annotation in medical image segmentation, previous studies, such as in [11], have investigated semi-supervised learning (SSL) methods to propagate the segmentation capabilities to unlabelled data. Nonetheless, the effectiveness of these approaches can be affected by multi-modal data, which present different features even on the same organ. A crucial step in multi-modal segmentation is image registration, which enables the transfer of the manual annotations that are typically only available on a single modality [16]. With the liver segmentation, recent research on fibrosis staging, like [4,8], demonstrated promising results on GED-enhanced MRI by investigating subregion multi-view features to minimise background interference of the entire scan. In fibrosis, patients often exhibit liver surface irregularities, lobar edge retraction, and subtle internal nodules [1], with MRI scans typically diffuse and widespread across the liver [12]. As a result, effective algorithms must capture not only local pixel intensity, but also capture the organ's complex shapes, textures, and directional features.

Motivated by these findings, we proposed an automated pipeline including multi-modal MRI registration, multi-modal liver segmentation, and fibrosis staging across all modalities using the features from segmented areas. In summary, in this study, we (i) extended the GED4 training dataset using mix-cases

Table 1. Data distribution of the Training dataset from the CARE-Liver 2025 track.

Vendor	Cases	Annotated Cases (GED4)	Fibrosis stage S1	S2	S3	S4
A	130	10	55	64	12	38
B1	170	10	39	29	11	91
B2	60	10	3	10	9	38
Total	**360**	**30**	**97**	**64**	**32**	**167**

data augmentation; (2) enabled multi-modal liver segmentation with generated pseudo-labels from GED4 annotations using a rigid co-registration method; (iii) applied nnUNet for liver segmentation across all the modalities provided in the track without using additional open-source datasets; (iv) proposed a fibrosis staging method using Random Forest classifiers based on STAD (Shape, Textural, Appearance, Directional) features derived from segmented regions-of-interest (ROIs). Our proposed method achieved top-tier performance in both LiSeg and LiFS tasks on the hold-out Validation dataset and demonstrated promising generalised capability on the hold-out out-of-distribution Test dataset.

2 Dataset

The study cohort of the CARE-Liver track involved 610 patients diagnosed with liver fibrosis. 360 patients from three vendors, labelled as A, B1, and B2, were provided as a multi-phase and multi-centre Training dataset. The Training data statistics are shown in Table 1. Each patient in the Training dataset has T2WI, DWI, and GED-enhanced dynamic MRIs. The GED-enhanced dynamic MRIs cover several key phases: non-contrast (T1WI), arterial (GED1), venous (GED2), delayed (GED3), and hepatobiliary (GED4).

However, it is challenging to perform tasks of LiSeg and LiFS due to the limited number of annotations and data imbalance. As shown in Table 1, the annotations are only available for GED4 data, and the number of annotated cases is limited to 10 cases in each vendor, less than 10% in total. Moreover, the distribution of cases from each vendor across the different fibrosis stages is significantly imbalanced, with 167 from S4, while only 32 from S3 in total. Additionally, MRI resolutions vary across different modalities, while the pre-alignments are not available, which makes sharing GED4 annotations directly difficult. Therefore, to expand the Training dataset, we applied data augmentation for the GED4 data and co-registration to other modalities, without utilising alternative open-source datasets.

2.1 Data Augmentation

We augmented annotated GED4 data by generating synthetic examples, using a structured vendor-wise instance mixing approach [13,15]. For each annotated

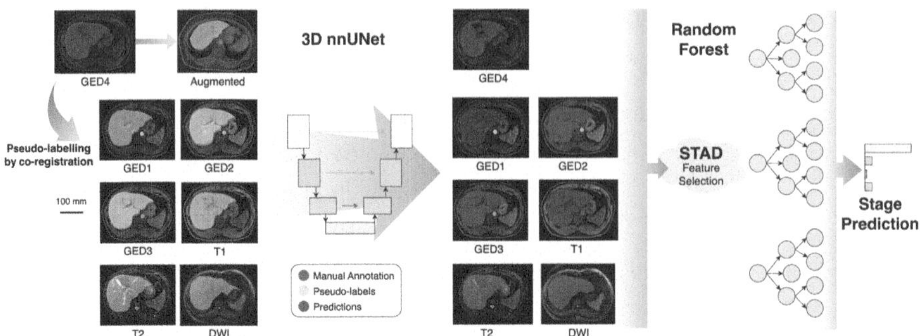

Fig. 1. The automated pipeline for liver segmentation and fibrosis staging. A 3D nnUNet was trained on the dataset involving the original annotated GED4 data, augmented GED4 data, and the registered multi-modality data. After that, the fibrosis staging was performed by the Random Forest classifiers based on the STAD (Shape, Texture, Appearance, Directional) features selected from the segmentation predictions.

GED4 sample as a source, we randomly selected the other five annotated samples within the same vendor as targets. Then, the source foreground was extracted and isotropically scaled to match the target foreground region spatially. At the end, the transformed source foreground replaced the target foreground. This method improved anatomical and intensity diversity while preserving realistic organ topology and sharp label boundaries. To avoid damaging the organ structure, we deliberately excluded other common augmentations like translation, rotation, Gaussian noise, and foreground-biased patch cropping.

2.2 Multi-modal Co-registration

To facilitate the multi-modal segmentation and fibrosis staging, we implemented rigid co-registration between manually annotated GED4 data and other modalities. The registration searched for a 3D Euler transformation along the translation, rotation, and scalling in the space, using mutual information (MI) as a metric optimised by a gradient descent algorithm. The registration was implemented utilising the SimpleITK Python package. Finally, the training dataset was expanded from the initial 30 annotated GED4 samples to a total of 354 multi-modal samples, incorporating both the original and augmented GED4 data.

3 Methods

The track of CARE-Liver 2025 involves two tasks of automated liver segmentation (LiSeg) and Multi-phase fibrosis staging (LiFS). Each task is further divided into the non-contrasted subtask (T1WI, T2WI, and DWI) and the contrast-enhanced subtask (GED 1 to 4). Therefore, we proposed a pipeline that can process all the tasks, streamlining the LiSeg and LiFS. Without using other open-source datasets, as shown in Fig. 1, we developed an automated method involving multi-modal liver segmentation and fibrosis staging based on the segmented liver regions.

3.1 LiSeg Task–Liver Segmentation

On the registered multi-modal samples and augmented GED4 samples, we applied the state-of-the-art 3D nnUNet [6] for liver segmentation. This method automates the biomedical image segmentation through network structure generation and training parameter selection based on the given training dataset. Before training the network, the dataset was pre-processed by an 8-bit conversion and data normalisation to prevent training bias, as the data types vary from each vendor and modality.

The network was optimised by Stochastic Gradient Descent (SGD) with the weighted soft Dice loss and Cross-Entropy loss, shown as in Equation 1.

$$\begin{aligned} L_{dc+ce} &= L_{soft\_Dice} + L_{Cross-Entropy} \\ &= -w_{dc} \frac{2\sum y_{pred} y_{true} + f_{smooth}}{\sum y_{pred} + \sum y_{true} + f_{smooth} + \epsilon} - w_{ce} \sum y_{true} \log y_{pred}, \end{aligned} \tag{1}$$

where the y_{pred} denotes the predictions from the segmentation model and y_{true} is the ground truths. f_{smooth} is the smoothing factor for the Dice score, with a default value of 1. The term ϵ, set to $1 \times e^{-8}$ by default, is set for numerical stability to prevent division-by-zero error. The weights w_{dc} and w_{ce} determine the relative contribution of the Dice loss and Cross-Entropy loss to the total loss, and both have a default value of 1.

3.2 LiFS Task–Fibrosis Stage Classification

The LiFS process began with feature selection, followed by stage classification using efficient Random Forest classifiers. The feature selection phase characterized the liver's macro-level morphologies and basic signal intensity within the segmented liver regions from the LiSeg task. Specifically, the features include:

- **Shape** features, such as volume, surface area, sphericity, and solidity, were computed to quantify geometric changes associated with fibrosis, like surface nodularity or parenchymal shrinking. Sphericity, for instance, measures how closely the liver's form resembles a perfect sphere, with deviations potentially indicating pathological alteration.
- **Texture** features were extracted to capture more complex patterns indicative of fibrotic tissue. The magnitude of the image gradient is computed to quantify local intensity changes and "edginess" within the tissue, reflecting the degree of structural irregularity. Moreover, texture is analysed using Gray-Level Co-occurrence Matrices (GLCM) on three orthogonal planes to assess the spatial relationship of voxels, with features like contrast revealing the tissue's coarseness.

- First-order **appearance** features were calculated from the distribution of voxel intensities within the liver mask. These include statistical moments like mean, standard deviation, skewness, and kurtosis, which reflect the overall tissue density and heterogeneity.
- **Directional** feature analysis involved computing eigenvalues from the structure tensor and Hessian matrix. The features, such as coherence and anisotropy, probe the underlying microstructural arrangement of the tissue by measuring local orientation and curvature, which are critical for detecting the organized patterns of fibrotic bands.

In general, the primary benefit of this comprehensive STAD feature extraction is its ability to generate a rich, multi-faceted quantitative signature of the liver. By combining simple morphological metrics with sophisticated, higher-order textural and directional features, it created a holistic profile capable of capturing subtle pathophysiological changes. In addition, to account for potential data variation across vendors, we further incorporated a flag indicating the scanner vendor.

These objective and explainable features are ideal for training robust Random Forest classifiers to accurately stage liver fibrosis without the risks associated with surgical biopsies. Ultimately, this approach paves the way for non-invasive diagnostics, enabling more frequent monitoring of disease progression and facilitating earlier detection and intervention.

4 Results and Discussion

In this section, we evaluated the model's performance on the hold-out Validation dataset and Test dataset from the CARE-Liver Track. Both datasets included samples from vendors, the same as the Training dataset, while the Test dataset introduced out-of-distribution data from a new vendor. For LiSeg and LiFS, we only trained and applied a single model for the tasks without ensembling.

4.1 Liver Segmentation

LiSeg aimed for segmentation on non-contrast modalities, including T1WI, T2WI, and DWI, and segmentation on contrast-enhanced modality, GED4. To facilitate the liver segmentation on multi-modal MRI images, we explored multiple configurations to train a 3D nnUNet. Due to the restricted access to the Validation and Test datasets, the Training dataset was split as training (Train-Train) and validation (Train-Val) based on a ratio of 4:1.

First, as shown in Fig. 2 (Ai.), we compared the models trained on annotated GED4 data only (Model-GED4) and on augmented data (Model-GED4-A), using identical training hyperparameters. The results show that Model-GED-A achieved better Dice scores on both Train-Train and Train-Val.

Second, after multi-modal registration, we trained a model on all the data involving GED4, augmented GED4, and registered data, named Model-All. Due

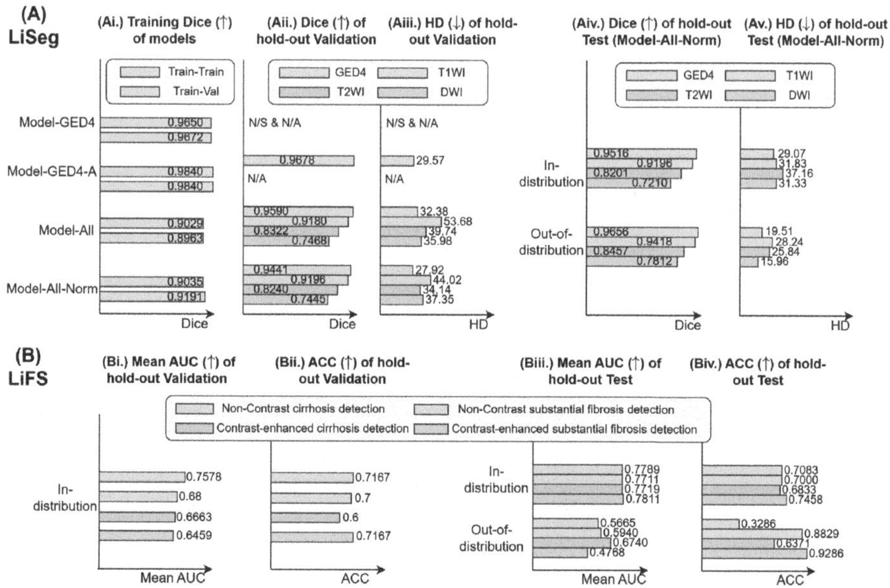

Fig. 2. Quantitative evaluation of the method on LiSeg and LiFS. (A) shows the Dice and Hausdorff distance (HD) of different model configurations on (Ai.) the Training dataset and (Aii.)(Aiii.) the hold-out Validation dataset. (Aiv.)(Av.) illustrates the Model-All-Norm model performance on the hold-out Test dataset. (B) indicates the AUC and ACC of the Model-All on (Bi.)(Bii.)the hold-out Validation dataset and (Biii.)(Biv.) the hold-out Test dataset. (N/S denotes Not Submitted to the scoring system, and N/A is Not Applicable).

to the data varying from intensity ranges and data types, we further trained a model (Model-All-Norm) on normalised data, which are 8-bit range of 0-255. By evaluating the Dice scores on the Training and Validation datasets, both models achieved a similar performance of a range ± 0.02 on all the MRI modalities. However, Model-All-Norm resulted in smaller Hausdorff Distances on GED4, T1WI, and T2WI. Therefore, we submitted the Model-All-Norm for the Test phase evaluation. It achieved better performance on Out-of-distribution data with $0.01 \sim 0.05$ Dice and $5 \sim 15$ HD improvements compared to the performance on In-distribution data, showing promising generalised segmentation capability.

Figure 3 shows the results of co-registration and the predictions from Model-All-Norm. In this example, rigid co-registration achieved good alignment for modalities with contrast similar to GED4, including T1WI, GED2, and GED3. However, the alignment was slightly shifted for the remaining modalities. Notably, T2WI and DWI demonstrate low contrast on the liver region and show different liver features, which makes co-registration and their pseudo-labels inaccurate. This introduced bias during model training, causing lower Dice on

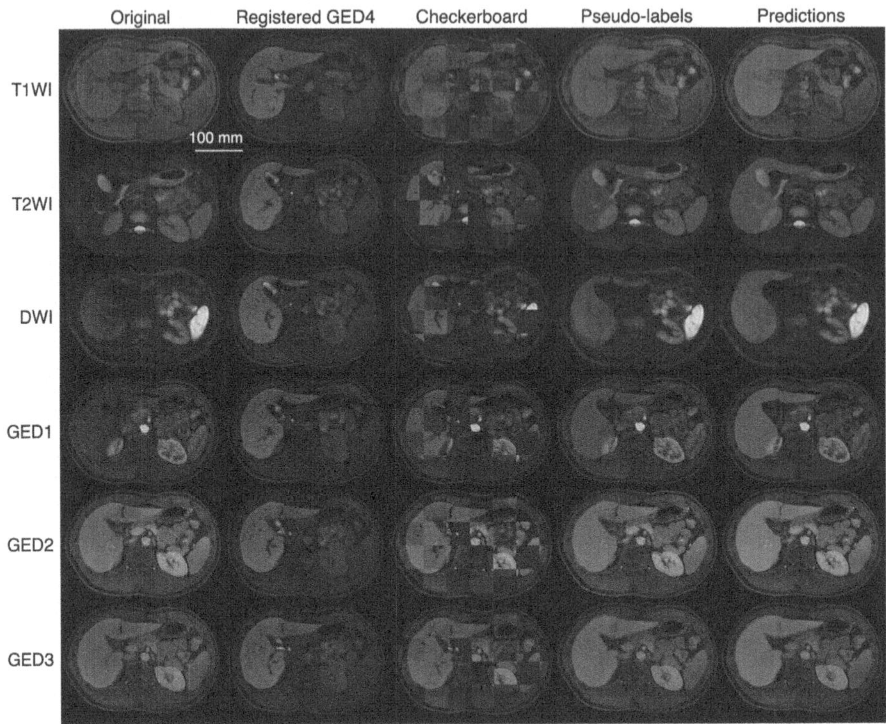

Fig. 3. Results of co-registration, pseudo-labelling, and corresponding predictions. All the modalities are from a randomly selected case with the 2D slices taken from the middle of the MRI volume along the z-axis.

both the hold-out Validation and Test datasets, with ~ 0.12 to 0.13 decrease compared to GED4 segmentation, while only ~ 0.05 decrease for T1WI.

4.2 Liver Fibrosis Staging

The LiFS aimed for two subtasks of cirrhosis detection (stage S4 vs. S1S3) and substantial fibrosis detection (Stages S2S4 vs. S1), evaluated separately on non-contrast and contrast-enhanced modalities. Using liver segmentation predictions on the Training dataset from Model-All, we isolated liver regions across various MRI modalities. From those regions, we extracted 32 STAD features, as illustrated in Fig. 4, and applied Random Forest classifiers on a train-validation split ratio of 4:1.

Figure 2 (B) demonstrates robust and consistent performance of our proposed model across both the hold-out Validation and in-distribution Test (which is also from vendors as Validation) datasets. Specifically, both metrics of mean Area Under the Curve (AUC) and Accuracy (ACC) improved on the Test dataset compared to those achieved in the Validation dataset. For example, the task of

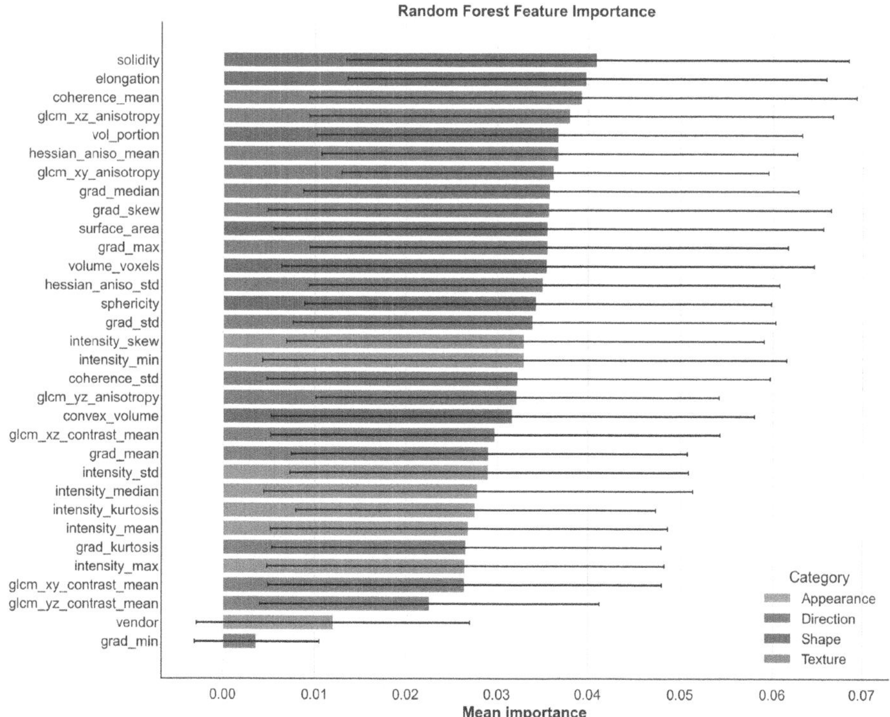

Fig. 4. Importance analysis of the features selected for Random Forest classifiers. Standard deviation is shown as the error bar in black.

Contrast-enhanced substantial fibrosis detection increased approximately 0.14 of the mean AUC, while the Contrast-enhanced cirrhosis detection increased nearly 0.09 on ACC.

When our model was presented with the out-of-distribution (OOD) Test dataset, the detection performance was impacted with decreases in the mean AUC metric among both modalities and tasks. Particularly, there was a drop to 0.4768 in contrast-enhanced substantial fibrosis detection compared to 0.7811 achieved in the in-distribution Test dataset. This highlighted the challenge of domain shift that often appears in medical image processing. However, the ACC of non-contrast and contrast-enhanced substantial fibrosis detection improved to 0.8829 and 0.9286, respectively, compared to an average of 0.7 and 0.72 on in-distribution data from Validation and Test. A decrease in mean AUC with an increase in ACC can indicate that some of the selected training features failed in OOD data. For example, variations in voxel intensity can adversely affect appearance-based features, potentially leading to detection errors, whereas other biologically consistent characteristics, like directional features, may provide compensation in some cases.

Therefore, we investigated the importance of the features used in the Random Forest classifiers, as shown in Fig. 4. The features were ranked by their mean importance score, with an error bar showing as standard deviation. The analysis results indicated that the shape-based and directional features are significant in the multi-modal fibrosis detection, with solidity and elongation emerging as the top predictive characteristics. Directional features, such as coherence (coherence_mean) and anisotropy (glcm_xz_anisotropy), also showed high importance, as they capture biological properties by assessing tissue orientation and curvature. Appearance-based features ranked lower in importance following some of the texture-based features. This feature importance analysis aligned with our fibrosis detection results on the hold-out Test dataset, further demonstrating that the feature selection process can be improved when considering the OOD data.

4.3 Discussion

One limitation that affects the performance of our proposed pipeline is the accuracy of the co-registration process. Inaccurate pseudo-labels can introduce bias during the segmentation training phase, making the model training difficult and leading overfitting problem. The error potentially impacts the feature selection process for the fibrosis staging task. In this study, we found that upsampling low-resolution data to higher-resolution data results in higher registration errors. Therefore, we registered annotated GED4 to other modalities due to the lower resolutions of other modalities, such as DWI, to improve the pseudo-labelling quality. To improve the registration and performance of downstream tasks, future work can include non-rigid co-registration methods that consider the detailed deformation during the registration process. Additionally, as shown in Fig. 3, the segmentation predictions can complementarily correct the pseudo-labels by filling the missing areas due to registration errors. Hence, fine-tuning the model on all Training dataset after performing an all-data inference might improve the segmentation performance, as in previous work [14].

Apart from the cumulative error from the registration and segmentation process, the fibrosis staging performance was also limited by the features selected. By accessing the performance on the hold-out Test dataset and the feature importance analysis, biologically consistent intrinsic features that display in multiple modalities were more reliable. Those features can make the classifiers more robust and generalisable. Therefore, in the future, more shape-based and directional features will be investigated and included in training the model with a reduction of intensity-based appearance features. In addition, although the Random Forest classifier provided interpretable features, it may underperform compared to recent deep learning approaches. The observed drop in mean AUC on out-of-distribution data highlights limitations in generalization, which likely stems from the reliance on handcrafted features. Our study's primary contribution lies in integrating multi-modal, real-world MRI data into a clinically interpretable framework, establishing a baseline for fibrosis staging in this context.

Future work could explore neural networkbased methods to improve generalization, particularly when larger annotated datasets become available.

5 Conclusion

In this study, we proposed an automated pipeline that integrates liver segmentation and fibrosis staging on multi-modal real-world clinical MRI images. Based on this pipeline, the nnUNet learned liver segmentation from multi-modal registered MRI images. The segmented regions, then, were used for STAD feature extraction and fibrosis stage classification through efficient Random Forest classifiers. The STAD features captured the fibrosis characteristics and features revealed from the real-world MRI images. The results demonstrated that our pipeline achieved top-tier performance on both LiSeg and LiFS tasks in CARE-Liver Track using limited data and annotations, without needing training on additional large open-source datasets. This work potentially presented novel insights for practical clinical MRI applications, particularly in scenarios involving multimodality and multi-task learning under limited annotations.

Competing interest statement The authors declare that they have no competing interests.

Acknowledgments. The authors acknowledge the use of the UCL Myriad High Performance Computing Facility (Myriad@UCL), and associated support services, in the completion of this work.

References

1. Aubé, C., Bazeries, P., Lebigot, J., Cartier, V., Boursier, J.: Liver fibrosis, cirrhosis, and cirrhosis-related nodules: imaging diagnosis and surveillance. Diagn. Interv. Imaging **98**(6), 455–468 (2017)
2. Czaja, A.: The prevention and reversal of hepatic fibrosis in autoimmune hepatitis. Alimentary Pharmacol. Therapeut. **39**(4), 385–406 (2014)
3. Devarbhavi, H., Asrani, S.K., Arab, J.P., Nartey, Y.A., Pose, E., Kamath, P.S.: Global burden of liver disease: 2023 update. J. Hepatol. **79**(2), 516–537 (2023)
4. Gao, Z., Liu, Y., Wu, F., Shi, N., Shi, Y., Zhuang, X.: A reliable and interpretable framework of multi-view learning for liver fibrosis staging. In: International Conference on Medical Image Computing and Computer-Assisted Intervention. pp. 178–188. Springer (2023)
5. Ginès, P., Krag, A., Abraldes, J.G., Solà, E., Fabrellas, N., Kamath, P.S.: Liver cirrhosis. Lancet **398**(10308), 1359–1376 (2021)
6. Isensee, F., Jaeger, P.F., Kohl, S.A., Petersen, J., Maier-Hein, K.H.: nnu-net: a self-configuring method for deep learning-based biomedical image segmentation. Nat. Methods **18**(2), 203–211 (2021)
7. Kazi, I.N., Kuo, L., Tsai, E.: Noninvasive methods for assessing liver fibrosis and steatosis. Gastroenterol. Hepatol. **20**(1), 21 (2024)

8. Liu, Y., Gao, Z., Shi, N., Wu, F., Shi, Y., Chen, Q., Zhuang, X.: Merit: Multi-view evidential learning for reliable and interpretable liver fibrosis staging. Med. Image Anal. **102**, 103507 (2025)
9. Oh, N., Kim, J.H., Rhu, J., Jeong, W.K., Choi, G.s., Kim, J.M., Joh, J.W.: Automated 3d liver segmentation from hepatobiliary phase mri for enhanced preoperative planning. Sci. Rep. **13**(1), 17605 (2023)
10. Wang, J., Peng, Y., Jing, S., Han, L., Li, T., Luo, J.: A deep-learning approach for segmentation of liver tumors in magnetic resonance imaging using unet++. BMC Cancer **23**(1), 1060 (2023)
11. Wu, F., Zhuang, X.: Minimizing estimated risks on unlabeled data: A new formulation for semi-supervised medical image segmentation. IEEE Trans. Pattern Anal. Mach. Intell. **45**(5), 6021–6036 (2022)
12. Yu, D., Li, X.H., He, X.L., Jia, X.B., Wang, Z.C., Yang, Z.H., Ren, A.H.: Mri findings of confluent hepatic fibrosis caused by different etiologies. BMC Gastroenterol. **25**(1), 512 (2025)
13. Yuan, K., Woods, H., Günar, Ü., Dominic, D., Wu, Y., Qiu, Z., Grant, S.G.: Prmix: Primary region mix augmentation and benchmark dataset for precise whole mouse brain anatomical delineation. NeuroImage 121881 (2026)
14. Zhang, H., Zhang, M., You, X., Gu, Y., Yang, G.Z.: Computing assessment for liver fibrosis staging using real-world mr images. In: MICCAI Challenge on Comprehensive Analysis and Computing of Real-World Medical Images. pp. 87–95. Springer (2025)
15. Zhang, X., Liu, C., Ou, N., Zeng, X., Zhuo, Z., Duan, Y., Xiong, X., Yu, Y., Liu, Z., Liu, Y., et al.: Carvemix: a simple data augmentation method for brain lesion segmentation. Neuroimage **271**, 120041 (2023)
16. Zhang, Y., Yang, J., Tian, J., Shi, Z., Zhong, C., Zhang, Y., He, Z.: Modality-aware mutual learning for multi-modal medical image segmentation. In: International conference on medical image computing and computer-assisted intervention. pp. 589–599. Springer (2021)

Multi-branch Attention Network for Liver Fibrosis Staging in Multi-phase MRI

Siqi Wang[1,2], Wentao Liu[1](✉), Qian Zeng[1], and Dong Han[1,2]

[1] CAS Center for Excellence in Nanoscience, National Center for Nanoscience and Technology, Beijing, China
liuwentao@nanoctr.cn

[2] University of Chinese Academy of Sciences, Beijing, China

Abstract. The accuracy of liver fibrosis staging is essential for disease management, treatment, and prognosis. The CARE 2025 challenge introduced the multi-phase liver fibrosis staging (LiFS) task, which aims to develop robust AI methods using multi-center, multi-phase magnetic resonance imaging (MRI) data and addresses variability in imaging protocols and scanner systems. In this task, we propose a multi-branch attention network, which consists of a multi-branch encoder, a branch-wise feature fusion module, and a lightweight attention-based bottleneck. First, MRI sequences are grouped into five modality-specific inputs and processed by separate pretrained encoders to independently extract intra-sequence representations of fibrosis-relevant features. Next, a branch-wise attention fusion module learns an adaptive set of weights to dynamically recalibrate the contribution of each branch, which can reduce the redundancy among branches. Furthermore, a lightweight bottleneck module integrates multi-head attention and learnable positional encoding, which capture both intra- and inter-sequence temporal features. The proposed method demonstrates strong robustness on the CARE 2025 validation and test sets, highlighting its potential for non-invasive liver fibrosis staging in complex real-world settings.

Keywords: Liver Fibrosis Staging · Multi-Phase MRI · Attention Mechanism

1 Introduction

Liver fibrosis staging plays a crucial role in monitoring disease progression, determining prognosis, and guiding treatment decisions in chronic liver disease [1, 2]. While liver biopsy remains the clinical gold standard, MRI-based imaging diagnosis is increasingly favored due to its lower cost and non-invasive nature [3].

In recent years, deep learning-based medical image classification has advanced rapidly [4]. Among these approaches, convolutional neural networks and Transformer-based methods have achieved remarkable success, as they can effectively capture both spatial features and contextual information from images [5, 6]. However, automatic LiFS still suffers from random sequence-missing patterns, inefficient multiphase feature fusion, and limited generalization on multi-center medical imaging data. CARE 2025

X. Zhuang et al. (Eds.): CARE 2025, LNCS 16257, pp. 247–255, 2026.
https://doi.org/10.1007/978-3-032-16271-7_23

extends the Liver Fibrosis Staging (LiFS) task that was initially introduced in CARE 2024, where fibrosis severity is clinically categorized into four stages (S1–S4). This track evaluates two clinically critical binary sub-tasks: cirrhosis detection (S1–S3 vs. S4) and substantial fibrosis detection (S1 vs. S2–S4). Compared with CARE 2024, CARE 2025 introduces 170 additional cases, which may enhance sample diversity and exacerbate class distribution shifts.

In CARE 2024, a 3DResNet-based framework processes each MRI sequence independently for classification or regression and then derives the overall staging score by averaging the individual sequence predictions [7]. While this framework achieves promising results, it fails to explicitly explore the correlation and complementarity across MRI sequences. In real clinical settings, MRI sequences acquired using different protocols provide multiple perspectives of liver features, some of which may exhibit temporal correlations, while others may be redundant. Methods that process each sequence independently may fail to effectively exploit these cross-sequence relationships.

In this paper, we propose a Multi-Branch Attention Network (MBAN) for liver fibrosis staging from multiphase MRI. Our approach comprises three core components: (1) a multi-branch encoder that independently processes each MRI sequence to learn intra-sequence features relevant to fibrosis; (2) a branch-wise attention fusion module that dynamically assigns diagnostic importance to each branch, thereby reducing redundancy and patient-specific variability; and (3) an attention-based lightweight bottleneck that captures inter-branch dependencies. Evaluated on the CARE 2025 LiFS dataset, the proposed method demonstrates robust performance under varying class distributions and highlights its potential as a reliable non-invasive tool for accurate liver fibrosis staging.

2 Method

2.1 Dataset

The study cohort consisted of 610 patients diagnosed with liver fibrosis, all of whom underwent multiphase MRI examinations. Compared with the CARE2024 cohort, 170 additional cases were included. The dataset was acquired using MRI scanners from three different vendors across four medical centers. The dataset consists of T2-weighted imaging (T2WI), diffusion-weighted imaging (DWI), and Gadolinium ethoxybenzyl diethylenetriamine pentaacetic acid (Gd-EOB-DTPA)-enhanced dynamic MRIs. The Gd-EOB-DTPA-enhanced dynamic MRIs cover the non-contrast phase (T1-weighted imaging, T1WI), arterial phase, venous phase, delayed phase, and hepatobiliary phase. Contrast-enhanced scans were performed based on the injection of the GD-EOB-DTPA agent. The arterial phase is captured 25 s after the contrast agent is injected. Subsequently, the portal phase is achieved 1 min later. After another 3 min, the delay phase is obtained, and finally, the hepatobiliary phase is reached 20 min thereafter.

All MRI sequences were spatially registered to a common anatomical space, after which each volume was resampled to 32 slices to ensure consistency across cases. Each slice was cropped and resized to a resolution of 192×192, resulting in an input shape of [32, 192, 192] per modality. Intensity values were normalized to zero mean and unit variance on a per-volume basis to reduce inter-scan variability. During training, standard data augmentation (random rotation, scaling, and flipping) was applied to improve robustness against anatomical and acquisition variations. The structure of the training, validation, and test sets is summarized in Table 1.

Table 1. The structure of CARE-LiFS dataset.

Training set			Validation set			Test set		
Vendor	Center	Cases	Vendor	Center	Cases	Vendor	Center	Cases
A	A	130	A	A	20	A	A	40
B	B1	170	B	B1	20	B	B1	40
B	B2	60	B	B2	20	B	B2	40
–	–	–	–	–	–	C (new)	C (new)	70

2.2 Model

The proposed Multi-Branch Attention Network (MBAN) comprise a multi-branch encoder, a branch-wise feature fusion module, and a lightweight attention-based bottleneck (see Fig. 1). Initially, multiple pre-trained encoders serve as individual branches, with each branch independently extracting primary features from its associated multi-sequence input. To reduce redundancy across different branches, an adaptive branch fusion module is introduced, where a set of weighting coefficients is learned to adaptively adjust the relative importance of each branch. Furthermore, a lightweight attention-based bottleneck is introduced to capture temporal dependencies within feature map. Instead of traditional RNN module, the attention-based transformer is used. These branch and spatial attention modules work sequentially to enhance the representations compressed by the encoder, capturing both inter- and intra-branch dependencies in feature space. Finaly, the Multi-layer Perceptron (MLP)-based classifier generates four classification scores, including S1 vs. non-S1 (S2-S4) and S4 vs. non-S4 (S1-S3).

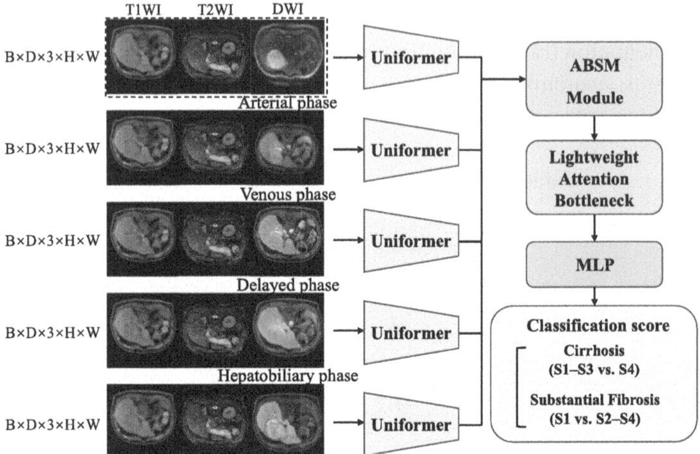

Fig. 1. The overall architecture of our multi-branch attention network (MBAN).

Multi-branch Encoder. Multi-sequence MRI comprises both non-contrast sequences and contrast-enhanced sequences. T1WI reflects tissue longitudinal relaxation. Fat appears hyperintense, while bile, blood, and ascites are hypointense [8]. T2WI reflects transverse relaxation. Fluids such as bile, cysts, and exudates are hyperintense, while fat is relatively hypointense [8]. T1WI and T2WI are routine components of liver MRI protocols and provide complementary structural and morphological infor-mation [9, 10]. DWI highlights areas of high cellularity and restricted diffusion and is particularly sensitive to early fibrosis [11]. Gd-EOB-DTPA-enhanced dynamic MRI provides multiple temporal phases (arterial, venous, delayed, and hepatobiliary), emphasizing perfusion patterns and vascular distribution [12]. DWI and Gd-EOB-DTPA-enhanced dynamic MRI provide complementary functional information. Therefore, T1WI and T2WI are used as shared inputs for each branch to ensure the basic anatomical information.

Specifically, T1WI and T2WI are paired with either DWI or dynamic Gd-EOB-DTPA sequences, resulting in five modality-specific three-channel inputs (see Fig. 1). Each branch is processed by a pre-trained UniFormer3D encoder, which models inter-slice correlations in a manner analogous to temporal frame processing in videos [13]. The UniFormer3D architecture consists of a 3D convolutional patch embedding module followed by multiple stages of transformer blocks. Each patch embedding layer applies strided 3D convolutions to reduce spatial resolution while expanding channel dimensions. The transformer blocks incorporate 3D positional embeddings, multi-head self-attention, feed-forward layers, and residual connections. A final LayerNorm layer normalizes the output feature map. During training, the UniFormer3D backbone is kept frozen to retain its pretrained representations. Multi-branch encoder can simultaneously leverage these complementary sources, enabling a more comprehensive and discriminative representation of fibrosis-related lesions compared with using non-contrast or contrast-enhanced sequences alone.

Adaptive branch squeeze-and-excitation module. Multi MRI-sequence branches provide complementary diagnostic clues. However, the feature fusion process often introduces redundant information. Inspired by Squeeze-and-Excitation Networks (SENet), we introduce an adaptive branch squeeze-and-excitation module (ABSM), which learns branch-wise attention weights by globally pooling concatenated multi-branch features and applying a lightweight 1D convolution (see Fig. 2) [14]. The at-tention weights adaptively assign branch importance based on global information, thereby highlighting informative branches while suppressing redundant ones.

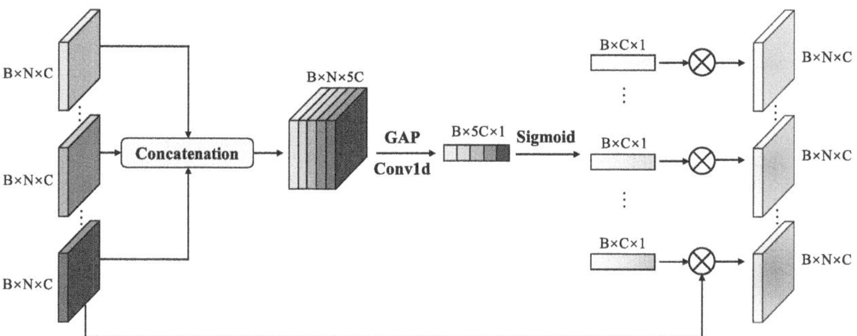

Fig. 2. A schematic illustration of the adaptive branch squeeze-and-excitation module (ABSM).

Lightweight Attention Bottleneck. We design a Lightweight Attention Bottleneck (LAB) module to further explore the fused feature maps from multiple branches (see Fig. 3). Specifically, the module first concatenates weighted feature sequences extracted from five modalities and incorporates learnable positional encodings to jointly model both temporal and modality-specific information. The concatenated features are then fed into a stack of lightweight Transformer blocks, where each block consists of a self-attention module, a feed-forward network, and a squeeze-and-excitation (SE) module. The LAB module captures both cross-branch dependencies and intra-sequence structural information, which enhances the representation of MRI features.

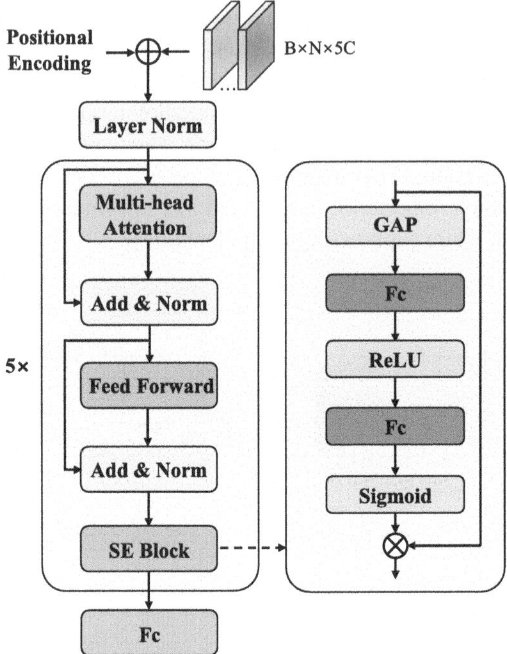

Fig. 3. A schematic illustration of the lightweight attention bottleneck (LAB).

3 Experiments

3.1 Experimental Setup

We conducted a series of experiments to evaluate the proposed method, in which each model was assessed using five-fold cross-validation for classification. In five-fold cross-validation, all subjects were randomly split into five equal subsets, and one subset served as the validation set, while the remaining four were used for training. The reported results are derived from the average metrics of all folds. Pytorch was used to train the models, based on the AdamW optimizer. The batch size was set to 16, and training was performed for up to 300 epochs with early stop (patience = 50 epoch). The initial learning rate was set to 0.0001, and a cosine annealing learning rate schedule was applied during training. The experiments were conducted on a workstation equipped with an NVIDIA Quadro RTX 8000 GPU (48 GB GDDR6 VRAM), Intel i9-10900K CPU, and 64 GB RAM.

To address variability in available MRI data, missing sequences were handled using a zero-imputation strategy, which ensured consistent input dimensions across subjects. For the loss function, we adopted a multi-task learning strategy. Each subtask was formulated as a binary classification, and the training objective was defined as the sum of two binary cross-entropy losses with logits (BCEWithLogitsLoss). This design enables balanced optimization across subtasks, improves multi-task robustness, and ensures numerical stability during training. Moreover, it aligns well with the evaluation metrics, thereby facilitating more effective performance improvements.

3.2 Results

Table 2 summarizes the ablation study results on the LiFS task, which compare different model variants to evaluate the impact of loss function, backbone pretraining, and adaptive fusion. In the LiQA challenge, the performance of liver staging in the LiFS task is evaluated using two metrics: Area Under the Receiver Operating Characteristic Curve (AUC) and Accuracy (ACC). The quantitative results of our method under these metrics are reported in Table 2, and all results are derived from the contrast-enhanced subtask.

The ablation study highlights the key components contributing to the performance of MBAN. Training UniFormer3D from scratch results in poor performance (AUC = 0.5682, 0.5985), which underscores the importance of our pretraining strategy. This observation reflects the inherent challenges of learning robust representations directly from limited medical imaging data, due to both small sample size and the complex nature of medical images. Replacing our loss with the standard four-class cross-entropy also yields inferior results (AUC = 0.6112, 0.6281), demonstrating the benefit of a task-specific loss. When ABSM is removed, the model achieves relatively high AUC (0.7215) on substantial fibrosis detection but reduced accuracy (68.33%), indicating that simple concatenation introduces redundancy and lowers stability.

Table 2. Quantitative performance of the proposed method on the validation set for LiFS task using five-fold cross-validation.

Method	Cirrhosis: S1–S3 vs. S4		Substantial fibrosis: S1 vs. S2–S4	
	AUC	ACC (%)	AUC	ACC (%)
Four-class cross-entropy loss	0.6112	56.67	0.6281	71.67
Non-pretrained uniformer	0.5682	53.33	0.5985	70.00
Without ABSM	0.6184	60.00	**0.7215**	68.33
Our MBAN	**0.6699**	**60.00**	0.7141	**73.33**

In contrast, the proposed MBAN outperforms most variants, achieving the highest cirrhosis detection AUC (0.6699) and the highest substantial fibrosis accuracy (73.33%) in the ablation study. The performance of MBAN is further validated on the test set under five-fold cross-validation (see Table 3). For in-distribution data, MBAN achieves AUC/ACC of 0.7831/72.50% for cirrhosis detection and 0.8450/80.83% for substantial fibrosis detection, demonstrating its robustness within the training distribution. For out-of-distribution data, MBAN achieves lower AUC/ACC in cirrhosis detection (0.6605/41.43%) but remains relatively high for substantial fibrosis (0.3723/82.86%), indicating limited generalization across domains. This is likely due to differences in scanner protocols, patient populations, and imaging quality between datasets. For future clinical deployment, strategies such as fine-tuning on site-specific data, domain adaptation, or federated learning across institutions could help mitigate these limitations. Overall, MBAN demonstrates strong predictive performance when applied to data with characteristics like the training set, highlighting its potential for clinical applications under controlled settings.

Table 3. Quantitative performance of the proposed method on the test set for LiFS task using five-fold cross-validation.

MBAN	In-distribution data (from vendors A, B1, B2)		Out-of-distribution data (from vendor C)	
	Cirrhosis: S1–S3 vs. S4	Substantial fibrosis: S1 vs. S2–S4	Cirrhosis: S1–S3 vs. S4	Substantial fibrosis: S1 vs. S2–S4
AUC	0.7831	0.8450	0.6605	0.3723
ACC	72.50%	80.83%	41.43%	82.86%

4 Conclusion

In this work, we propose a Multi-Branch Attention Network (MBAN) for liver fibrosis staging from multiphase MRI. The framework integrates a multi-branch encoder, an adaptive branch-wise fusion module, and a lightweight attention bottleneck to capture both intra-sequence and inter-sequence dependencies while reducing redundancy. Ablation studies and five-fold cross-validation on the CARE 2025 LiFS dataset demonstrate that MBAN outperforms most baseline variants, particularly in substantial fibrosis detection, and exhibits strong generalization on in-distribution data. The results also highlight challenges in cross-vendor generalization, emphasizing the importance of domain-aware design. Overall, MBAN provides a reliable and effective tool for non-invasive liver fibrosis assessment, offering potential support for clinical decision-making.

Disclosure of Interests. The authors have no competing interests to declare that are relevant to the content of this article.

References

1. Huang, D.Q., et al.: Global epidemiology of cirrhosis–aetiology, trends and predictions. Nat. Rev. Gastroenterol. Hepatol. **20**(6), 388–398 (2023). https://doi.org/10.1038/s41575-023-00759-2
2. Bataller, R., Brenner, D.A.: Liver fibrosis. J. Clin. Invest. **115**(2), 209–218 (2005). https://doi.org/10.1172/JCI24282
3. Zheng, S., He, K., Zhang, L., Li, M., Zhang, H., Gao, P.: Conventional and artificial intelligence-based computed tomography and magnetic resonance imaging quantitative techniques for non-invasive liver fibrosis staging. Eur. J. Radiol. **165**, 110912 (2023). https://doi.org/10.1016/j.ejrad.2023.110912
4. Zhou, L.Q., et al.: Artificial intelligence in medical imaging of the liver. World J. Gastroenterol. **25**(6), 672–682 (2019). https://doi.org/10.3748/wjg.v25.i6.672
5. Mei, X., et al.: Interstitial lung disease diagnosis and prognosis using an AI system integrating longitudinal data. Nat. Commun. **14**(1), 2272 (2023). https://doi.org/10.1038/s41467-023-37720-5
6. Zeng, W., et al.: Microscopic hyperspectral image classification based on fusion transformer with parallel CNN. IEEE J. Biomed. Health Inform. **27**(6), 2910–2921 (2023). https://doi.org/10.1109/JBHI.2023.3253722

7. Zhang, H., Zhang, M., You, X., Gu, Y., Yang, GZ.: Computing assessment for liver fibrosis staging using real-world MR images. In: Comprehensive Analysis and Computing of Real-World Medical Images (CARE 2024). pp. 87–95 (2025). https://doi.org/10.1007/978-3-031-87009-5_9
8. Yu, D., et al.: MRI findings of confluent hepatic fibrosis caused by different etiologies. BMC Gastroenterol. **25**(1), 512 (2025). https://doi.org/10.1186/s12876-025-04101-9
9. Xue, S., et al.: T1/T2 mapping as a non-invasive method for evaluating liver fibrosis based on correlation of biomarkers: a preclinical study. BMC Gastroenterol. **25**, 122 (2025). https://doi.org/10.1186/s12876-025-03701-9
10. Chen, Z., et al.: A novel radiomics signature based on T2-weighted imaging accurately predicts hepatic inflammation in individuals with biopsy-proven nonalcoholic fatty liver disease: a derivation and independent validation study. Hepatobiliary Surg. Nutr. **11**(2), 212–226 (2022). https://doi.org/10.21037/hbsn-21-23
11. Galea, N., Cantisani, V., Taouli, B.: Liver lesion detection and characterization: role of diffusion-weighted imaging. J. Magn. Reson. Imaging **37**(6), 1260–1276 (2013). https://doi.org/10.1002/jmri.23947
12. Ichikawa, S., Goshima, S.: Clinical significance of liver MR imaging. Magn. Reson. Med. Sci. **22**(2), 157–175 (2023). https://doi.org/10.2463/mrms.rev.2022-0100
13. Li, K., et al.: UniFormer: unifying convolution and self-attention for visual recognition. IEEE Trans. Pattern Anal. Mach. Intell. **45**(10), 12581–12600 (2023). https://doi.org/10.1109/TPAMI.2023.3282631
14. Hu, J., Shen, L., Sun, G.: Squeeze-and-excitation networks. In: Proceedings of the IEEE/CVF Conference on Computer Vision and Pattern Recognition (CVPR), pp. 7132–7141 (2018). https://doi.org/10.1109/CVPR.2018.00745

Author Index

X. Zhuang et al. (Eds.): CARE 2025, LNCS 16257, pp. 257–258, 2026.
https://doi.org/10.1007/978-3-032-16271-7

The manufacturer's authorised representative in the EU is Springer Nature Customer Service Centre GmbH, Europaplatz 3, 69115 Heidelberg, Germany. If you have any concerns regarding our products, please contact ProductSafety@springernature.com

Printed and bound by CPI Group (UK) Ltd, Croydon, CR0 4YY
07/07/2026
02160906-0005